PEDIATRIC NUTRITION
IN
HEALTH AND DISEASE

PEDIATRIC NUTRITION
IN
HEALTH AND DISEASE

Madhu Sharma RD
Senior Dietician
Department of Dietetics
Postgraduate Institute of Medical Education and Research (PGIMER)
Chandigarh, India

Foreword
BNS Walia

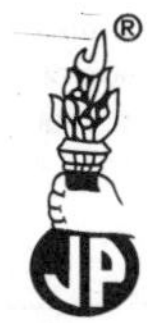

JAYPEE BROTHERS MEDICAL PUBLISHERS (P) LTD

New Delhi • London • Philadelphia • Panama

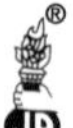

Jaypee Brothers Medical Publishers (P) Ltd

Headquarters

Jaypee Brothers Medical Publishers (P) Ltd
4838/24, Ansari Road, Daryaganj
New Delhi 110 002, India
Phone: +91-11-43574357
Fax: +91-11-43574314
Email: jaypee@jaypeebrothers.com

Overseas Offices

J.P. Medical Ltd
83 Victoria Street, London
SW1H 0HW (UK)
Phone: +44-2031708910
Fax: +02-03-0086180
Email: info@jpmedpub.com

Jaypee-Highlights Medical Publishers Inc.
City of Knowledge, Bld. 237, Clayton
Panama City, Panama
Phone: + 507-301-0496
Fax: + 507-301-0499
Email: cservice@jphmedical.com

Jaypee Brothers Medical Publishers Ltd
The Bourse
111 South Independence Mall East
Suite 835, Philadelphia, PA 19106, USA
Phone: + 267-519-9789
Email: joe.rusko@jaypeebrothers.com

Jaypee Brothers Medical Publishers (P) Ltd
17/1-B Babar Road, Block-B, Shaymali
Mohammadpur, Dhaka-1207
Bangladesh
Mobile: +08801912003485
Email: jaypeedhaka@gmail.com

Jaypee Brothers Medical Publishers (P) Ltd
Shorakhute, Kathmandu
Nepal
Phone: +00977-9841528578
Email: jaypee.nepal@gmail.com

Website: www.jaypeebrothers.com
Website: www.jaypeedigital.com

Pediatric Nutrition in Health and Disease

First Edition: **2013**

ISBN 978-93-5090-330-8

Printed at Rajkamal Electric Press, Plot No. 2, Phase-IV, Kundli, Haryana.

Dedicated to

The memory of my late parents

Shanti Nath and Bijeshwar Nath
and my late husband

AC Sharma
for their blessings and motivation in achieving my goal

Foreword

The value of food as a healer of disease was well recognized by healers of the past. Hippocrates is reported to have said, *leave your drugs in the chemist's pot, if you can heal the patient with food.* When few drugs were available for treatment of disease about sixty years ago, every doctor, *hakim* or *vaid* used to provide extensive instructions to patients regarding what foods to take or restrict in order to get well. Somehow as the medical armamentarium expanded, we have seen the emphasis on nutritional advice dwindle considerably over the years.

The subject of clinical nutrition appears so simple, that everyone thinks that he/she knows everything. Yet, this is far from true, as the subject does not receive adequate emphasis in the training of doctors and nurses. It is a result of health professionals in general, inclined to minimize the importance of nutrition as a therapeutic tool. In the last fifty years, physiologic studies, research on the impact of good nutrition in immune functions of the body and in promotion of healing have been better appreciated, culminating in the statement made by Jean Carper, 'Food is the breakthrough drug of the 21st century.'

The current emphasis on holistic medicine includes use of therapeutic diets in treatment of patients, whereas, in some conditions like galactosemia and other metabolic disorders and malnutrition, appropriate diets may be the only drug required to be administered. In numerous situations like chronic illnesses, cancer, congenital heart disease, Type II diabetes, kidney diseases, diet modification is equally important to patient's chances of recovery.

The present volume follows the same style of presentation in which the author first dwells on normal nutrition, the basic nutrient requirements of children right from infancy to adolescence and nutritional demands in specific conditions like different activities or lifestyle followed under varied conditions. Subsequently, the reader is led to more diverse settings like different pathological disturbances, metabolic, renal, cardiac and other systemic diseases likely to be encountered among the pediatric population. Finally, the author sets out to advise the routes of administration of dietetic formulae, which are appropriate for the relevant clinical state of the disease.

As in the previous two texts published by the author, the advice is based on sound nutritional principles and current knowledge of the subject; the exhaustive list of references provided at the end of each chapter reveals, the study and hard work that has been undertaken for compilation of each chapter. The book is a treasure house of advice on basic and therapeutic management of a sick child, knowledge of the principles of therapeutic diets and how to apply those while treating patients, which would make the reader a more effective healer. Chapters on Nutritional Management of Cancer and Bone Marrow Transplant in Children, Nutritional Management of Pediatric Heart Disease, Management of Severe Acute Malnutrition, and Probiotics—Role in Child Health and Role of Other Micronutrients in Children, all deal with a clinician's current concerns. Chapters on Maternal Nutrition in Pregnancy and Lactation, and Nutrition for Premature Infants are very informative and add to the value of the book.

The present book should be of equal value for general practitioners, pediatricians, nurses and dieticians. I know of no other creative dealing with the subject of normal and therapeutic nutrition for children, which covers the subject so simply and succinctly.

BNS Walia
Emeritus Professor Pediatrics
Former Director
Postgraduate Institute of Medical Education and Research (PGIMER)
Chandigarh, India

Preface

Besides air and water, one thing that is 'a must' for survival of any living being from birth is food and along with this comes the role of optimal nutrition. In case of humans, the role of nutrition comes into focus even before birth, since it is well recognized that optimum outcome of a pregnancy is based on optimum nutrition during the antenatal period. Keeping this in mind, the initial chapters of the book are devoted to maternal nutrition besides that for the infants and children.

The earlier part of the book deals with nutritional management of children in healthy children, their needs and requirements through various phases of their growth, starting from infancy to the adolescent period. In 2010, the Indian Council of Medical Research (ICMR) updated certain standards for the nutritional assessment and requirements at various stages, which have also been incorporated in this compilation. More and more children are actively participating in sports and related performances, which alter their nutritional demands considerably. These children need to be counseled appropriately, so as to maintain a healthy balance between physical output and diet intake, thereby, enhancing their performance. This aspect has been dealt with explicitly in this book. The issue of maintaining a vegetarian eating pattern is of great concern for many parents, who may be confused regarding how best to meet the nutritional demands of their growing child, without compromising their religious sentiments. This issue has been explored herein, giving details of how to choose and plan a healthy diet for their kids.

Other aspects like food allergies, which are commonly encountered among children, the role of important micronutrients like fat soluble vitamin A and minerals like iron and calcium in the diet, and how the nutritional status can impact the onset of infections or vice versa, all have been covered in this compilation.

Obesity and malnutrition are two extreme conditions, which are seen to exist side-by-side. How nutritional management and counseling can help prevent and restore health has been dealt with extensively in this book. Illness, be it of any kind, can adversely affect the nutritional status of children, who are vulnerable to even minor setbacks on their physical status. The second-half of the book deals with various diseases ranging from the gastrointestinal tract, liver, kidneys, heart and Type I diabetes mellitus to some of the more acute problems like cancer and HIV infections, and how appropriate nutritional management can help tide over the difficult phases of the disease, thereby, helping in rehabilitation to the normal state. Finally, there are certain not so common diseases, yet encountered in sizeable numbers especially in referral hospitals, which have been touched upon like some of the metabolic diseases, cystic fibrosis, hypoglycemia and storage disorders.

It may be noted that all issues discussed herein ranging from health to disease, have been tackled so that it would be of benefit for the students from colleges and hospitals dealing with children. The author hopes that this book would serve as a useful guide for all students of nutrition and dietetics, medicine and nursing. It can well be a part of libraries of all medical and nursing institutes and home science colleges where nutrition and dietetics form a major component of the syllabi. It would not be an exaggeration to expect that this book would also find a place in the book shelves of all practitioners involved with child care.

Madhu Sharma

Acknowledgments

No work is complete without the support of the team involved in its achievement; and so is true in the compilation of this humble attempt of mine to expand on my earlier books on Pediatric Nutrition. I am indebted to my readers, students, well wishers and publishers in particular who encouraged and inspired me to strive to achieve greater heights. Above all, but for the ever-inspiring advice and constant support and blessings, that I received by my mentor Professor BNS Walia from time to time, this book could never have seen the light of the day.

Contents

SECTION 1: BASIC NUTRITION

SECTION 2: NUTRITION IN DISEASE

SECTION 1

Basic Nutrition

Chapter 1: Functions of Food
Chapter 2: Nutrient Requirements
Chapter 3: Nutritional Assessment of Children
Chapter 4: Maternal Nutrition in Pregnancy and Lactation
Chapter 5: Nutrition for Premature Infants
Chapter 6: Feeding of Infants (0–6 months)
Chapter 7: Nutrition for Older Children
Chapter 8: Nutrition for the Adolescent
Chapter 9: Nutrition for the Athlete Child
Chapter 10: Interaction of Nutrition and Infection in Children
Chapter 11: Vegetarianism in Children
Chapter 12: Food Allergies and Intolerances
Chapter 13: Vitamin A Deficiency in Children
Chapter 14: Nutritional Anemia in Children
Chapter 15: Iodine Deficiency Disorders in Children
Chapter 16: Zinc in Infant Nutrition
Chapter 17: Role of Other Micronutrients in Children
Chapter 18: Nutrition Counseling—Role in Children
Chapter 19: Probiotics—Role in Child Health
Chapter 20: Nutrition for Dental Health in Children

1 Functions of Food

BALANCED DIET

"Proper diet can become an instrument for maintaining health and cultivating increased levels of awareness"

Chinese proverb
Master Mantak Chia

All of us know and have heard so often of a 'Balanced Diet' and tend to believe it is a Healthy Diet. But, unfortunately they are actually confusing the two entities-rather 'using' it as synonyms. A 'balanced diet' is one which provides us with all the nutrients (present in a wide range of foods) in the right proportion and the right amount. It will also provide a regular supply of vitamins, minerals and other nutrients, ensuring optimum health and vitality. Optimum health means less illness and health complications.

A 'healthy' diet plan is mainly a consumption of natural, fresh and wholesome foods for each meal of the day. Such foods may be low in fats, sodium and refined sugars. The difference is, a healthy diet plan provides us with 'some nutrients', but the balanced diet plan provides all 'essential nutrients'.

A combination of both healthy and balanced diet plan can help achieve the following:

- a variety in the diet
- provide more grain, fresh fruits and vegetables to provide energy
- low fat intake-especially saturated fats
- reduce sugar intake
- lower salt intake
- provide optimum health and vitality to remain active
- mental well being
- ability to withstand on going ageing process with minimum functional impairment
- ability to combat disease, like.
  a. resisting infections, i.e. providing immunity
  b. preventing onset of degenerative diseases and cancer
  c. resisting the effect of environmental toxins and pollutants.

There is a wide variety of foods consumed by us over the whole day. Some of them may not be consumed daily or there are some which might be consumed in greater proportions compared to certain other types of food. All these foods have some role to play in our health-directly or indirectly. Based on the functions of various foods and the nutrients provided by them, these can be classified into three main types as given in Table 1.1.

Now based on these functions, foods are further classified into groups depending upon the main nutrients provided by them. Some experts have classified them into seven groups, where in fruits were grouped apart from vegetables. Others grouped

TABLE 1.1: Functions of food

Food function	Nutrients provided
Energy providing	Carbohydrates, fats
Body building	Proteins
Protective	Vitamins, minerals, fiber

meat and other animal foods as a separate group from pulses, but grouped fruits with vegetables. But most experts have classified food into five basic groups as given in Table 1.2.[1] These food groups can be used as:

1. *Tools for nutritional assessment and screening*: A brief dietary history can give us an idea of the inadequacies of any nutrient from any of the groups and thus provide a hint of the possible deficiency if any.
2. *Tool for nutritional counseling*: It can serve as a guide for nutrition education by any health care providers.
3. *Food labeling and surveillance*: Food groups can be used for food labeling and for nutrition surveillance system.

Cereals and millets like wheat flour, rice, maize, bajra, etc. are basically the staple food item of any Indian meal. Besides providing energy which is their main function, also provides proteins and other minerals and vitamins. These are a good source of fiber too.

Pulses comprise a variety of dals, which are an important component of any Indian diet. These are a rich source of proteins, almost double those of cereals (24%). Soyabeans of course are the highest source of proteins amounting to almost 40%. These are also good substitutes for vegetarian diets with respect to protein contents. *Besides these are also rich in certain other important nutrients like phytoestrogens*

Pulses and cereals are generally consumed in combination in most Indian households and this is very important in order to enhance the bioavailability of proteins. The amino acid lysine is deficient in cereals but rich in pulses. On the other hand cereals are a good source of methionine but deficient in

TABLE 1.2: Food groups and their nutrients

Food groups	Major nutrients
Cereal and millets	Energy, iron and B group vitamins
Pulses and Legumes Nuts and Oilseeds	Proteins, energy, B group vitamins
Milk, Egg and Flesh Foods	Proteins, calcium, vitamin A
Vegetables and Fruits	Vitamins, minerals, fiber
Fats and sugars	Energy, essential fatty acids (fats only)

lysine. Therefore, when consumed in combination, the deficit of each food is complemented by each other, thereby improving the quality of total proteins consumed. The role of pulses is mainly body building with of course good energy content. For nonvegetarians, meat, chicken fish and eggs are an excellent source of high biological value proteins. However, unlike pulses these are poor source of fiber.

Milk and milk products are a group by themselves and rich in proteins besides being a useful source of calcium for all age groups. The proteins of milk (casein) are of high biological value and considered as first class quality. Their basic role is that of body building apart from the protective role by virtue of its being rich in fat soluble vitamins like A and D.

Green leafy vegetables and fruits are mainly protective foods due to their mineral and vitamin content besides also being a good source of fiber. They are however low in calories and proteins. Vitamins like A, E and C are also considered as antioxidants, therefore a good helping of these foods in the diet can protect the body from free radical produced consequent to various metabolic actions. Fiber in the diet is a very important component of food to keep the gastrointestinal tract in action and also helps control hyperglycemia and hyperlipidemia.

Fats and oils and sugars are basically high caloric foods used as a part of the ingredients of any food preparation and termed as energy giving foods as they are calorie dense. Fats are twice as high in calories compared to sugars.

A judicious use of foods chosen from all the food groups (as per sex and age requirements) will take care of the requirements of all macronutrients, i.e. proteins, fats and carbohydrates, as also the micronutrients which include all vitamins, minerals trace elements and fiber (Fig. 1.1). Illustrates the typical food pyramid for any healthy individual. The amounts of each food group can vary depending upon the age and sex of the individual. Overall, a balanced diet should provide around 60%–70% of total calories from carbohydrates, 10%–20% from proteins and 20%–25% of total calories from fat.

The segments of the pyramid depict the ratio of the different food groups that need to be consumed in any balanced diet. Cereals and millets are shown

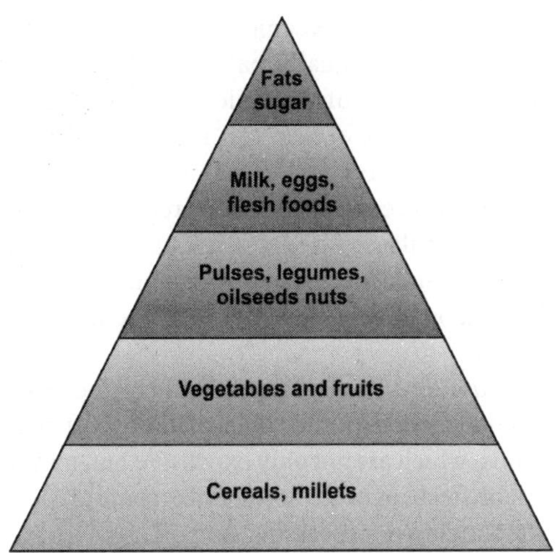

FIGURE 1.1: The food pyramid

to be consumed in the maximum ratio followed by vegetables and fruits, pulses and nuts, milk and other flesh foods and lastly the fats and sugars which need to be consumed in the least ratio.

A balanced diet may be planned and calculated using the simple exchange list for portion size and nutrient content of all food groups as given in Table 1.3.[2]

Principles of Planning a Balanced Diet

While planning a balanced diet there are certain important criteria to keep in mind. These apply to the family as a whole, but in the case of a child special points need to be considered:

a. *Meeting the nutritional requirements*: A menu providing adequate nutrients from all the food groups, which includes macro and micro nutrients.
b. *Meal pattern should fulfill family needs*: The menu should be such that members of different age groups and sex need to be accounted for. The requirements of a 5-year-old girl would be different from those of her adolescent sib, which again would differ for another sib who is an adult in the family and perhaps a sports person.
c. *Meal planning should be time sparing*: Any meal planning should be such that the housewife is not left to spend long hours cooking or the recipes are such that they involve a great deal of effort time and energy.
d. *Economic considerations*: The meal planned is based on the economic factors to a large extent. Low cost nutritious recipes can be counseled to families with limited resources, like utilizing the seasonal foods available judiciously can be healthier then spending more on foods not easily available or difficult to procure.
e. *Prevention of maximum nutrient losses*: Meal planning should involve recipes and techniques which do not involve excessive nutrient losses, e.g. too much of frying or boiling involved in recipes, though may be delicious, but may result in maximum losses especially of the water soluble

TABLE 1.3: Nutrient exchange list for portion size of various food groups

Food groups	G/portion	Energy (kcals)	Protein (g)	Carbohydrate (g)	Fat (g)
Cereals/Millets	30	100	3.0	20	0.8
Pulses	30	100	6.0	15	0.7
Egg	50	85	7.0	-	7.0
Meat/Chicken/Fish	50	100	9.0	-	7.0
Milk (toned)	100	70	3.0	5.0	3.0
Roots/Tubers	100	80	1.3	18.0	-
Green Leafy Veg.	100	45	3.6	-	0.4
Other Vegetables	100	30	1.7	-	0.2
Fruits	100	40	-	10.0	-
Sugar	5	20	-	5.0	-
Fats/Oils	5	45	-	-	5.0

Source: NIN[2]

vitamins or fat soluble vitamins in case of frying for long duration. Cooking methods involving pressure cooking, baking or micro-wave cooking can save time, nutrient losses and also retain maximum flavor of the food itself. Sprouting, malting or fermenting processes can enhance certain nutrients in the meals.

f. *Likes and dislikes*: Although meal planning should consider nutrient quality and balance of all nutrients, etc. it is equally important to consider the individual likes and dislikes of the child. he recipes can be modified to appeal to their taste or some other substitutes may be offered instead.

g. *Variety:* Variety is not only the spice of life as is said, but also helps break monotony in the meals from day to day. Recipes may be modified or substituted for equally balanced alternatives so that the interest of the child is maintained. This can specially be of help for 'fussy eaters'.

h. *Meals should give satiety*: If a meal is prepared taking into account all the food groups, comprising cereals, pulses, fats, etc. it can provide more satiety than just cereal alone or some vegetables. Spaced out meals are better than one time heavy meals.

i. *Availability of foods*: Meals should include locally available foods rather than planning off season foods, which are not only expensive but, may also not be fresh, or need more cumbersome procedure for cooking or processing it.

REFERENCES

1. BVS Thimayamma and Swaran Pasricha. Balanced Diet *In* Textbook of Human Nutrition, eds by MS Bamji, N Prahlad Rao, Vinodini Reddy,1996.
2. Nutrient Requirements and Recommended Dietary Allowances for Indians. A report of the expert group of the Indian Council of Medical Research. New Delhi, Indian Council of Medical Research, 2010.

2 Nutrient Requirements

Nutrient requirements of any individual are based on their age, sex and activity. These nutrient requirements are met by a combination of various foods obtained from the five food groups discussed earlier.

A detailed list of nutrient requirements for each group including special conditions like pregnancy and lactation have been compiled by the Nutrition Expert Committee, Indian Council of Medical Research (ICMR), India (2010) as given in Table 2.1.[1]

The requirements for vitamins for each group are shown in Table 2.2.[1] These requirements represent the optimum amount of each nutrient provided in a day's diet to support optimum health and maintain good nutrition through each stage of one's life.

Since the life cycle of an infant actually begins from the womb, it would be prudent to first discuss the optimum nutritional requirements of a mother to be, i.e. during the pregnancy stage.

NUTRITIONAL REQUIREMENTS DURING PREGNANCY AND LACTATION

It would not be an exaggeration to state that the foundation of a healthy baby at birth is in fact laid during the adolescent stage of a girl who eventually is going to be the 'future mother'. Therefore it becomes important that due attention be given to the nutritional requirements of a girl right from her adolescence. However, in this chapter, we shall begin by first discussing the requirements of a woman during pregnancy and lactation.

During the first 8 weeks of prenatal period, the fetal organs are being formed. The second half is crucial because the major gain in weight of the fetus takes place during that period. Consequently, the demands for the building material for new or added tissues steps up markedly. These additional requirements have to be made up by increased/improved diet. The increased dietary requirements also take into account the growth of certain tissues like the mammary glands and accessory tissues supporting the fetus.

Numerous studies from our own country conducted by various researchers have time and again established the importance of a good nutritionally complete diet of the mother during her pregnancy on the birth weight of the new born.[2–4]

Energy

Indian Council of Medical Research (ICMR) recommendations for a pregnant woman from the second trimester onwards is 350 calories/day, for a pregnancy weight gain between 10–12 kg, which corresponds to the WHO recommends an addition of 150 cal/day in the first trimester and 350 cal/day in the last 2 trimesters.[5] For the breast feeding mother, an additional energy requirement during exclusive breast feeding (first 6 months) would be 600 kcals and for partial breast feeding during 7–12 months, it would be 520 kcals approximately.[1]

Protein

Protein requirement increases greatly during the second half of pregnancy by about 23 g/day over

TABLE 2.1: Summary of Recommended Dietary Allowances (RDA) for energy, protein, fat and minerals for Indians (2010)

Group	Activity/Age	Body weight (kg)	Net energy (Kcal/d)	Protein (g)/d	Visible Fat (g/d)	Calcium (mg/d)	Iron (mg/d)	Zinc (mg/d)	Magnesium (mg/d)
Men	Sedentary work	60	2320	60	26	600	17	12	340
	Moderate work		2730		30				
	Heavy work		3490		40				
Women	Sedentary work	55	1900	55	20	600	21	10	310
	Moderate work		230		25				
	Heavy work		2850		30				
	Pregnant		(+) 350	78	30	1200	35	12	
	Lactating 0–6 m		(+) 600	74	30		21		
	6–12 m		(+) 520	68	30				
Infant	0–6 months	5.4	92 kcal/kg/d	1.16 g/kg/d		500	46 µg/kg/d		30
	6–12 months	8.4	80 kcal/kg/d	1.69 g/kg/d	19		5	—	45
Children	1–3 years	12.9	1060	16.7	27	600	9	5	50
	4–6 years	18.0	1350	20	25		13	7	70
	7–9 years	25.1	1690	29.5	30		16	8	100
Boys	10–12 years	34.3	2190	39.9	35	800	21	9	120
Girls	10–12 years	35.0	2010	40.4	35	800	27	9	160
Boys	13–15 years	47.6	2750	54.3	45	800	32	11	165
Girls	13–15 years	46.6	2330	51.9	40	800	27	11	210
Boys	16–17 years	55.4	3020	61.5	50	800	28	12	195
Girls	16–17 years	52.1	2440	55.5	35	800	26	12	235

Refer. ICMR, 2010

TABLE 2.2: Summary of Recommended Dietary Allowances (RDA) for water soluble and fat soluble vitamins for Indians (2010)

Group	Category/Age	Body weight (kg)	Vitamin A (μg/d)								
			Retinol	β-carotene	Thiamine (mg/dl)	Riboflavin (mg/dl)	Niacin equivalent (mg/dl)	Vitamin B_6 (mg/d)	Ascorbic Acid (mg/d)	Dietary folate (μg/d)	Vitamin B_{12} (μg/d)
	Sedentary work				1.2	1.4	16				
Men	Moderate work	60	600	4800	1.4	1.6	18	2.0	40	200	1.0
	Heavy work				1.7	2.1	21				
	Sedentary work				1.0	1.1	12				
	Moderate work		600	4800	1.1	1.3	14	2.0	40	200	1.0
	Heavy work				1.4	1.7	16				
Women	Pregnant	55	800	6400	+0.2	+0.3	+2	2.5	60	500	1.2
	Lactating 0–6 m		950	7600	+0.3	+0.4	+4	2.5	80	300	1.5
	6–12 m				+0.2	+0.3	+3	2.5			
Infants	0–6 months	5.4	350	—	0.2	0.3	710 μg/kg	0.1	25	25	0.2
	6–12 months	8.4		2800	0.3	0.4	650 μg/kg	0.4			
	1–3 years	12.9	400	3200	0.5	0.6	8	0.9		80	
Children	4–6 years	18.0			0.7	0.8	11	0.9	40	100	0.2–1.0
	7–9 years	25.1	600	4800	0.8	1.0	13	1.6		120	
Boys	10–12 years	34.3			1.1	1.3	15	1.6	40	140	0.2–1.0
Girls	10–12 years	35.0			1.0	1.3	15	1.6			
Boys	13–15 years	47.6			1.4	1.6	16	2.0	40	150	0.2–1.0
Girls	13–15 years	46.6	600	4800	1.2	1.4	14	2.0			
Boys	16–17 years	55.4			1.5	1.8	17	2.0	40	200	0.2–1.0
Girls	16–17 years	52.1			1.0	1.2	14	2.0			

Refer. ICMR, 2010

and above the normal RDA, for 10 kg weight gain. This increased requirement is calculated on the basis of protein deposition in the fetus, plus the needs of the mother herself which are increased to account for the enlargement of certain of her own body tissues during the prenatal period. The quality of protein should be of high quality for optimal utilization. During lactation, based on the optimum milk volume of 850 ml per day, WHO has suggested an extra protein intake of about 16 g/day during the first 6 months of lactation, 12 g/day during the second 6 months and 11 g/day thereafter.[5] ICMR recommendations (2010) are 18.5 g/day for first 6 months and 12.5 g/day from 6–12 months. It may be borne in mind that these values have been computed in terms of mixed vegetable protein of relative net protein utilization (NPU) of 65.[1]

Calcium

Calcium is an integral component of the skeletal system and naturally routinely prescribed for all pregnant and nursing mothers. As per the ICMR recommendations an extra intake of 600 mgs is advised in addition to that required for normal individuals.[1] This works out to be 1200 mgs/day. The role of adequate calcium also helps minimize problems like osteoporosis in later age among the women, which is so frequently encountered by most in their mid forties. Of course calcium supplement also helps provide adequate stores to the rapidly developing skeletal growth of the fetus.

Iron

Iron deficiency anemia is very common among most of the Indian women especially during pregnancy. Very often the mothers to be are already anemic before their conception and if on an already poor reserve of iron in the body, the burden of a pregnancy is thrust upon, the brunt is borne both by the mother herself and also the growing fetus. The mother lands into severe anemia and the fetal growth too is affected resulting in low birth weight babies. Studies have demonstrated that maternal hemoglobin (Hb) levels have been related to perinatal and neonatal mortality.[6] Bhargava et al have shown that severe anemia is associated with higher Hb and ferritin values in the fetus and a significant decrease in birth weight and gestational age.[7] The iron requirement as recommended by the ICMR expert group, 2010, is laid down as 35 mg/d.[1]

Folic Acid

Along with iron, folic acid deficiency also is widely present among most Indian women. This leads to a condition called megaloblastic anemia. It is well established that good stores of folic acid during the pre and perinatal period help prevent neural tube defects.[8] Besides, folic acid deficiency has also shown to affect the birth weight of the new born.[9] Therefore, it is routinely given at all antenatal centers along with iron supplements.

Iodine

The role of iodine in prevention of hypothyroidism and cretinism is well known especially during pregnancy. This is evident from the fact that following the Iodized Salt Program in India nation wide, the incidence of neonatal hypothyroidism has markedly decreased[10] (see Chapter 15 also).

Studies from Nutrition Foundation of India have identified 197 districts out of 457 in India as endemic zones for iodine deficiency[11] thereby emphasizing the role of iodine fortification in diets of the vulnerable groups of our population, the expectant mothers and children.

The role of other micronutrients, zinc, B_6, magnesium, selenium and copper is ill defined and no conclusive data are available to support supplementation during pregnancy and lactation.

Vitamins

Fat Soluble Vitamins

During pregnancy there is no extra requirement of vitamin A and is similar to that of a normal adult woman. But during lactation period, the needs are slightly increased, taking into account the content present in breast milk. Hence an additional 350 micro grams/day have been recommended.[1]

Water Soluble Vitamins

Since the requirements of thiamine, riboflavin and niacin are dependent upon the amount of calories consumed or required; all these vitamins of the B group are increased proportionately as seen in Table.[2]

However, the requirement of vitamin C, though unchanged during pregnancy, does increase twofold during lactation to compensate for that secreted in breast milk.[5]

NUTRITIONAL REQUIREMENTS OF INFANTS, CHILDREN AND ADOLESCENTS

Fluids

Fluid requirement for neonates are as shown in Table 2.3.

For older children the holiday and segar formula is used as for energy requirements (Table 2.5). Incase of an illness associated with fever, the requirement may be increased by 10% for every 10 degree centigrade of fever.

Energy

The growth pattern of infants during the first year of life follows a pattern of rise and fall. It is most rapid during the first 3 months after birth. Then the velocity of weight gain slows down from 4–9 months after which there is a rise again the end of the first year of life. The energy requirement of infants has been computed by various expert groups at various times. FAO/WHO in 1973, recommended intakes[12] ranging from 120 calories per kg. body weight from the first 3 months and decreasing gradually to 110 by 6–9 months and then increasing to 112 by the end of the first year of life. But again in 1985,[13] the same group brought down these levels to 116 cal/kg in the first 3 months to 95 cal/kg between 6–9 months and again increasing it to 101 cal by the end of the first year of life. However, the recommendations by the ICMR expert group, 2010 have based the current estimate of energy requirements of infants which is about 11%–20% lower than the 1988 estimates as given in Table 2.4.[1] It was also emphasized by this group that in case of malnourished children, the recommendations should be on the basis of actual age and not the existing body weight. This would help in their catch up growth.

For children and adolescents, the recommendations are based on healthy boys and girls, who have attained the 95th percentile of weight for age and have a moderate activity level as given in Table 2.5.

However, there are other authors who have devised more simple and practical formula for calculating the energy requirements of children which is also referred to as 'bedside' estimates for these requirements.[14] This estimate has been based on the assumption that a one year old child requires 1000 calories and then for every increase of age by one year 100 calories are added on yearly till puberty. This estimate works out to be lower than recommended by ICMR, but then this can be considered as minimum requirement. This

TABLE 2.3: Fluid requirement of neonates

Day of life	Fluid volume (ml/kg/d)
1	60
2	70
3	80
4	90
5	100
6	110
7	onwards 120

Source: ICMR[1], 2010

TABLE 2.4: Recommended energy requirements of infants (0–12 months)

Age	Boys			Girls		
Months	Weight (kg)	Energy Kcals/day	Kcals/ kg/d	Weight (kg)	Energy Kcals/d	Kcals/ kg/d
0–1	4.58	520	115	4.35	460	105
1–2	5.50	570	105	5.14	520	100
2–3	6.28	600	95	5.82	550	95
3–4	6.28	570	80	6.41	540	85
4–5	7.48	610	80	6.92	570	80
5–6	7.93	640	80	7.35	600	80
6–7	8.30	650	80	7.71	600	80
7–8	8.62	680	80	8.03	630	80
8–9	8.89	700	80	8.31	650	80
9–10	9.13	730	80	8.55	680	80
10–11	9.37	750	80	8.78	690	80
11–12	9.62	780	80	9.0	710	80

Refer. ICMR, 2010

TABLE 2.5: Energy requirements of Indian children and adolescents

Age (years)	Boys			Girls		
	Wt. (kg)	Kcals /d	Kcals/ kg/d	Wt. (kg)	Kcals/ kg/d	Kcals /d
1–2	10.3	910	85	10.2	830	80
2–3	13.3	1120	85	12.7	1030	80
3–4	15.3	1230	80	15.0	1150	75
4–5	16.5	1290	80	16.0	1200	75
5–6	18.2	1390	80	17.7	1290	75
6–7	20.4	1510	75	20.0	1400	70
7–8	22.7	1630	70	22.3	1510	70
8–9	25.2	1750	70	25.0	1630	65
9–10	28.0	1890	70	27.6	1740	65
10–11	30.8	2030	65	31.2	1880	60
11–12	34.1	2180	65	34.8	2010	60
12–13	38.0	2370	60	39.0	2140	55
14–15	48.0	2760	60	47.1	2340	50
15–16	51.5	2890	55	49.4	2390	50
16–17	54.3	2980	55	51.3	2430	45
17–18	56.5	3060	55	52.8	2450	45

Refer. ICMR, 2010

TABLE 2.6: Holiday and Segar formula

Upto 10 kg	100 calories/kg.
10–20 kg	1000 + 50 Kcal for each kg above 10 kg
Above 10 kg	1500 + 20 Kcal in excess above 20 kg

implies that beginning from one year if the calorie requirement is 1000, then for every subsequent year it would be 1100, 1200 and so on till twelve years when it would be 2100. After that for adolescent boys it can be taken as 2400 and for adolescent girl it would be 2100 calories.

Another quick way of calculating has been given by Holiday and Segar Formula as given in Table 2.6.[14]

Proteins

Protein requirements for infants are derived from the estimate of protein content of breast milk and the volume of milk consumed by healthy infants growing normally. Studies from Gopalan on Indian mothers have shown that this requirement is about 2.0 g/kg. during the first two weeks which falls to around 1.1 g/kg at 94 weeks.[15] Beyond 6 months, breast milk is not adequate to sustain normal growth of an infant; supplements in the form of vegetable proteins have to be added to breast milk.

The ICMR Expert Committee, 2010 has recommended the safe level of protein for infants as calculated on the basis of the sum of maintenance requirement and the protein deposition rate (growth

TABLE 2.7: Protein requirement and dietary allowances

Age group	g/kg/d	g/d	g/kg/d	g/d
Infants (months)				
6–9	1.69	13.4		
9–12	1.69	14.9		
Preschool Children (y)	Boys		Girls	
1–2	1.47	15.1	1.47	14.1
2–3	1.25	16.0	1.25	15.1
3–4	1.16	17.2	1.16	17.8
4–5	1.11	18.3	1.09	19.3
School Children (y)	Boys		Girls	
5–6	1.09	19.8	1.9	19.3
6–7	1.15	23.5	1.15	23.0
7–8	1.17	26.6	1.17	26.0
8–9	1.18	29.7	1.18	32.6
9–10	1.18	33.0	1.18	32.6
Adolescents (y)	Boys		Girls	
10–11	1.18	36.3	1.18	36.8
11–12	1.16	39.6	1.15	40.0
12–13	1.15	43.7	1.14	44.5
13–14	1.15	43.7	1.13	49.0
14–15	1.14	54.7	1.12	52.8
15–16	1.13	58.2	1.09	53.8
16–17	1.12	60.8	1.07	54.9
17–18	1.10	62.2	1.06	56.0

Refer. ICMR, 2010.

adjusted for 66% efficiency of utilization as shown in Table 2.7. These levels are lower than those provided by the 1985 FAO/WHO consultation.

Fats

Fats are an important component of any Indian diet and provide a major percent of calories. Besides contributing to the calorie density of a diet, fats also help make the food palatable. Fats are made up of fatty acids which are mainly saturated or unsaturated. The unsaturated fats are further classified into mono and polyunsaturated fatty acids. Saturated fats are the ones which solidify at room temperature and include palmitic and stearic acid like ghee, hydrogenated fats and coconut oil. However, these are poor sources of essential fatty acids. The polyunsaturated fatty acids include linoleic acid (omega 6) and linolenic acid (omega 3), both of which are not synthesized in the body and hence have to be provided in the diet. These are termed as essential fatty acids like safflower, sunflower, corn and soya oils and contain almost 50%–70% of the essential fatty acids. Groundnut oil has about 25% essential fatty acids (EFA). An important point to bear in mind is that the omega 6 and omega 3 fatty acids need to be maintained in a desirable ratio of around 5–10. A ratio beyond 10 can produce adverse affects like inflammatory diseases and respiratory problems like asthma. All refined oils are a good source of linoleic acid, but may be too low in linolenic acid, thereby disturbing the ratio. Oils like mustard and ghee have a balanced ratio of omega 6 and omega 3 and hence considered desirable in appropriate ratio. The ideal ratio of the three types of the fats should be one each of saturated fats polyunsaturated fats (PUFA) and monounsaturated fats (MUFA). A normally breast fed infant receives nearly 70 grams of fat per day of which 10% is linoleic acid, and 1% is linolenic acid.[1] there by taking care of the requirements of EFA of an infant which is about 6% of total energy. The recommendations of fat as given by ICMR are as given in Table 2.8.

Infants: The fat content of human milk is relatively constant at 3%–4% by weight and delivers 50%–60% of energy. Infant formulae milk should have fat and individual fatty acid contents (including arachidonic acid and docosahexaenoic acid) similar to levels of human milk. Preterm infants have a higher requirement for arachidonic acid (AA) and docosahexaenoic acid (DHA).

A typical Indian mixed diet based on cereals, pulses and vegetables provides approximately 10%–15% of fat as invisible fat. Based on this fact, the recommended the recommended level of visible fat is restricted to about 20% of total energy provided by the diet. In any case the total fat intake should not exceed 30% of the total energy due to adverse affects on the cardiovascular system.

By the second half of the first year of life the percent of fat can be increased to 35% of energy

TABLE 2.8: Recommendations for dietary fat intake in infants and children

Age group	Physical activity	Minimum intake %energy	Invisible fat (foods) %energy	Visible fat (cooking oil)	
				%energy	g/d
Infants	0–6 months 7–24 months	40–60 35*	Human Milk 10†	Human milk 25	25
Children	3–6 years 7–9 years	25 25	10 10	15 15	25 30
Boys	10–12 years	25	10	15	35
	13–15 years	25	10	15	45
	16–17 years	25	10	15	50
Girls	10–12 years	25	10	15	35
	13–15 years	25	10	15	40
	16–17 years	25	10	15	35

Refer. ICMR, 2010

*gradually reduce depending on physical activity
†human milk/infant formula + complementary foods

gradually depending on the physical activity. Babies can derive a mix of breast feeds and complementary food between 6–24 months which should provide with at least 3%–4.5% energy.

Beyond 2 years to adolescence (17 years) the fat intake should be approximately 25% of energy to maintain growth, for which the minimum level of visible fat should range between 25–30 grams per day in the diets of children and adolescents.

Vitamins

Fat Soluble Vitamins

These vitamins are stored in the liver and the body reserves can be utilized from day to day. These are not easily destroyed by heat unlike the water soluble vitamins. Generally it is the deficiency of vitamin A and occasionally vitamin D which are encountered among children in the form of night blindness, bitot's spots, (vitamin A) or rickets (vitamin D). However, the other two vitamin deficiency and K are not generally seen and hence no specific recommendations are made for different age groups. Recently vitamin E has been emphasized for its role as an antioxidant in many disease conditions in therapeutic doses. ICMR has recommended 0.8 mg per gm of EFA in food. No such recommendation has been laid down for vitamin K.

Vitamin A: The recommended intake of vitamin A for infants and children in terms of retinol and beta carotene as determined by ICMR are given in Table 2.9.[1] The requirement in early infancy is 50 micro grams/kg, based on the retinol content of breast milk of well nourished mothers.[16] This requirement is proportional to the growth rate of children at different stages.

Vitamin D: This vitamin is considered as a pro-hormone in the formation of bones and calcium absorption. The required amount is generally met by adequate exposure to sunlight. Estimates suggest that only 5 minutes of exposure to sunlight is adequate to meet the daily requirements.

Water Soluble Vitamins

As these vitamins are not stored in the body these need to be provided on a daily basis from dietary source.

Vitamin C: This vitamin has an important role to play in prevention of scurvy. The recommended doses for infants and children are shown in Table 2.2.

B Complex Vitamins: This group includes vitamin B_1 (thiamine), B_2 (riboflavin), B_6 (pyridoxine), niacin, B_{12} and folate. Niacin is a derivative from tryptophan, an essential amino acid. 60 mg of tryptophan is equivalent to 1mg of niacin. The RDA for B_1 and B_2 are computed on the basis of total calorie consumption or ideal calorie requirement as seen in Table 2.2.

Folic Acid and B_{12}: These are mainly involved in hemopoiesis, the deficiency of which can lead to megaloblastic anemia. The recommended intakes are shown in Table 2.2.

Calcium and Phosphorus

Calcium and phosphorus are an important components of a diet for infants and children due to their role in formation of strong skeletal system besides good dental health. Calcium in ionic form plays a crucial role in transmission of nerve impulses. On the other hand, phosphorus is an important constituent of nucleic acids and phospholipids involved in cellular metabolism. As in the case of EFA ratio, the Ca:P ratio also is important to be maintained at a desirable level of 1:1 in case of children and in infants 1:1.5. Table 2.10 gives the recommended intakes of calcium

TABLE 2.9: Recommended intake of vitamin A for children

Group	Age	Retinol (I.U)	β-carotene (μg)*
Infants	0–6 month 6–12 months	350	- 2100
Children	1–6 years 7–9 years	400 600	3200 4800
Adolescents	10–17 years	600	4800

Refer. ICMR, 2010
*Conversion ratio of 1:8 is used.

TABLE 2.10: Recommended intakes for calcium for children

Category	Age	Calcium (mg/d)	Phosphorus (mg/d)
Infants		800	750
Children	1–9 years 10–17 years	600 800	600 800

Refer. ICMR, 2010

and phosphorus for children up to 18 years.[1] No recommendation has been fixed for phosphorus on the assumption that a mixed Indian diet can provide sufficient content to cater to the daily body needs.

Iron

The iron needs of an infant are taken care of by the breast milk up to 6 months of life. Beyond that milk, whether breast or cow's milk, both are inadequate to sustain the increasing demands of the child. Though breast milk too is not a very good source of iron, the needs of the infant are taken care of by the maternal reserves deposited during the course of the mother's pregnancy. At birth the infant has about 80 mgs of iron/kg body weight or total of 270 mgs. The maternal iron stores are used up by the infant by 6 months after which there is no reserve store until about 2 years. During childhood the iron stores build up to 5 mg/kg, and remain so until menarche in the females. In males there is further increase of 12 mg to 15 mg/kg between 15 and 30 years.[1]

After 6 months, if the child is fed exclusively either on breast milk or cow's milk, or even predominantly formula milk, the reserve iron stores get gradually depleted. In this situation if no dietary source is provided, the child begins to show signs of anemia. Therefore it is very important that from 6 months onwards, the child's feeds are supplemented with cereals, pulses and vegetables gradually over a period of time. Formula fed babies may have an adequate store of iron as most of the baby milk formulae are fortified with important minerals and vitamins. The RDA for iron requirements of infants and children are as given in Table 2.1.

REFERENCES

1. Nutrient Requirements and Recommended Dietary Allowances for Indians. A Report of the Expert Group of the Indian Council of Medical Research. New Delhi, Indian Council of Medical Research. 2010.
2. Venkatachalam PS. Maternal nutritional status and it's effect on the new born Bull WHO. 1962;26:203-11.
3. Bhargava SK, Bhargava V, Kumar S, et al. Maternal nutrition and fetal growth retardation. J Trop Pediatr. 1983;29:48-150.
4. Devi RR, Agarwal KN. Maternal nutrition and fetal growth. Ind J Pediatr. 1984;51:443-9.
5. Leela Raman and Veena Shatrugna Nutrition in Pregnancy and lactation In: Textbook of Human Nutrition ed. by Mahtab S Bamji, N Prahlad Rao, Vinodni Reddy. 1996.
6. Rathi S, Khosla A, Sharma N, et al. Pregnancy outcome in severe anemia. J Obst Gynec India. 1987;4:478-80.
7. Bhargava M, Kumar R, Iyer PU, et al. Effect of maternal anemia and iron depletion on fetal iron stores, birth weight and gestation Acta Pediatr Scand. 1989;78: 321-22.
8. MRC Vitamins Study Research Group: Prevention of neural tube defects. Results of the Medical Research Council Vitamin Study. Lancet. 1991;338:131-7.
9. Iyengar L, Rajalakshmi K. Effect of folic acid supplement on birth weight of infants. Am J Obstet Gynec. 1975;122:332-36.
10. Kochupillai N. The impact of iodine deficiency on human resource development. Prog Food Nutr Sci. 1989;13:1-15.
11. Vir S. Control of iodine deficiency in India Bull NFI. 1994;15(2).
12. Energy and Protein Requirements. Report of a Joint FAO/WHO Expert Committee. WHO Technical Report Series No. 522. Geneva, World Health Organization. 1973.
13. Energy and Protein requirements. Report of a Joint FAO/WHO/UNU Expert Consultation. WHO Technical Report Series 724. Geneva, World Health Organization. 1985.
14. KE Elizabeth. Applied Nutrition, In Nutrition and Child Development, 3rd ed, Paras Medical Publisher, Hyderabad. 2004.
15. Gopalan C. Protein requirement of breast fed poor infants. J Trop Pediatr. 1956;2:89.
16. BS Narsinga Rao. Nutrient Requirements and Recommended Allowances in Textbook of Human Nutrition, Ed. Mahtab S Bamji, N Pralhad Rao, Vinodini Reddy. Published by Oxford & IBH Publishing Co Pvt Ltd. 1996.

3 Nutritional Assessment of Children

In order to plan any dietary regime for a child or any individual, it is important to first have an idea of his/her pre-existing condition. For this, the child is assessed for his nutritional status which may include various parameters depending upon what circumstances and where he is managed. Ideally nutritional assessment is the first step towards the management of a child brought in a hospital. This gives us an idea of his pre-existing condition, besides the clinical picture that might be presented to us upon admission or may be in the out patient clinic also. Based on this assessment, the further course of action is planned.

The four main parameters generally used for nutritional assessment of a child in a hospital are:

- Anthropometry
- Dietary
- Clinical
- Biochemical.

Besides these there are other parameters like radiological, morphological and epidemiological which are beyond the scope of present discussion. We shall look into the 4 parameters listed above in detail:

ANTHROPOMETRY

This is perhaps the first step undertaken when a child is presented for any medical management. The various parameters covered under this give a fair idea of the nutritional status of the child.

However, it is important that measurements taken to assess anthropometry be very accurate and done by trained personnel using certain accepted standard techniques. In case of children, the parameters so assessed are compared to standard 'growth charts'. The weights and heights are plotted against the curve on these charts and depending upon where they fall, the level of nutritional status can be evaluated. The equipments used for the measurements also should be precise and free from errors. The tools used to cover anthropometry are:

Weight: Weight is a useful tool to evaluate the nutritional status of children of all age groups, from birth to adolescence. The weighing scale should be accurate. The commonly used scales are the ones using a beam. Care should be taken to set the pointer at zero at resting phase and should be moving freely. The surface where the scale is placed should be flat and even. Readings are taken in kilograms. The accuracy should be to the nearest 500 grams for older children and for smaller children up to 100 grams. Electronic scales are commonly used in many centers and are more accurate. Ideally weight should be taken with minimum clothing and without shoes. Small children can be made to sit on the scale designed for them, while older children can be made to stand on the platform weighing scale.

The weights so measured are compared to some appropriate reference standards for his age, over a period of time which is done using the growth charts (Figs 3.1 to 3.6). The references internationally accepted are those by Combined National Center for Health Statistics (NCHS) and Center for Disease Control (CDS) Task Force, which have been published by WHO in 1983,[1] also referred as WHO standards. The fiftieth centile of Harvard Standards

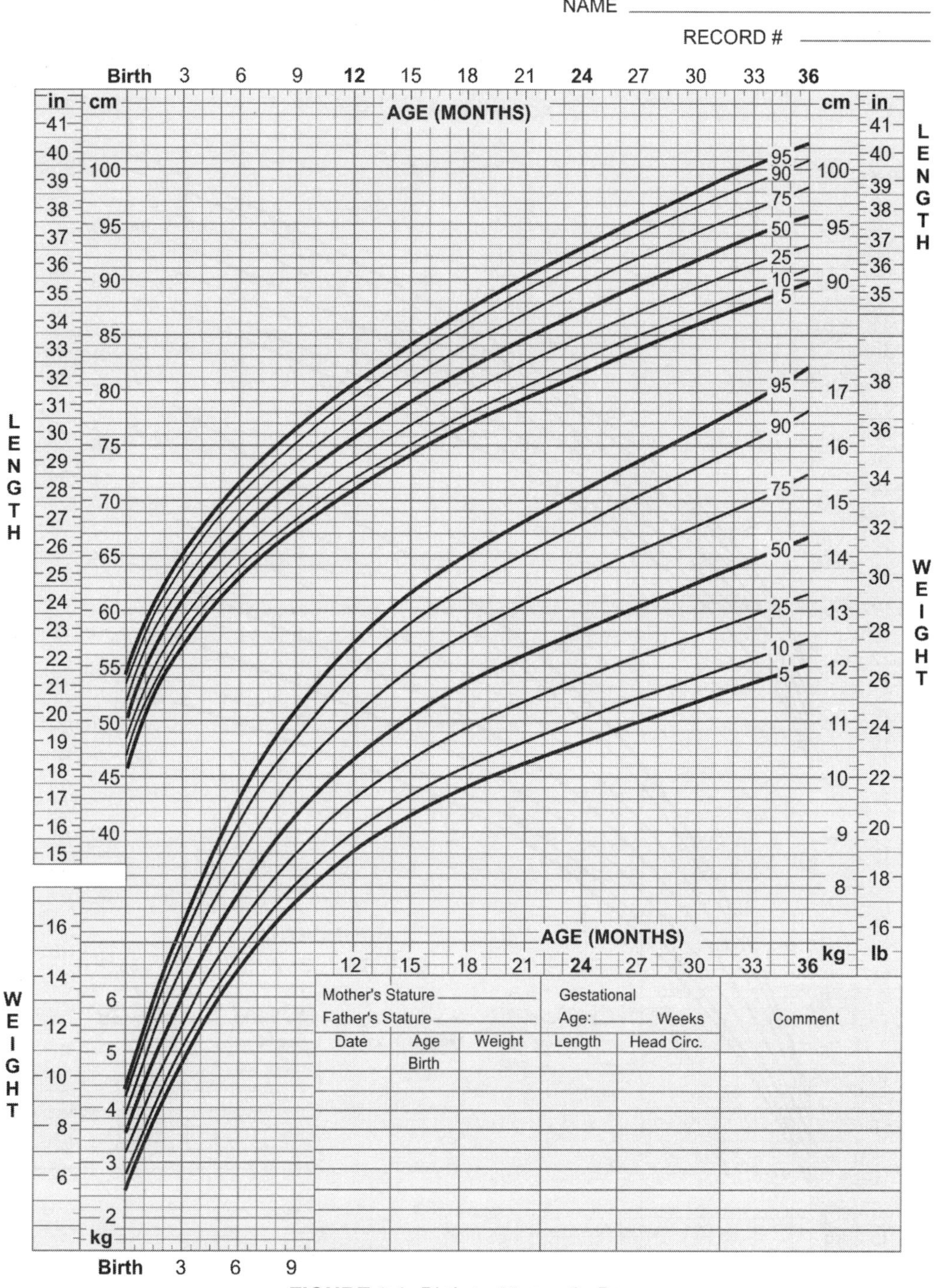

FIGURE 3.1: Birth to 36 month: Boys length-for-age and weight-for-age percentiles

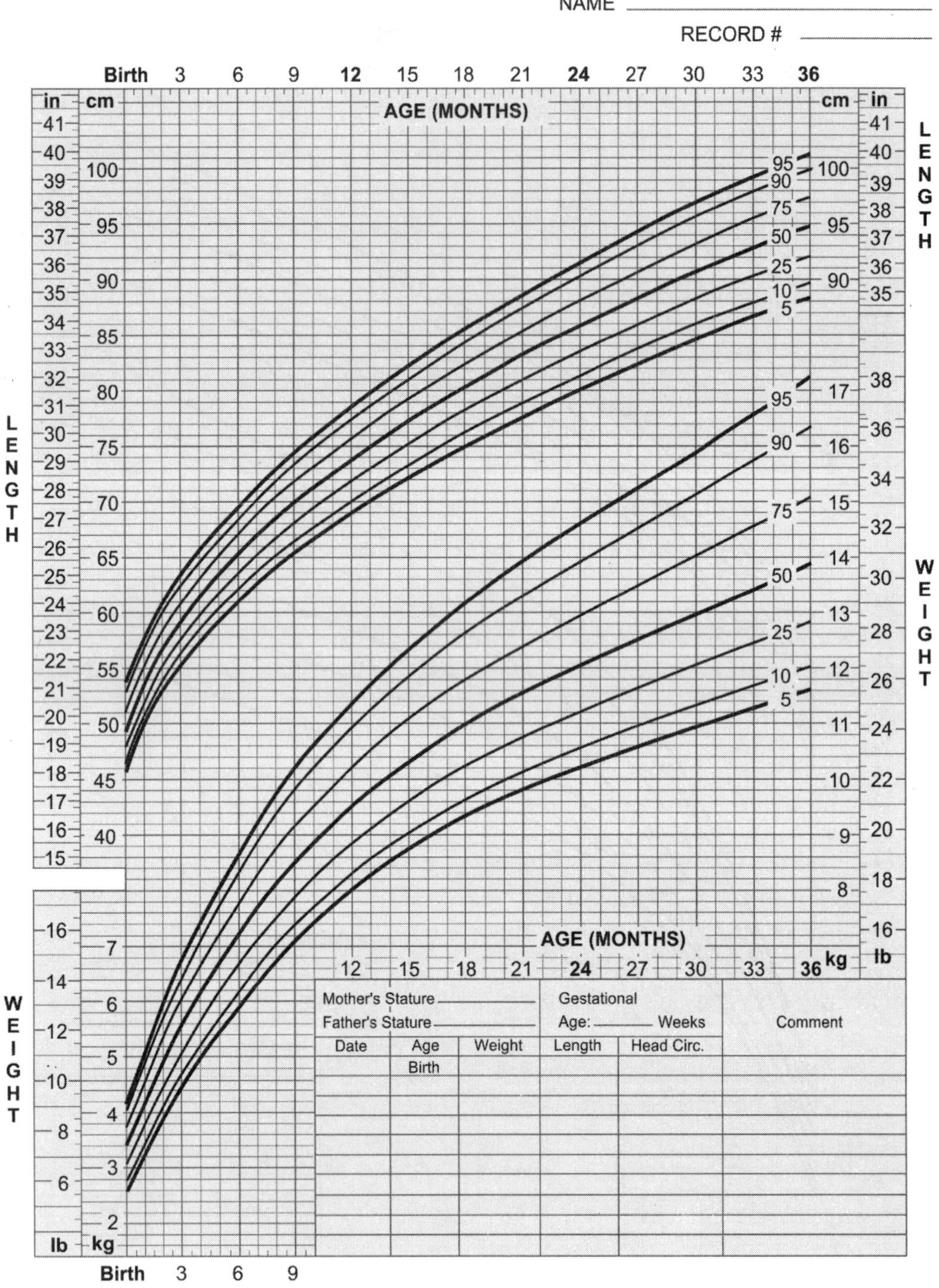

FIGURE 3.2: Birth to 36 month: Boys length-for-age and weight-for-age percentiles

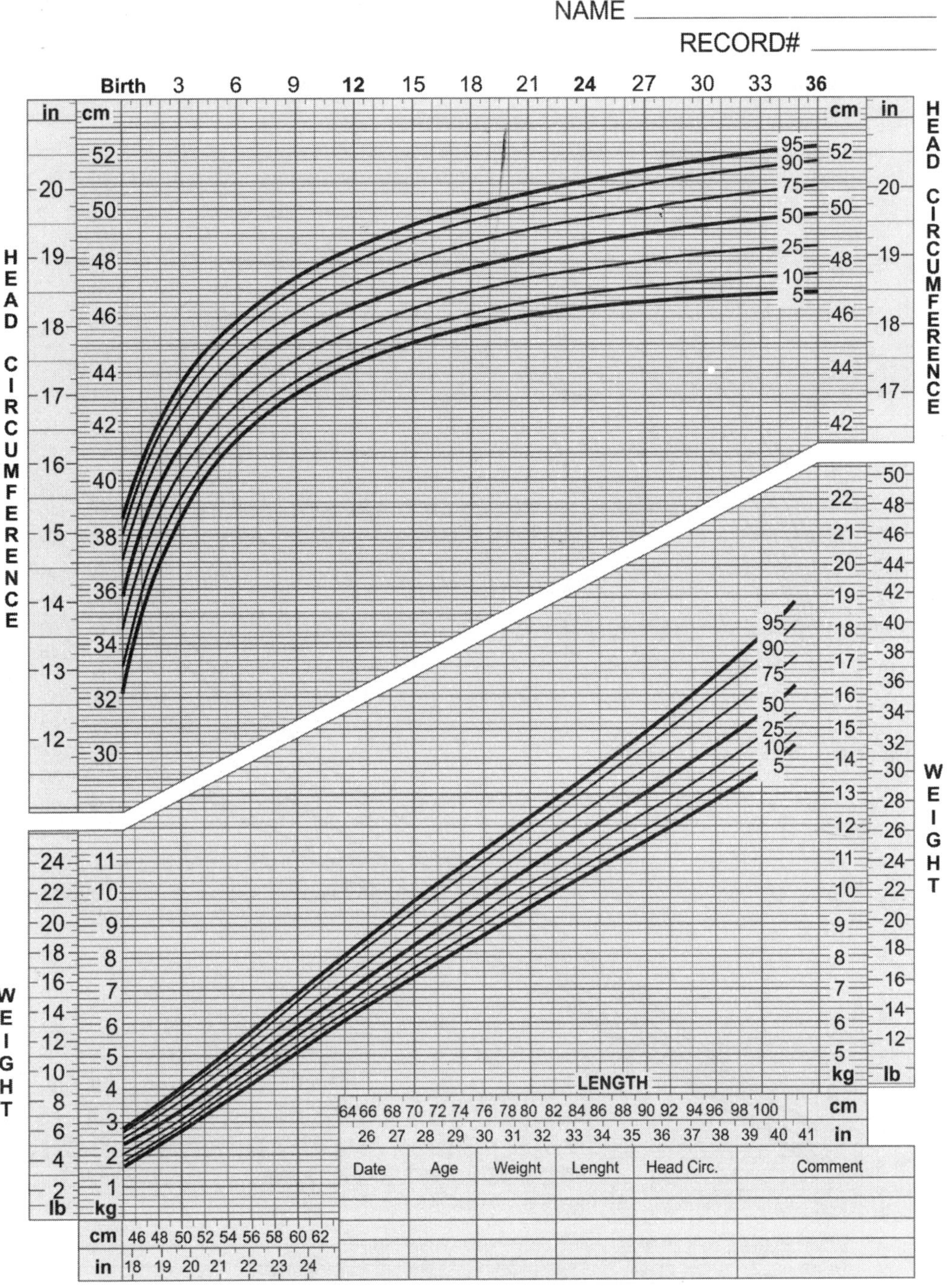

FIGURE 3.3: Birth to 36 month: Boys
Length-for-age and Weight-for-age percentiles

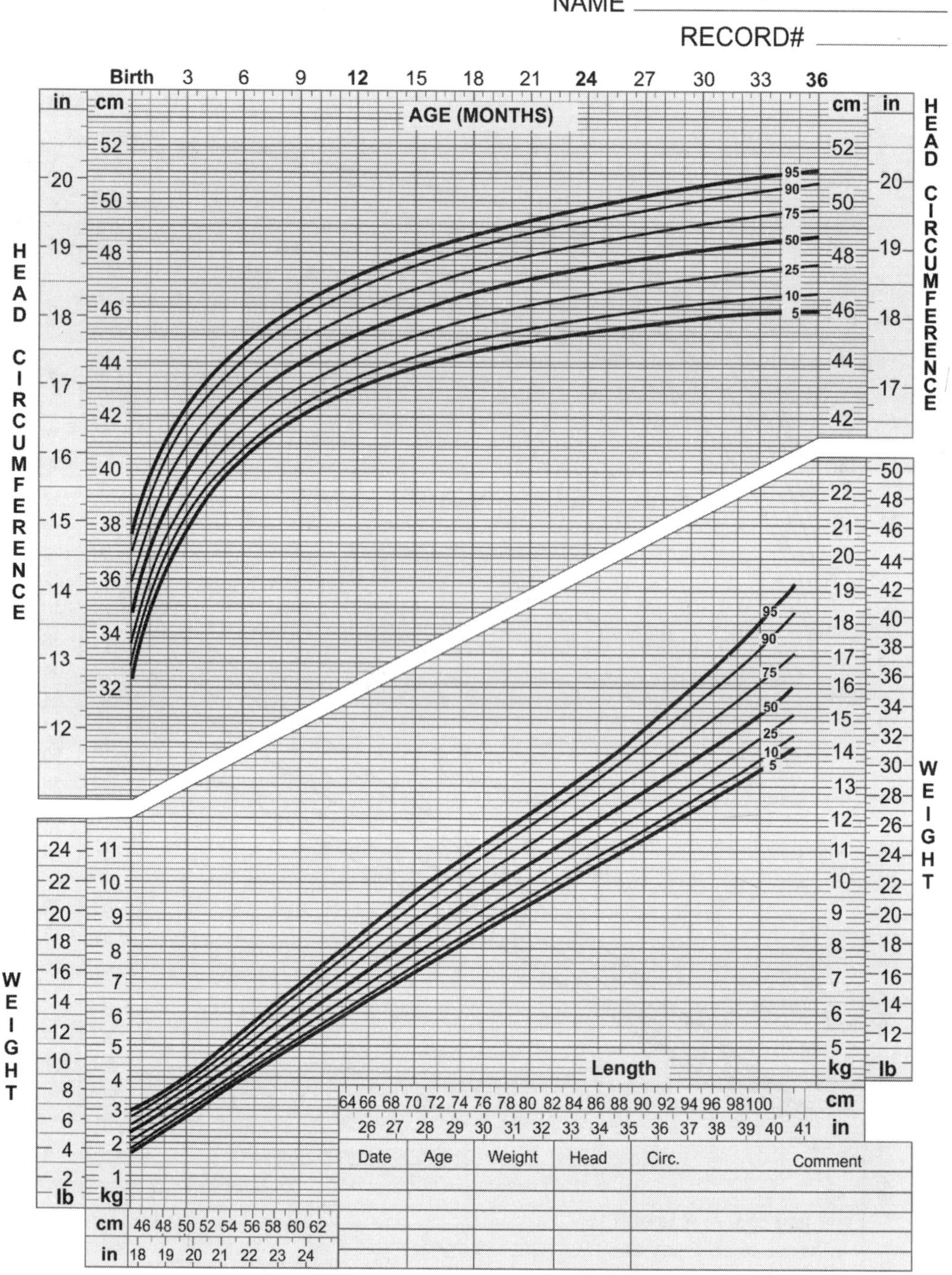

FIGURE 3.4: Birth to 36 month: Girls
head circumference-for-age and weight-for-age percentiles

NAME ____________

RECORD# ________

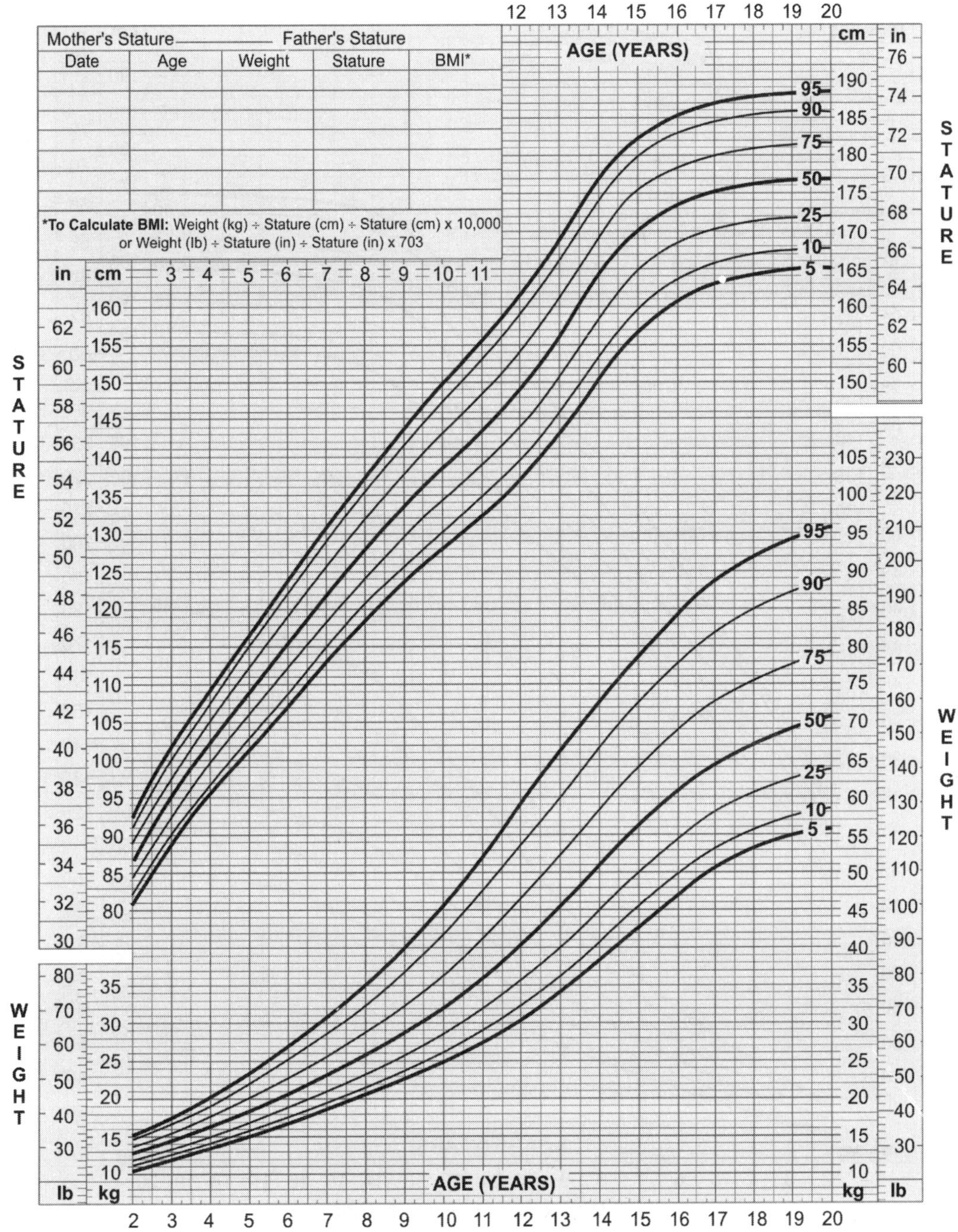

Mother's Stature		Father's Stature		
Date	Age	Weight	Stature	BMI*

*To Calculate BMI: Weight (kg) ÷ Stature (cm) ÷ Stature (cm) x 10,000 or Weight (lb) ÷ Stature (in) ÷ Stature (in) x 703

FIGURE 3.5: 2 to 20 years: Boys

Stature-for-age and weight-for-age percentiles

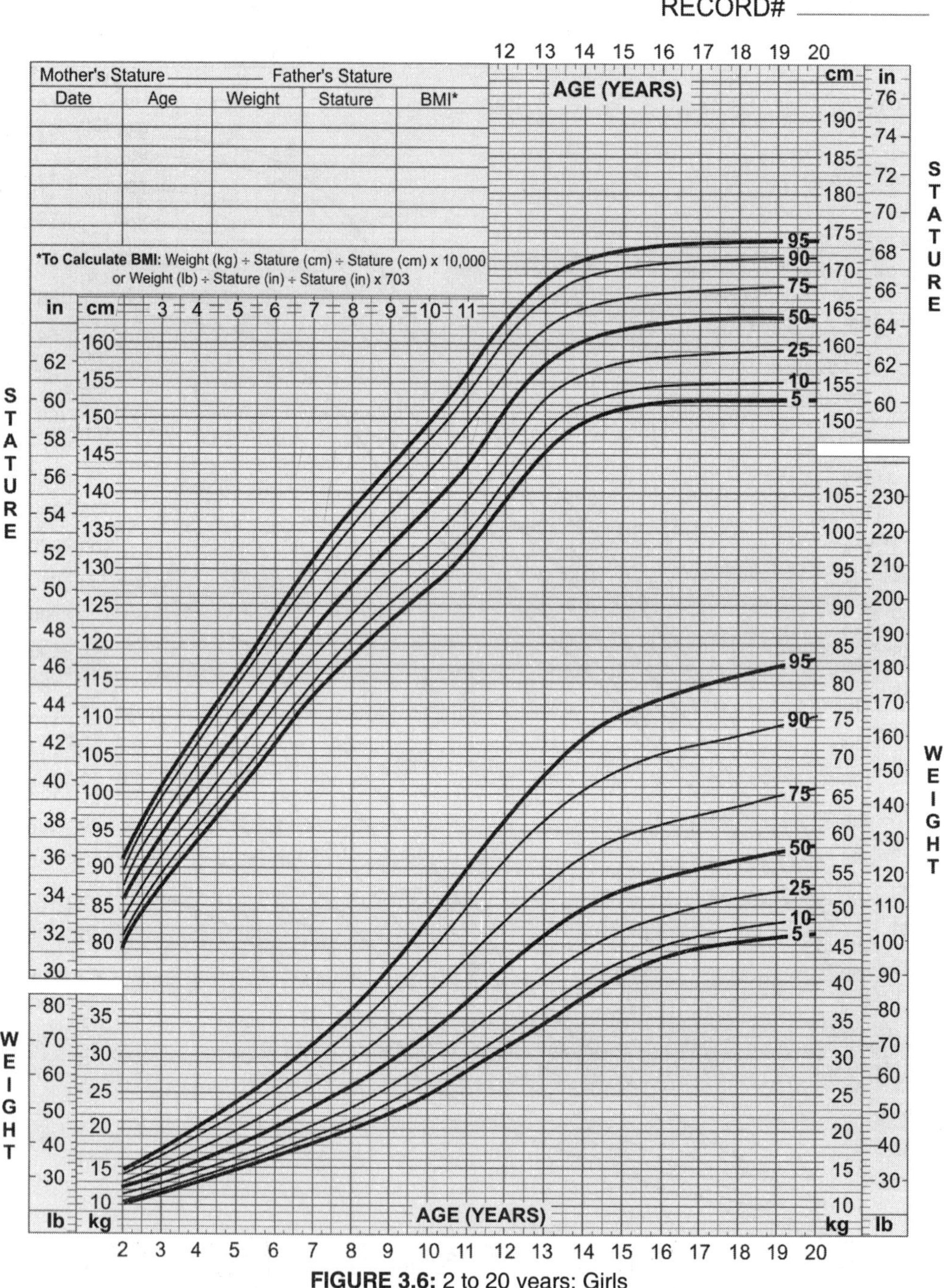

FIGURE 3.6: 2 to 20 years: Girls
Stature-for-age and weight-for-age percentiles

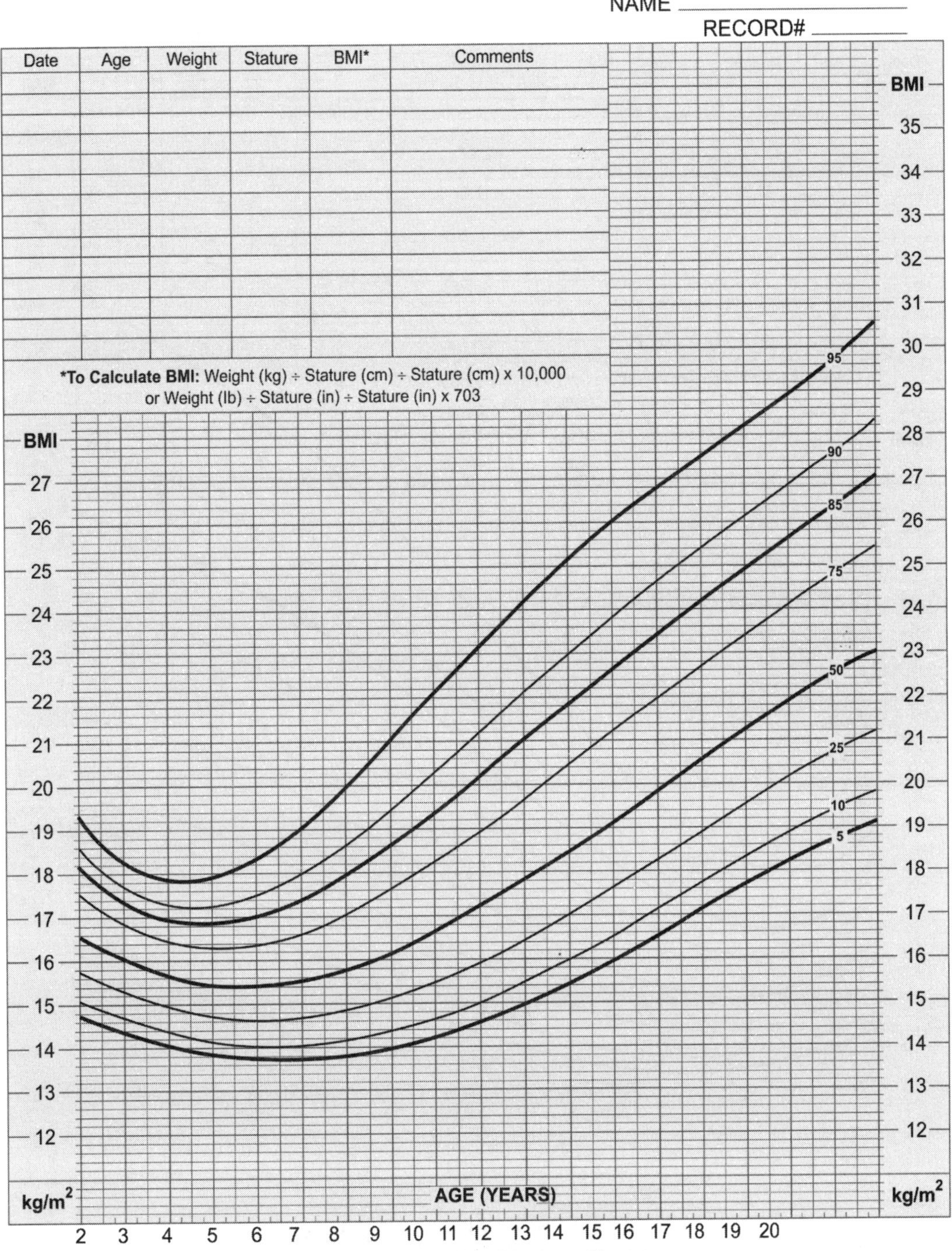

FIGURE 3.7: 2 to 20 years: Boys
Body mass index-for-age percentiles

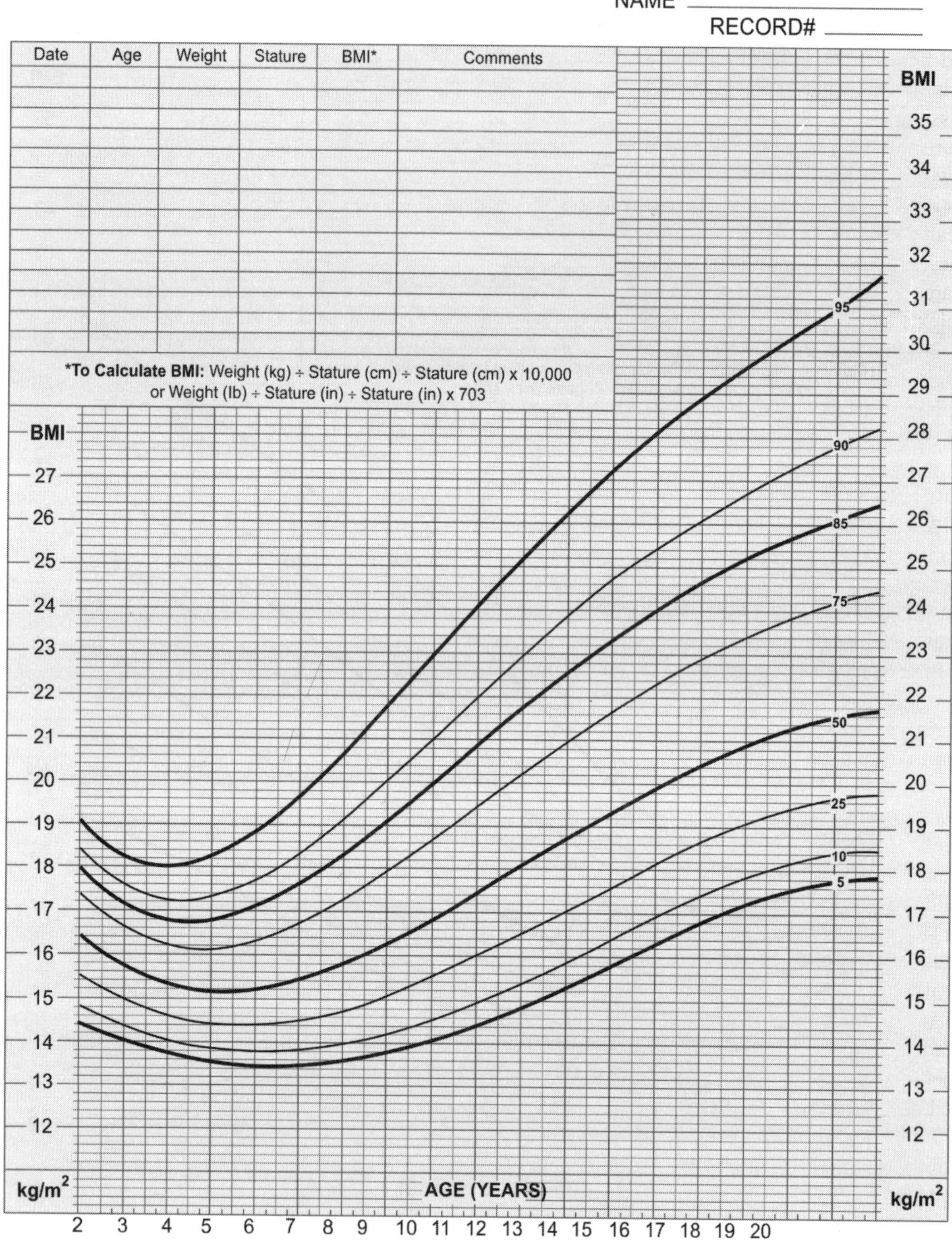

FIGURE 3.8: 2 to 20 years: Girls
Body mass index-for-age percentiles

was taken as 100 percent and references are available for weight for age, height for age, weight for height and head circumference separately for boys and girls. Based on these reference standards, a child was classified as normal or malnourished. However, these charts are not much popular now after a new set of new growth charts were brought out in 2000 by the National Center for Chronic Disease Prevention and Health Promotion, referred to as the CDC charts. These are a revised version of the 1977 NCHS growth charts.[2] These charts consist of percentiles related to weight, length and head circumference for infants (0–36 months) and percentiles related to weight, height and BMI for children (2–19 years).

The new CDC charts now include an assessment for BMI (Figs 3.7 to 3.8). These are based primarily on data gathered through National Health and Nutrition Examination Survey (NHANES), the only survey that collects data from actual physical examination on a cross section of people from all over the United States. The new BMI growth charts can be used clinically beginning at 2 years of age, when an accurate stature can be obtained.

In order to revise the growth charts, the NHANES survey conducted from 1988 through 1994, contained more than 8000 children aged 2 months to six years. The data showed that in the past two decades, the number of overweight children and teens has doubled. It was hoped that these new charts will be used to identify overweight children and teens for intervention at an early age. Moreover, the new CDC charts track children through 19 years of age, two years longer than the 1977 NCHS charts. The revised head circumference charts also show some significant differences when compared to the earlier ones. Compared to the original infant charts that were based on primarily formula fed infants, the revised growth charts for infants contain a better mix of both breast and formula fed infants in the US population.

There are different classifications used by different workers to categorize children as normal or malnourished. For malnutrition, further classifications have been made to differentiate between varying degrees of malnutrition from mild to severe. The most widely used are the Gomez classification and the Indian Academy of Pediatrics (IAP) classification.[3,4] as given in Tables 3.1 and 3.2.

TABLE 3.1: The Gomez classification

% Expected	Classification	Category of Nutritional Status weight-for-age
> 90%	Normal	Normal
76–90	Mild malnutrition	1st degree malnutrition
61–75	Moderate malnutrition	2nd degree malnutrition
< 60	Severe malnutrition	3rd degree malnutrition

TABLE 3.2: The IAP classification

%of Expected Weight (weight-for-age)	Nutritional Classification*
> 80%	Normal
71–80	Grade 1
61–70	Grade 2
51–50	Grade 3 (severe malnutrition)
< 50	Grade 4 (severe malnutrition)

*If coexisting edema of nutritional origin, the letter K is suffixed along with grade of malnutrition to denote kwashiorkor

Height/length: In case of infants and children up to age 1–2 years, the length can be measured placing the child lying down using a horizontal measuring rod or an infantometer. The child is made to lie down flat on the back with the head just touching against the fixed end with a vertical board. The legs are stretched with the knees pressed together and the other mobile end (foot end) is made to touch the heels with feet at right angles. This procedure requires at least two people to take the measurements. The accuracy is usually up to 0.5 cm. It may be worth mentioning here that height for any age may not always be a correct indicator of the nutritional status of a growing child. But it does definitely give an idea of any past or chronic malnutrition. Height is largely genetically predisposed also; therefore such factors may reflect possible variations in any age group.

Weight for height: Weight for height is age independent. This criterion may not give a true picture of nutrition of a child since height measured at a given time may not always co-related to the weight for height standard. In case a child has the desired weight for height but his linear growth is inadequate, it would be wrong to term this child as normal, even though his actual growth is inadequate. Therefore height for age also needs to be accounted for along with weight for height. This criteria had been proposed by Seoane and Lytham Table 3.3.[5] This criteria has been found

TABLE 3.3: Seoane and Lytham classification

Nutrition Status	Height-for-age (cms)	weight-for-age (kgs)	Weight-for-height (cms)
Normal	Normal	Normal	Normal
Past chronic malnutrition	Low	Low	Normal
Current short duration malnutrition	Normal	Low	Low
Current long duration malnutrition	Low	Low	Low

to be better than other criteria as reviewed by Sastry and Vijayraghvan.[6]

Growth pattern: This refers to the height and weight velocity from 1–18 years of age.

Weight: The mean birth weight of an Indian child is 2.7 kg to 2.9 kgs. An infant normally gains 25–30 grams per day till 3 months; then doubles by five months; triples by one year and becomes four times his/her birth weight by two years. After 2 years of age, there is an increase of 1.5–3 kg in weight every year till preadolescent age.

Height/Lengh: The average length of a child at birth is 50 cm. Thereafter the growth rate is 14 cm in the first 6 months. By the end of first year there is an addition of 25 cm. Another addition of 12.5 cm is made by the end of two years and then between 2–3 years there is an increase of 7.5 cm. On an average the child gains about 5–6 cms height each year after 3 years of age along the percentile band achieved by 2–3 years.

There is a period of growth spurt during adolescence when the increase is 9–10 cms in height and a weight gain of 8–10 kg. In girls the growth spurt occurs between 10–12 years while in boys it occurs 2 years later.

During the first 12–24 months after birth there is maximum postnatal growth velocity wherein the infants seek their own curve. By 2–3 years the child's stature reflects his/her own genetic endowment rather than mother' size.

Mid arm circumference (MAC): This measure-ment is made on a nondominant arm, midway between the acromial and olecranon processes, with the arm hanging relaxed. Measurements are done using a simple flexible measuring tape, gently without applying any pressure. This reading should be taken to the nearest 0.1 cm. MAC co-related well with weight for height. The cut off points used to determine malnutrition using this criterion are:

Normal	14.00 cm
Mild/Acute malnutrition	12.4–14 cm
Severe malnutrition	< 12.5 cm

Head circumference: This is also referred as occipitofrontal circumference (OFC) which is measured using a flexible measuring tape being firmly placed over the most prominent region of the occipital and frontal crests. The measurement is taken accurately to the nearest 0.1 cm. However, this parameter is of value for children up to about 2 years only, since by this age the increase in head circumference is usually complete.

Chest circumference: This measurement is also done using a flexible tape and is taken at the level of the nipple, with the child sitting, midway between inspiration and expiration. In infancy the OFC is more than the chest circumference, but by one year of age, both are almost equal, after which the chest circumference takes over the head circumference. In malnourished children, this ratio of OFC to chest continues to be >1, i.e. OFC continuing to be more than chest circumference.

Triceps skinfold (TSF): This is done using a Harpenden skinfold caliper and is calculated to the nearest millimeter. This measurement is made on the back of the nondominant arm mid way between the acrmial and the olecranon process, with the arm hanging relaxed.

Midarm-muscle circumference: This is derived by using the MAC and the TSF using the following equation: MAMC (cm) = MAC (cm) – TSF (mm) × 0.314.

Mid parental height (MPH): This criterion is not usually used as a routine. However, where the child is presented with growth retardation or short stature, this formula proves to be a helpful tool. The estimate for boys and girls is done as follows:

$$\text{Boys} = \frac{\text{Father's height (cms)} + \text{Mother's height} + 13}{2}$$

$$\text{Girls} = \frac{\text{Father's height (cms)} + \text{Mother's height} - 13}{2}$$

The values obtained for all the above measurements are compared to percentiles based on the child's age and sex as given in the growth charts. Values of less than 5% are indicative of significant malnutrition where as above 95th percentile denote over nutrition or obesity.

Apart from all the above parameters used to assess nutritional status, there are certain criteria made use of for quick bed side evaluation of the child's status. This formula is referred to as the Weech's formula or the NCHS criteria. In this formula, the expected weight is based on the assumption that *birth weight doubles by 5 months and triples by 1 year (10 kg) and quadruples by 2 years (12 kg). Thereafter, add 2 kg per year for children up to 6 years of age, and beyond that add 3 kg per year till puberty. Similarly, for height also, assuming birth length to be 50 cm, it becomes 75 cm, at 1 year and 87.5 cm by 2 years. Birth length doubles by 4 years, after which 6 cm per year is added on till puberty. Birth length triples by 12 years.*

For head circumference, at birth it is considered 35 cm. It increases to 40 cm by 3 months, 45 cm by 9 months, 47 cm by 1 year, 49 cm by 2 years and 50 cm, by 3 years. The approximate increase is 2.0 cm per month in the first 3 months, 1 cm per month in the next 3 months and 0.5 cm per month in the next 6 months.[6] These bed side calculations are summarized in Table 3.4.

TABLE 3.4: Bedside calculation for weight*, height**, head circumstances

Age (years)	Weight (kg)	Height (cm)	Head circumference (cm)
Birth	3	50	33–35
3/12	5	60	39–40
6/12	7	66	42–44
9/12	9	71	44–45
1	10	75	45–47
2	12	87	47–49
3	14	94	49–50
4	16	100	50–51
5	18	106	50–52
6	20	112	51–52
7	23	118	
8	26	124	
9	29	130	
10	32	136	
11	35	142	
12	38	150	

Refer. 6

*Add 2 kg/year in 1–6 years of age and add 3 kg/year thereafter till puberty.

**Add 6 cm/year after 2 years of age till puberty

Table 3.5 shows formulae for calculating average weight, height and head circumference in children from birth to 12 years.[7]

TABLE 3.5: Formula for average weight, height and head circumference in children (birth to 12 years)

Age	Weight (kg)
Birth	3
3–12 months	$\frac{\text{Age (month)} + 9}{2}$
1–6 years	Age (year) × 2 + 8
7–12 years	$\frac{\text{Age (month)} \times 7 - 5}{2}$
Height	**cm**
Birth	50
3 months	60
6 months	66
1 year	75
2–12 years	Age (year) × 6 + 77
Head circumference	**cm**
Birth	35
Infant	$\frac{\text{Length (cm)}}{2} + 9.5 \pm 2.5$
3 months	40
6 months	43
1 year	47
2 years	49
3 years	50
4 years	50.4
5 years	50.8

Refer. 7

Body mass index (BMI): This is a measure of body fatness expressed in relation to body weight and height. It is calculated as weight (kg)/height $(m)^2$. Certain cut off values have been fixed for defining under nutrition or over nutrition. BMI changes with age. At birth, the median is about 13 kg/m^2, increasing to 17 at one year and then decreasing to 15 at 6 years and gradually increasing to 21 by adulthood.

In recent years BMI has received increased attention for pediatric use. In 1994, an expert committee charged with developing guidelines for overweight in adolescent preventive services (ages 11–21 years) recommended that BMI be used routinely to screen overweight adolescents. In addition, in 1997 an expert committee on the assessment and treatment of obesity concluded that BMI should be used to screen for overweight children, ages 2 years and older, using BMI curves from the revised growth charts. BMI can also be used to characterize underweight (though no expert guidelines exist for the classification of underweight based on BMI).[8]

However, most studies have shown that even though BMI above 18.5 is regarded as normal, most of our adolescents falling below 13 years have a BMI > 18.5. It was felt by certain workers that BMI < 15 indicated under nutrition or chronic energy deficiency (CED) and < 13 indicates severe malnutrition. The upper value of 22 has been fixed as cut off for over weight and 25 for obesity in young adolescents during the growth period. These values are similar to those fixed by IOTF standards. Elizabeth[9] has developed another set of growth charts taking into consideration weight, height and BMI instead of age, sex, pubertal growth and parental status. These are called the ELIZ Health Path for adolescent children (EHPAC) as given in Figs 3.9 and 3.10. These charts have the advantage of plotting weight and height in the same chart, doing away with actually calculating BMI. They also denote various curves denoting normal, under nutrition, over

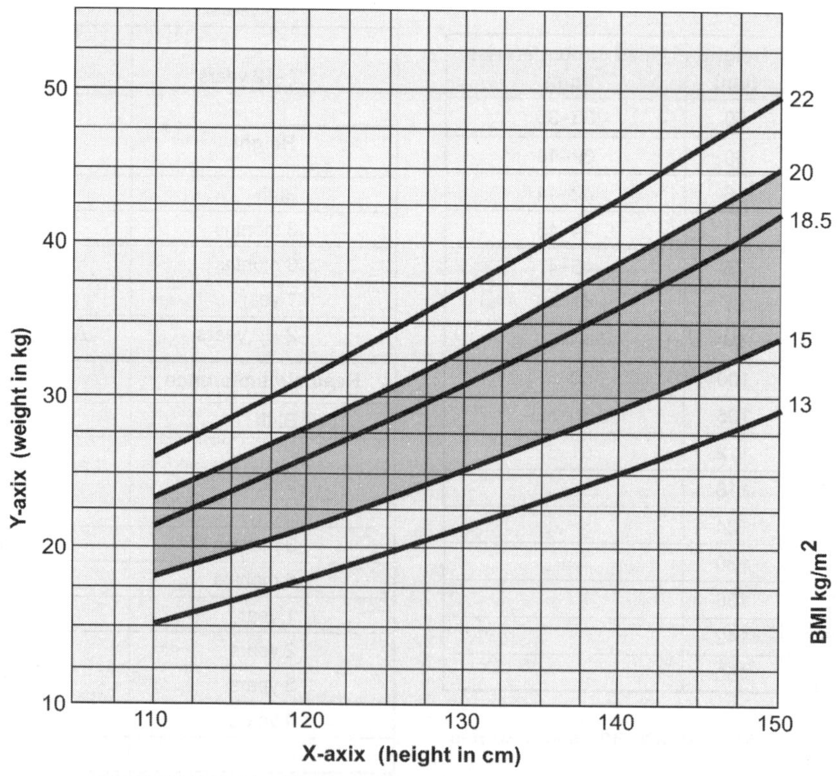

FIGURE 3.9: The ELIZ health path for older children (EHPOC)
(*Source*: KE Elizabeth in Nutrition and Child Development, 2004)

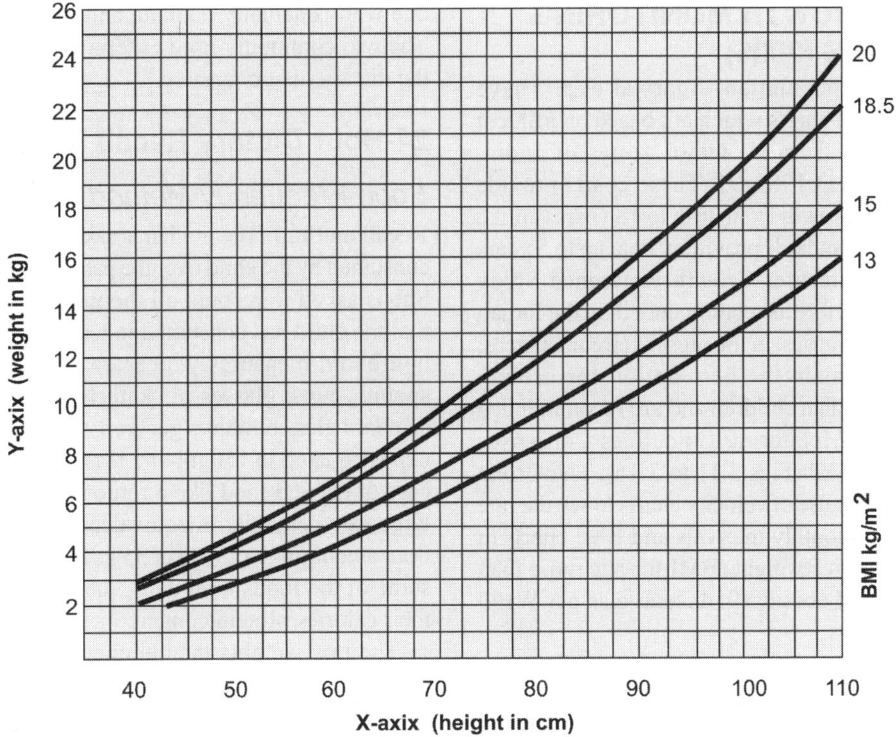

FIGURE 3.10: The ELIZ health path for under five children (EHPUC)
(*Source*: KE Elizabeth in Nutrition and Child Development, 2004)

weight and obesity. These charts are a helpful tool for a child or adolescent to actually realize where he/ she stands vis a vis their stature, i.e., whether they fall in the normal range or are inclined to obesity, or are in fact under weight, where as they must be considering themselves above normal. They should bear in mind that this is their last chance for improving their nutritional stature and come at par within the desired range. This is particularly true for the present generation youngsters who are unduly conscious of their figures or on the other end those who are quite unmindful of their over weight condition.

Plot the height on X-axis and weight on Y-axis. Mark the meeting point and project the point along or parallel to the dotted line and directly read the BMI from right margin.

Readings in shaded are in normal range.

Readings < 15 indicate underweight
Reading > 20 indicate overweight
Readings > 22 indicate obesity

Plot the height on X-axis and weight on Y-axis. Mark the meeting point and project the point along or parallel to the dotted line and directly read the BMI from right margin.

(0–1 years) between 40–70 cm

Readings in shaded area are in normal range
Readings < 13 indicate underweight
Reading > 15 indicate overweight
Readings > 18.5 indicate obesity.

(1–5 years) between 70–110 cm

Readings in shaded area are in normal range
Readings < 15 indicate underweight
Reading > 18.5 indicate overweight
Readings > 20 indicate obesity.

THE IAP GROWTH MONITORING GUIDELINES (2006)

For the Indian population, Agarwal et al[10] have compiled growth charts which are based on affluent urban children from all major zones of India, measured between 1989–91. These charts provide information on growth from birth to 18 years (unlike the new WHO standards providing data up to 5 years as per the Multicenter Growth Reference Study (MGRS).[11] Therefore as recommended by the Indian Academy of Pediatrics, in the present circumstances, these charts remain the best option for growth monitoring in Indian children and are recommended by the Growth Monitoring Guidelines Consensus Meeting of the IAP (Figs 3.11 to 3.16). The Group also recommends use of velocity charts to see the rate of growth at 6 monthly intervals and BMI charts to help in guiding overweight (BMI for age more than 85th centile) and obesity (95th centile as per WHO recommendations.

DIETARY ASSESSMENT

After assessing the anthropometry, the next step to evaluate the nutritional status is to do the dietary assessment. This can be done in two ways. One is the qualitative intake and the other is the quantitative aspect. Qualitative assessment is done mainly to get information on the type of food consumed in a particular population or section of population with regard to their social or cultural background and food practices. These methods are more relevant in institutions or group of population for survey studies. The other being the quantitative evaluation which deals with the actual amounts of different foods consumed in terms of cooked and raw amounts and subsequently, the nutrients derived from these foods. These intakes are then assessed in terms of their adequacy vis a vis the RDA for any particular group of population. It is this aspect of the dietary evaluation which is relevant in the present context. In order to know whether the child's intake in terms of macro-and micro-nutrients is adequate or not, a detailed dietary history needs to be elicited from the mother. In our country the mother is the best source of providing the information, since she is the only one who is actually cooking and feeding the child. The two commonly used criteria used for assessing the dietary history are:

24-Hour Dietary Recall Method

Food Frequency Method

Recall method: The mother is asked to recall the diet consumed by the child over the past 24 hours in detail. She is asked to recount all the ingredients or foods that the child has consumed in terms of quantitative household measures which are standardized like spoons, cups, glasses or 'katoris'. For instance, a standard glass tumblers generally of 200 ml, or a tea cup is equated to 150 ml or a teaspoon is of 5 ml. In case of cooked food like a roti of small, medium or large size generally is equivalent to raw weight of flour amounting to 25, 30 or 35 g. Table 3.6 represents some of the foods used daily, their portion size and their calories/protein content.[10]

The raw weights then elicited from the cooked portions, the nutritive value of various macro- and micronutrients can be calculated using the standard ICMR reference Tables.[13]

We can also make use of the Food Exchange (Table 3.7), to calculate the nutrients, mainly the macronutrients. By this method, portion size of the main food groups are so fixed so that one exchange equates to 100 calories. The amount of food consumed can be assessed in terms of number of exchanges and the approximate calories derived from those foods can be calculated, e.g. one medium roti which is equivalent to about 30 g is of around 100 calories. Similarly, one medium katori of cooked dal equates to about 30 g which again equates to roughly 100 calories. The protein content of the different food exchanges can also be fixed for easy reference (Table 3.8).

This method may not be 100% accurate, but will suffice for bed side calculation of a child's intake and thereby assess his/her nutritional status. It can give us an idea whether the child's intake in terms of the macro-or micronutrients are adequate or not. These estimates can be co-related with their clinical, anthropometry or biochemical parameters, thereby giving a fair idea of the nutritional status of the child.

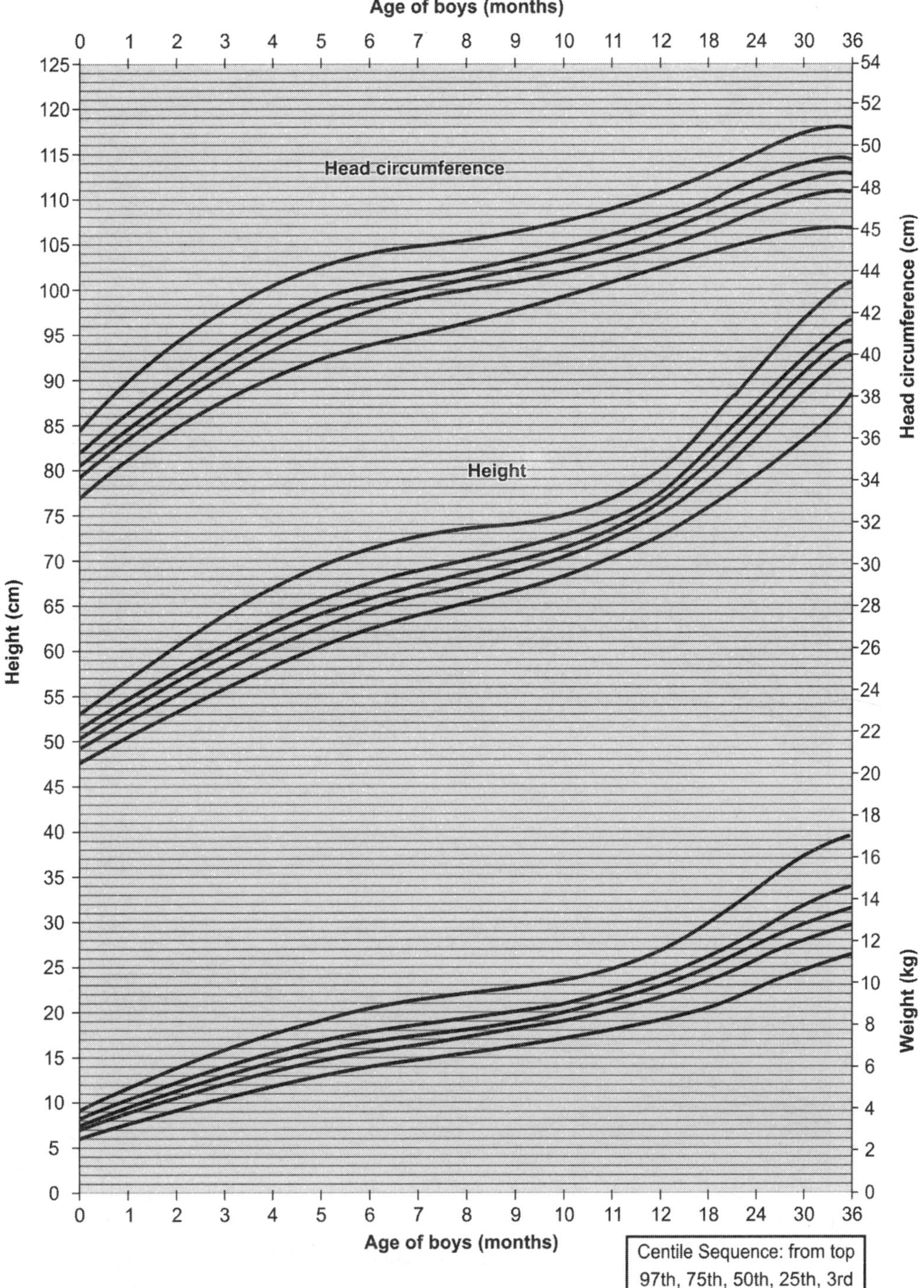

FIGURE 3.11: Height, weight and head circumference for boys 0–36 months. Redesigned by Agarwal KN, Agarwal DK, Bansal AK for the Indian Academy of Pediatrics[10]

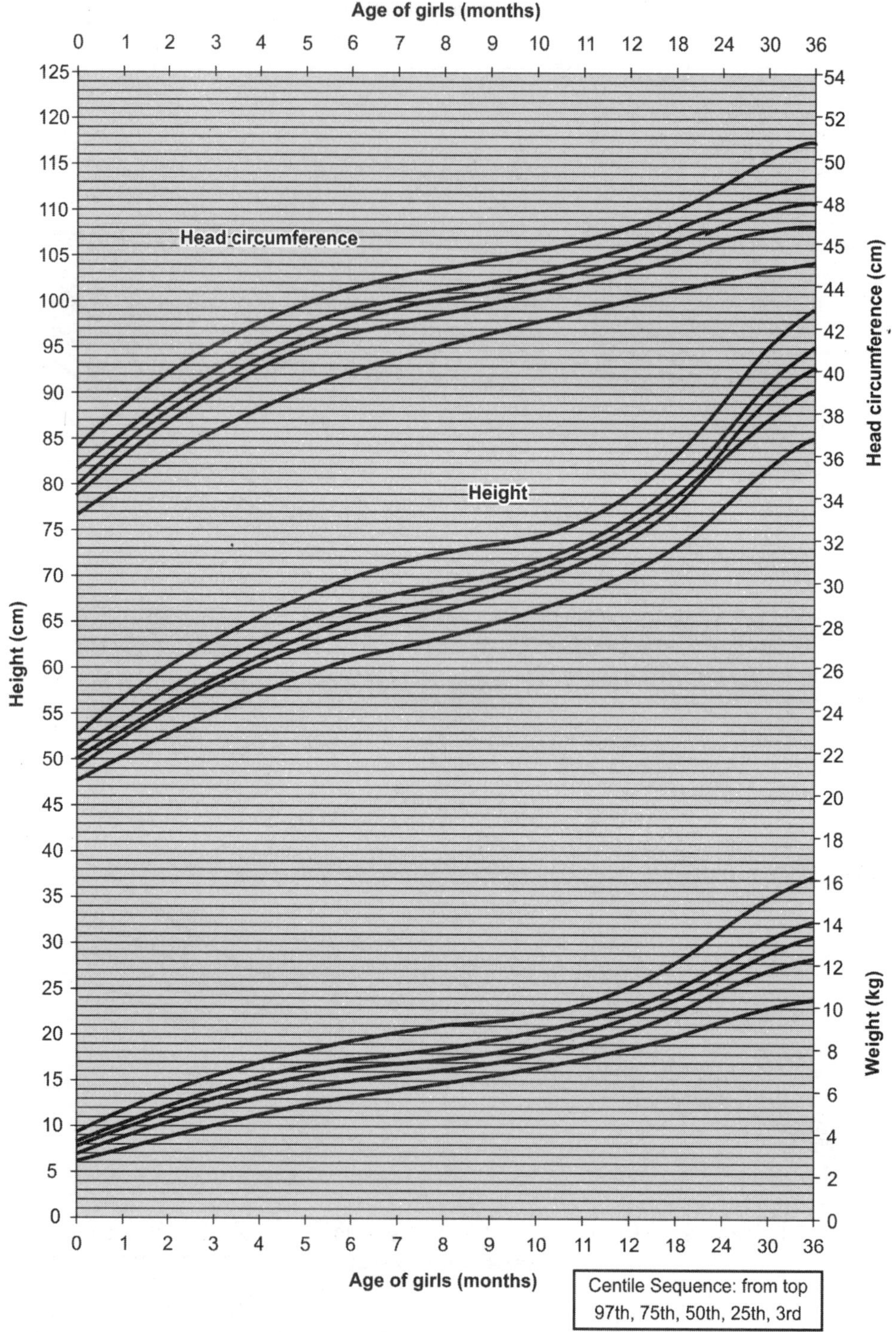

FIGURE 3.12: Height, weight and head circumference for girls 0–36 months. Redesigned by Agarwal KN, Agarwal DK, Bansal AK for the Indian Academy of Pediatrics[10]

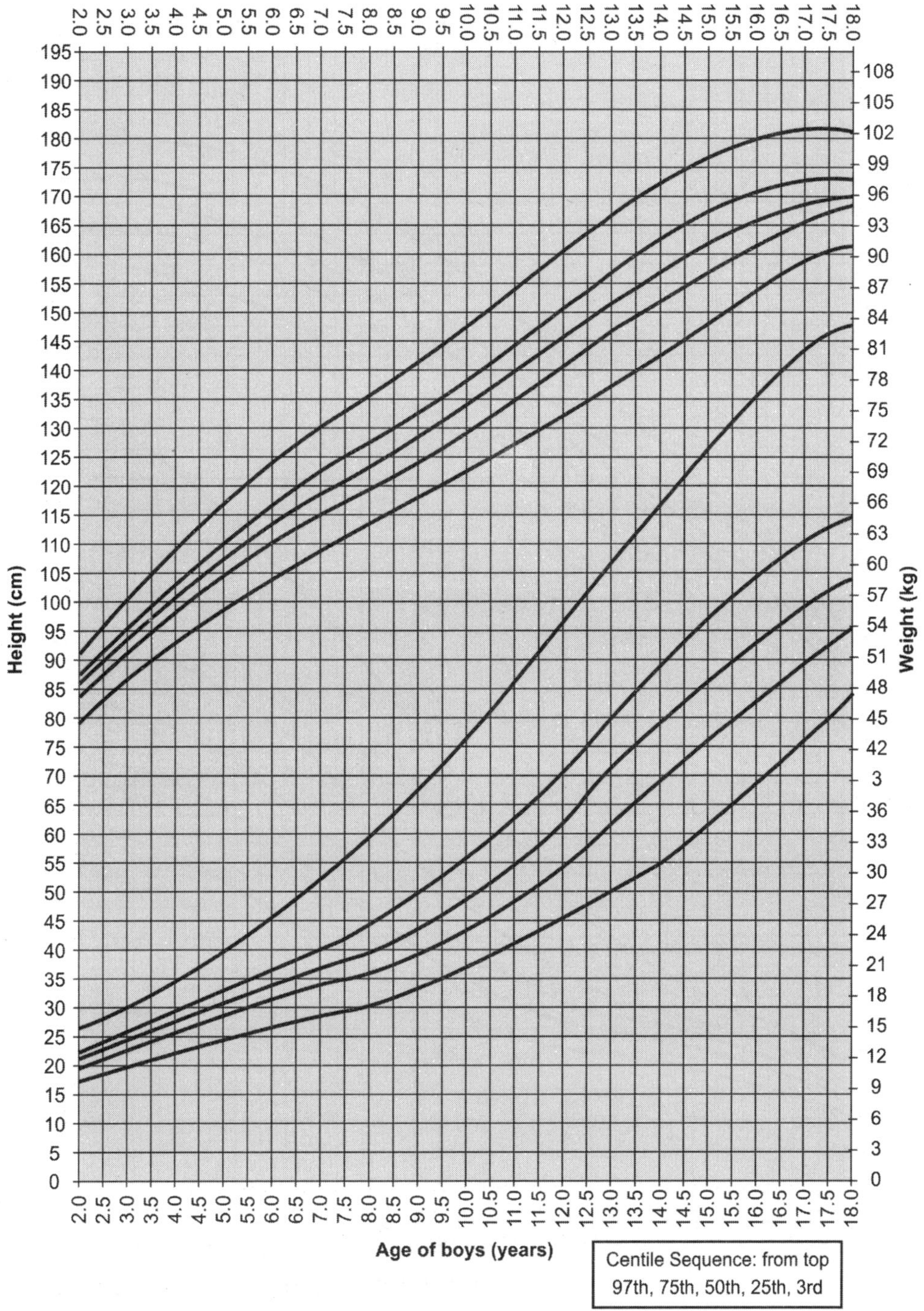

FIGURE 3.13: Height and weight for boys 2–18 years. Redesigned by Agarwal KN, Agarwal DK, Bansal AK for the Indian Academy of Pediatrics[10]

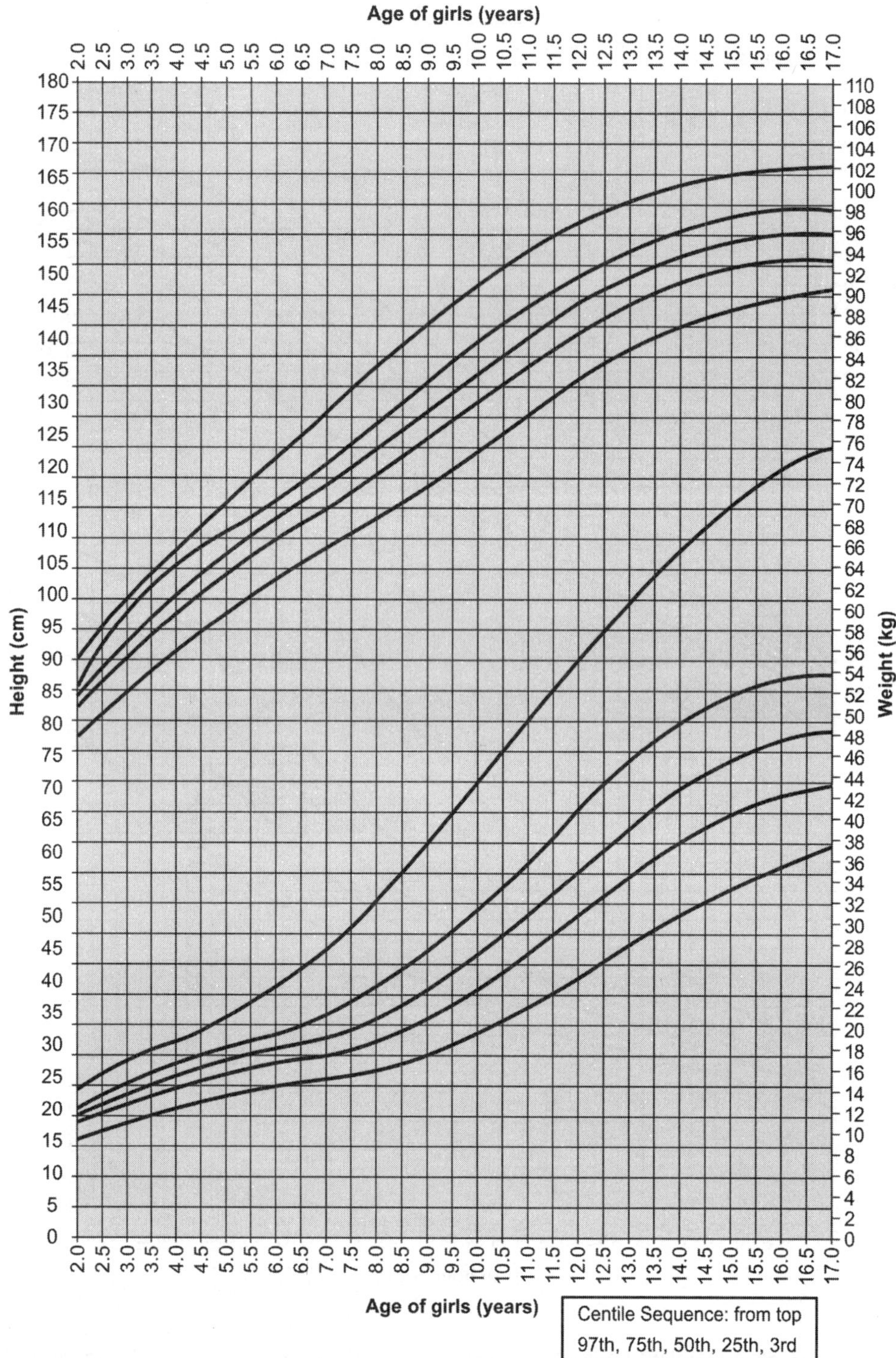

FIGURE 3.14: Height and weight for girls from 2–17 years. Redesigned by Agarwal KN, Agarwal DK, Bansal AK for the Indian Academy of Pediatrics[10]

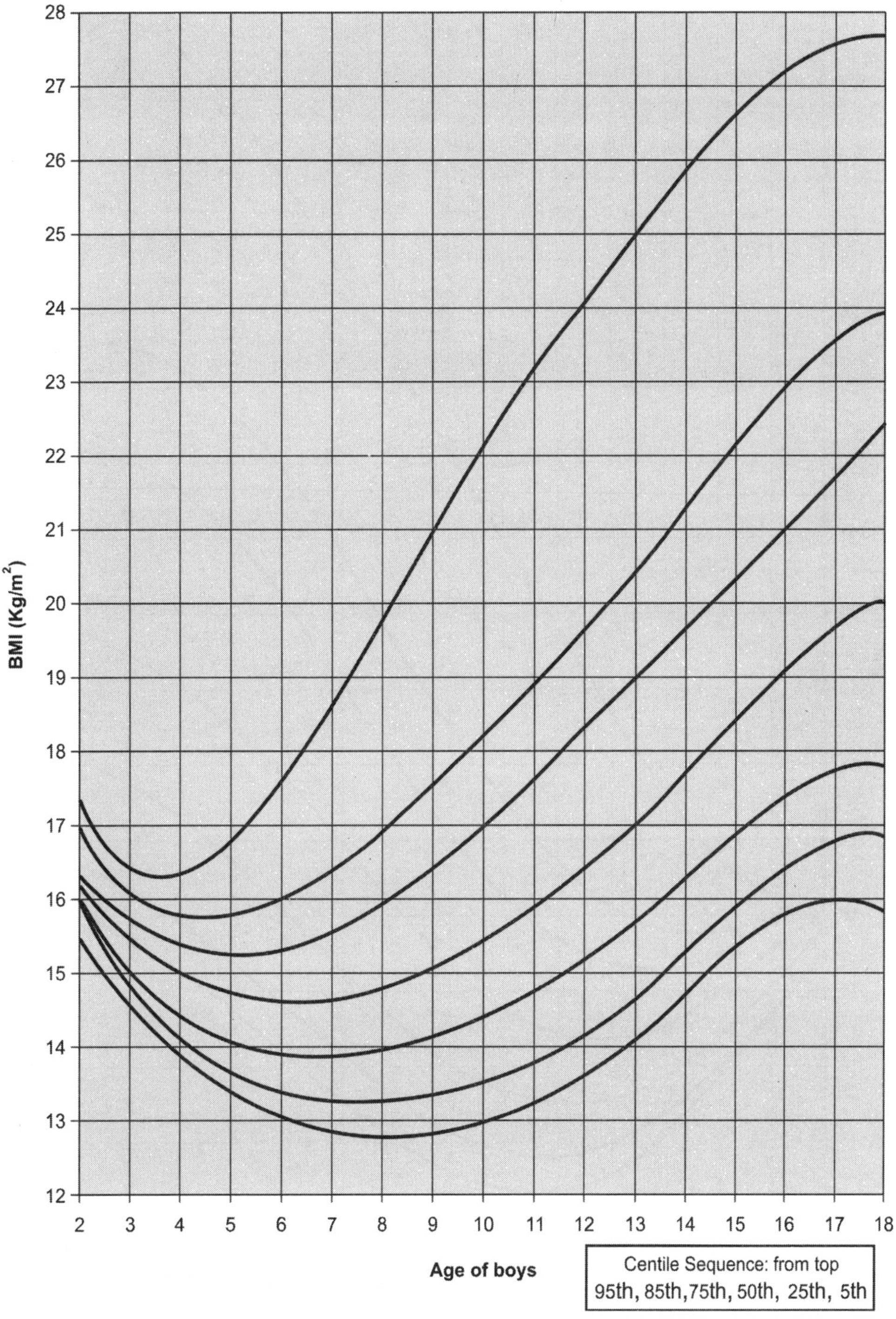

FIGURE 3.15: Body mass index for boys 2–18 years. Redesigned by Agarwal KN, Agarwal DK, Bansal AK for the Indian Academy of Pediatrics[12]

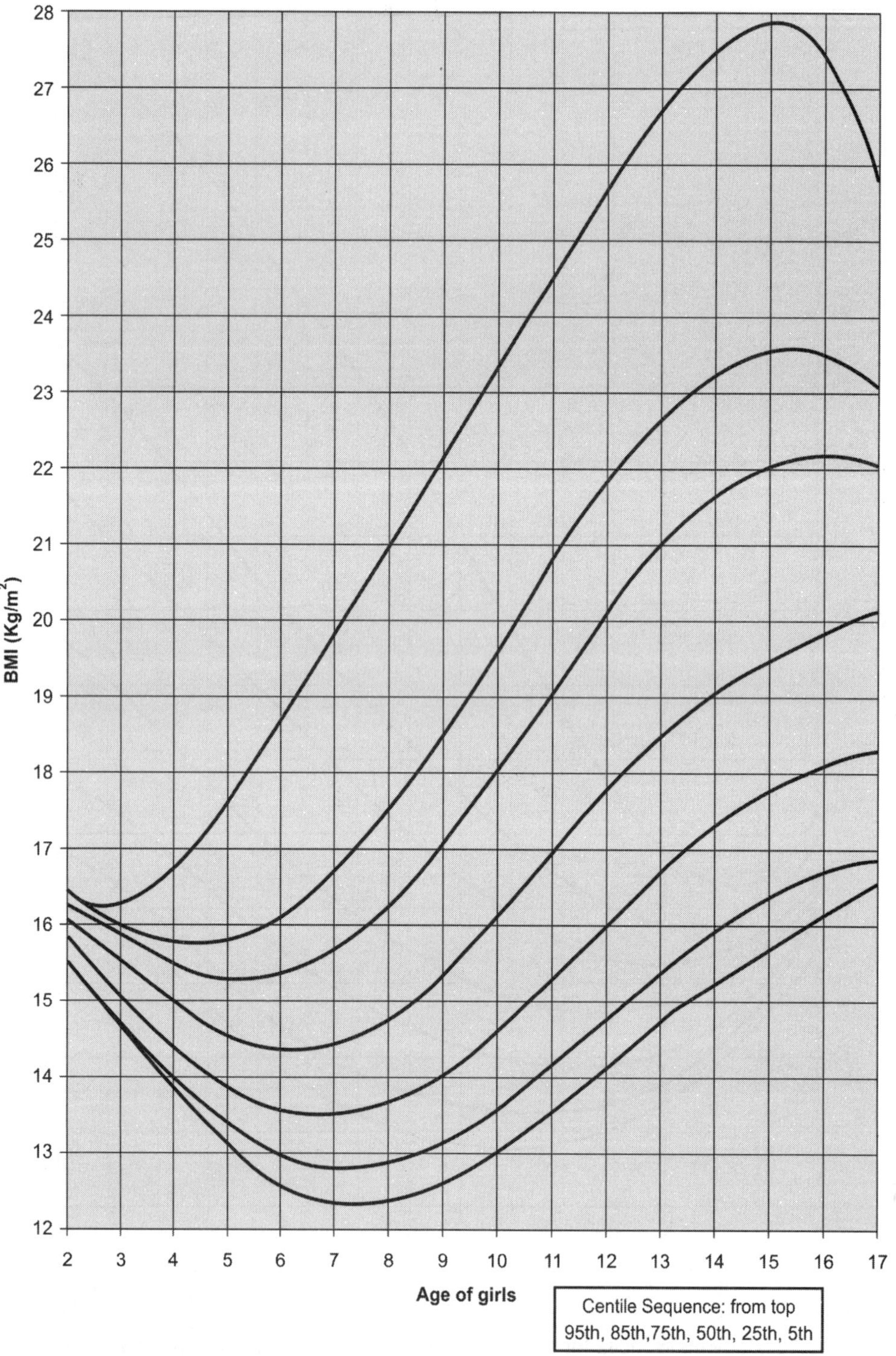

FIGURE 3.16: Body mass index for girls 2–17 years Redesigned by Agarwal KN, Agarwal DK, Bansal AK for the Indian Academy Pediatrics[12]

TABLE 3.6: Nutritive values of common household measures of cooked foods

Foods	Measure (Cooked)	Volume/ Amt. (Raw)	Energy	Protein g	Fat g	Carbohydrate g
Buffalo Milk (ml)	1 glass	250 gm	292.5	10.75	16.25	12.5
Cows Milk (ml)	1 glass	250 gm	167.5	8	10.25	11
Paneer	1 cube	25 gm	66	4.6	5.2	0.3
Skimmed Milk	1 cup	250	72.5	6.25	0.25	11.5
Paneer (Buffalo)	1 cube	25 gm	73	3.35	5.2	0.3
Curd Toned milk	1 cup	100 gm	60	3	4	3
Roti (small)	1	25 gm	85.25	3	0.42	17.35
Roti (big)	1	30 gm	102.3	3.63	0.41	20.82
Dal (wash)	1 katori	30 gm	105	17.7	0.74	6.87
Dal (whole)	1katori	30 gm	105.5	15.5	1.47	7.55
Vegetable	1	100 gm	23	1.3	0.2	4
Leafy Vegetable		100 gm	42.8	4.2	0.92	4.52
Root Vegetable		100 gm	57.71	1.1	0.2	13
Banana	1 med	100 gm	11.6	1.2	0.3	27.2
Apple	1 med	100 gm	59	0.2	0.5	13.4
Citrus Fruit	1 med	100 gm	46	0.8	0.4	9.78
Egg	1	50 gm	86	6.6	6.6	–
Chicken	–	100 gm	109	26.0	0.6	–
Fish	–	100 gm	104	18	1.9	3.65
Mutton (with bone)	–	100 gm	118	21.4	3.6	–
(Vegetable oil)	1 tsp	5 ml	45		5	
Butter	1 tsp	10 gm	73		8	
Cream	1 tsp	5 gm	10		1.0	
Sugar	1 tsp	5 gm	20			5
Honey	1 tsp	5 ml	16			4
Brown Bread	1 slice	15 gm	36.6	1.32	0.21	7.35
White Bread	1 slice	15 gm	36.75	1.17	0.11	7.79
Biscuit (Marie)	2 no.		56		1	
Biscuit (Good day)	2 no.		100		6	

TABLE 3.7: Food Exchange Table I

Cereal exchange (100 calories)	Meat Exchange (80 calories)	Milk Exchange (100 calories)
Chapati—1 (Flour—30 gm)	Egg—one	Cow's milk—1 cup (150 cc)
Bread—2 slices	Fish—90 gm	Toned milk—1 cup (150 cc)
Rice— 25 gm (Raw)	Chicken—100 gm	Buffalo's milk—½ cup
= 65 gm (cooked)	Meat—50 gm	Sk. Milk—3½ cups
(2/3 cooked katories)	Paneer—20 gm	Curd—3½ cups
Country porridge—20 gm	Curd toned milk—150 gm	(200 gm)
Oatmeal porridge—20 gm	Dall—30 gm	Butter milk—600 cc
Dal—85 gm (cooked)	(1 katori cooked)	

Fruit exchange per (50 calories in each portion)

Items	Quantity	Weight	Items	Quantity	Weight
Apple Big	1/2	80 gm	Orange	1 medium	100 gm
Small	1				
Mausami	1 medium	125 gm	Lemon	2 medium	100 gm
Papaya	1/4	150 gm	Pear	1 medium	100 gm
Arhu	2 medium	100 gm	Alocha	4 to 5	100 gm
Kharbuja	1/4 slice	300 gm	Guava	1	80 gm
Lichi	2 to 3	80 gm	Jamun	6 to 7	80 gm
Loquate	5 to 6	120 gm			

Refer. 13

TABLE 3.8: Food Exchange Table II

Foods	Exchange	Calories	Protein g	Cholesterol g	Fats g	Carbohydrates mg	Fe g	Fibre g
Cereals	1(30 g)	100	3.5	20	-	48	4.9	1.9
	(25 g)	80	3.0	17	-	45	4.0	1.5
Pulses	1(25 g)	80	5.0	15	-	75	3.8	1.5
	(30 g)	100	7.0	20		80	4.0	2.0
Vegetables								
Group A	100 g	16	1.0	3.0	-	25	0.5	1.0
Group B	100 g	36	2.0	7.0	-	28	0.75	1.5
Fruits	100 g	40–50	-	10–15	-	15	0.5	1.4
Milk	1(250 ml)	165	8.0	11	8.0	300	0.5	-
Meat/egg								
Egg	40 G							
Chicken	40 G (1 MED)							
Fish	40 G	80	6.0	-	6.0	60	2.1	-
Cheese	30 G							
Paneer	35 G							
Liver(sheep)	35–40 G							
Fats/oils								
Oil/ghee	1 TSP (5 ml)							
Cream	2 TSP (10 g)	45			5.0			
Butter	1 TSP (5 g)	40	-	-		-	-	-
Dry fruit	6 PCS (8–10 g)	45			5			

Refer. 13

For more accurate estimates required in surveys over a larger population, the same recall method is used but with more details. Besides eliciting the quantitative and qualitative intake, the volume of total cooked food is recorded too. Using the standardized measures, the distribution of the food by all family members is also recorded. The nutritive values are calculated from the raw weight of food stuffs using the formula:

Individual intake (volume) =

$$\frac{\text{Individual intake (volume)}}{\text{Total cooked quantity (volume)}} \times \text{raw amount}$$

Ideally, this method of 24 hour recall should be done on three consecutive days and the mean of the three days can give a fair idea of the actual diet take. Care should be taken to avoid feasting and fasting days in order to have a true picture. The advantage of this method is that it is useful in quick recapitulation of one's habitual diet and also gives an idea of extreme variations that might occur.

Food frequency method: In this method, the frequency of different foods consumed over a given period (daily, weekly, fortnightly, monthly correlated) is recorded and this information can be co-related with the 24 hour recall information, to give a more accurate picture of the child's intake. For this a questionnaire is prepared enlisting all foods that are possibly consumed at different frequencies and intervals and intakes recorded (Table 3.9). Whereever required, the total cooked volume of food and its distribution among the number of family members is recorded from which the intake of an individual is derived. For foodstuffs like fats, where it is difficult to quantify individually, a better way is to record the total consumption of all types of oil, ghee, etc. on monthly basis among a fixed number of family members. The individual intake can be calculated by dividing the total fat consumed (lts.) per month by number of members and the figure so derived, divided by 30 would give the amount consumed by one member per day.

This method has the advantage of providing information where evidence is required of an association of a child's existing nutritional status with diet in general rather than any specific nutrient.

TABLE 3.9: Food consumption frequency questionnaire

Foods	Amt. g/ml	Daily	3-4/wk	1-2/wk	2-3/mth.	1/mth.	Rarely
Cereals:							
Wheat flour							
Rice							
Sooji							
Bread							
Other							
Pulses							
Green leafy vegetables							
Other vegetables							
Root vegetables							
Fruit							
Milk							
Curd/Paneer							
Eggs							
Chicken/Meat							
Oil/Ghee/Butter							
Sugar							
Sweets							
Savoury							
Chips							
Cold Drinks							
Biscuits							
Cake/Pastry							
Ice Cream							
Noodles							
Pizza/Burger							
Fried snacks							

Questionnaire method: This method involves recording the diet history but without an interviewer being involved. Here the questionnaire is distributed or posted to the respondents who in turn fill them up and return or post it back to the interviewer. But this method is not applicable for assessing the nutritional status of children in a hospital setting or in the out patient clinic. Moreover, this method also requires the respondent, the mother in this case, to be literate enough to be able to comprehend and fill up the form correctly and independently. However, it can be used to collect data on large scale samples in short periods with limited resources.

Biochemical method: Besides anthropometry and dietary history, biochemical parameters are also used to co-related with the available information and the given clinical picture. Blood and urine samples are the most commonly used specimens used to determine the level of the required nutrients. These parameters can depict deficiency or any abnormality in absorption or utilization of any particular nutrient which can further be co-related clinically, e.g. hemogram showing levels of Hb. can demonstrate prescence or absence of anemia which most often is related to iron deficiency in the diet. Serum lipid profile can give an idea of the levels of total cholesterol, HDL, triglycerides, etc. denoting hypercholesterolemia which can be co-related with dietary intake of fats.

Serum albumin levels are commonly used to assess protein energy malnutrition. Serum albumin and transferrin levels reflect long term changes in the nutritional status, serum retinol binding protein and thyroxine binding prealbumin show more rapid changes. These values are mostly of use to monitor protein status during convalescence. Table 3.10 presents guidelines to interpret serum albumin in protein energy malnutrition in children.[14]

CLINICAL ASSESSMENT

Clinical signs to assess nutritional status have been used but are always co-related with biochemical or anthropometric status also. These signs can

TABLE 3.10: Serum albumin levels in children with PEM

Age	Serum Albumin (g/100 ml)		
	Deficit (high risk)	Low Medium risk	Acceptable low risk
0–11 months	-	< 2.5	< 2.5
1–5 years	< 2.8	< 3.0	> 3.0
6–12 years	2.8	2.8–3.4	> 3.5

Refer. 14

manifest as marginal changes which may be short term. However, independently this assessment is not considered a very useful tool. The various organs by which we can assess nutritional status clinically are the eyes, skin oral cavity dental history and the skeletal system. Presence of bitot spots in the eyes can be related to Vitamin A deficiency, or pallor of the under side of the eyelids can be co-related to iron deficiency anemia. Koilonychia (spoon shaped nails) are also indicative of anemia. Cracks at the corners of the mouth are suggestive of thiamine deficiency or loss of papilla on the tongue can help identify deficiency of vitamin B_2 or riboflavin. Similarly, bleeding or inflammed gums may suggest deficiency of vitamin C, presenting as scurvy. On examining a child, appearance of bow legs or beading of ribs may indicate rickets, deficiency of vitamin D.

Overall appearance of a child showing wasting with or without edema can immediately be associated with protein energy malnutrition. Flag sign of the hair showing color change can also be associated with protein deficiency in the form of kwashiorkor. Edema of the feet in certain hepatic disorders is also a sign of protein depletion.

Dietary Assessment of Infants and Toddlers

Assessing the intake of an infant on breast feeds or formula feeds or both is an important tool of assessing developmental milestones that support rapid changes in food habits and nutrient intakes. These milestones are based on the development of infant feeding skills as shown in Table 3.11.[15]

Dietary Assessment Techniques

In the case of infants on breast feed or formula feeds various techniques have been defined by various workers:

TABLE 3.11: Development of infant feeding skills

Chronological age	Feeding skills
0–1 month	Suckling and sucking reflexes Frequent feedings of > 8–12/24 hours Only thin liquid tolerated
1–3 months	Volume increase up to (150–200 ml/feed) Frequency drops to 4–8/24 hours Sucking pattern allows thin liquids to be swallowed
4–6 months	Cannot swallow lumpy feeds, but pureed foods swallowed (150–200 ml/feed), with 4–5 feeds/d(may vary in breast fed infants) Interest in munching, biting and new tastes Can hold bottle (if bottle fed)
7–9 months	Self-feeding with hand emerges Munching and biting emerges. Indicates hunger and satiety clearly
10–12 months	Likes self feeding with hands Spoon feeding emerges Drinks from an open cup Sitting position for eating Enjoys chopped or easily chewed foods with lumps

Refer. 15

1. *Collection of breast milk sample*: This method is used to investigate the nutrient content of milk and assess level of exposure of infant population to certain environmental chemicals. Guidelines for collection and storage of human milk have been laid down by the technical workshop on Human Milk Surveillance and Research on Environmental Chemicals in the US[16] as under:
   a. Milk sample should not be an undue burden on the mother, nor compromise the nutritional status of the infant.
   b. The time elapsed since the feeding on the breast to be pumped, should be at least 2 hours.
   c. Provide standardized collection and storage containers composed of natural material.
   d. For each collection the mother should:
      - Wash the breast with a mild soap and rinse with distilled water.
      - Express milk using breast pump till milk flow declines to a drip.

- Add collected milk to a storage container kept in home freezer until the required volume is obtained.
- Transport milk to the laboratory in a cooler with dry ice to keep samples frozen.

2. *Test weighing*: This method involves weighing the infant immediately before and after feeding without change of clothing or diapers and recording the gain in weight of the infant in grams to be the net milk intake (in ml). An alternate approach in breast fed infants involves weighing the mother before and after each feed.[17]
3. *Doubly labelled water (DLW)*: This method involves carefully administering a DLW dose to the infant and collecting samples of urine or saliva at base line and over the subsequent 5–15 days. This method has the advantage of being noninvasive and requires no special equipment.[18]
4. *Direct observation*: This method involves observing the duration of each feed in breast fed infants. For exclusively breast fed infants, milk intake is approximately 780 ml while for an infant on breast milk and formula, i.e. above 7 months it is assumed to be 600 ml.[19]

REFERENCES

1. World Health Organisation, Measuring change in nutritional status, Geneva, WHO. 1983.
2. Center for Disease Control and Prevention, National Center for Health Statistics, CDC Growth charts: United States, http://www.cdc.gov/growth charts/May 30. 2000.
3. Gomez F, Ramos, Galvan R, et al. Mortality in second and third degree malnutrition. J Trop Pediatr. 1956;2:77-83.
4. Nutrition Sub committee of the Indian Academy of Pediatrics, Report. Ind Pediatr. 1971;17:98-104.
5. Seoane N, Lytham MC. Nutritional anthropometry in the identification of malnutrition childhood. J Trop Pediatr. 1971;17:98-104.
6. Sastry JG, Vijayaraghvan K. Use of anthropometry in grading malnutrition in children. Ind J Med Res. 1973;61:1225-32.
7. Elizabeth KE, Normal growth in children. In: Nutrition and Child development, 3rd edn. Paras Publishers, Hyderabad. 2004.
8. US Department of Health and Human services, Centers for Disease control and Prevention: National Health Statistics, Division of data Services, Hyattsville MD. 2000.
9. Elizabeth KE, Normal growth of children, In: Nutrition and Child Development, 3rd edn. Paras Medical Publishers, Hyderabad. 2004.
10. Agarwal DK, Agarwal KN, Upadhyay SK, et al. Physical and sexual growth pattern of affluent Indian children from 6-18 years of age. Indian Pediatr. 1992;29:1203-82.
11. WHO (MGRS) Charts : http://www.who.int/childgrowth/standards/en/.
12. Agarwal KN, Saxena A, Bansal AK, et al. Physical Growth assessment in adolescence. Indian Pediatrics 2001;38:1217-1235.
13. Gopaln C, Rama Sastri BV, Balasubramnian SC. Nutritive Value of Indian Foods, National Institute of Nutrition, Indian Council of Medical Research, Hyderabad, 2002.
14. Sauberlich HE, Dowdy RP, Skala JH. Laboratory tests for the assessment of nutritional status. CRC Critical Reviews in Clinical Laboratory Sciences. 1973;4:215-340.
15. Ryan AS, Wenjun Z and Acosta A. Breast feeding continues to increase in the new millennium. Pediatrics. 2002;110:1103-09.
16. Lovelady CA, Devey KG. Picciano MF and Dermen A. Guidelines for collection of human milk samples for monitoring and research of environmental chemicals. J Toxicol Environ Health. 2002;65:1881-91.
17. Montandon CM, Wills C, Gaza C, et al. Formula intake of 1 and 4 month old infants. J Pediatr Gastroenetrol Nutr. 1986;5:434-38.
18. Meier PP, Engstrom JL, Fleming BA, et al. Estimating milk intake of hospitalized preterm infants who breast feed. J Hum Lact. 1996;12:21-26.
19. Devaney B, Kalb L, Briefel R. Feeding Infants and Toddlers Study: Overview of the Study Design, 2000 J Am Diet Assoc. 2004;104:S8-S13.

4 Maternal Nutrition in Pregnancy and Lactation

INTRODUCTION

Maternal nutrition not only influences the health and well being of the mother but also has intermediate and long-term effects on the development and health of the infant.[1] The fact that maternal nutrition during the antenatal period directly influences the fetal outcome has well been recognized. When a precursory study into the link between nutrition and pregnancy was done in a series of women who consumed minimal amounts over the 8-week period, it was discovered that they had a higher mortality or disorder rate concerning their off spring than women who ate regularly since children born to well fed mothers had less restriction within the womb.[2] Pregnancy and lactation are times of heightened vulnerability. The threat of malnutrition begins in the womb and continues through the life cycle. A mother who was malnourished as a fetus, young child or adolescent, is more likely to enter pregnancy stunted and malnourished. Her compromised nutritional status affects the health and nutrition of her own children. Growth faltering earlier in life leaves women permanently at risk of obstetric complications and delivering low birth weight babies.

PRECONCEPTION NUTRITION

It is estimated that a woman planning for a pregnancy be prepared even before the conceptual stage, which is known as the perinatal period. It requires a mother to be in good nutritional state prior to conception and that this state be maintained throughout pregnancy, labor and the period after birth. A mother well nourished before conception, will encounter fewer premature births and produce healthier babies.

The most important factor in prepregnancy nutrition is ensuring that the mother is healthy and without any major factors, which could worsen the chances of conception, like anorexia or bulimia, both of which can hinder conception. The minimum basal metabolic index (BMI) of 20.8 is a positive factor for preconception stage. Gaining weight restores fertility and a body fat content of at least 22% is necessary for a normal ovulatory function and menstruation.[3] On the other hand the same is true for obese women with a BMI of more than 30, which is a direct result of decrementing amounts of insulin activity and sex hormones may reduce the viability of the ovum. If a woman planning to conceive needs to gain or lose weight, it is recommended to be done gradually. The ideal weight of a woman planning to conceive is thought to be optimal at BMI between 20–26. This together with good diet and nutrition before pregnancy, would also maximize the reserves of micronutrients which are required during pregnancy.[4]

Some nutrients are considered to be beneficial for the pregnancy state and it is recommended that the standard dosage of these is followed as per the RDA:

- Magnesium and zinc supplements for the binding of hormones at the receptor sites.

- Folic acid supplement or dietary requirement of foods containing it for regular growth of the follicle.
- Regular vitamin D supplement decreases the chances of deficiency in adolescence. It has an important role in reducing the incidence of rickets with pelvic malformations which can hamper normal delivery.
- Vitamin B_{12} is known to reduce chances of infertility and ill health.
- Omega 3 fatty acids help in prevention of premature delivery and low birth weight.[3] Good dietary sources are oily fish, flax seeds, walnuts and pumpkin seeds.

NUTRITION DURING PREGNANCY

The post conception stage and the weeks following it are the most vulnerable, being the period when fetal development occurs within the womb. The energy needed for the organ and system development is derived from those present in the mother's circulation and around the lining of the womb. During the early stages the placenta is not formed and hence the transport of nutrients from the mother to the embryo is not possible. Therefore it is important that the mother's diet is healthy comprising all the essential nutrients so that the embryo is not deficient in these components. Diets should be rich in folic acid and iron to prevent neural tube defects.

Nutritional Recommendations During Pregnancy

Energy

Energy requirements during pregnancy are variable due to the energy sparing adaptations which protect the mother or fetus from nutritional strains.[5] Energy supplements in pregnancy have been shown to have variable effects on birth outcome, with more obvious benefit in women who are nutritionally at risk during this stage. The National Institute of Nutrition (NIN), (ICMR) group has worked out the recommendations of various nutrients for the pregnant and lactating mothers. Based on the prepregnancy weight of 55 kg, 'the additional energy requirements' of an Indian woman as per the recommendations of NIN are:[6]

	12 kg increase	10 kg increase
1st trimester	85 kcals	70 kcals
2nd trimester	+ 280 kcals	+ 230 kcals
3rd trimester	+ 470 kcals	+ 390 kcals

Therefore an average recommendation of 350 kcals/d through the second and third trimesters, as additional requirement during pregnancy (for an Indian woman of 55 kg body weight and pregnancy weight gain between 10–12 kg) may be made.

Proteins

Protein intakes to meet the average requirements of women during pregnancy, have been worked out by NIN by rounding off high quality protein for 10 kg gestational weight gain. These are 1, 7 and 23 g/d in 1st, 2nd and 3rd trimesters respectively.[6] A balanced energy/protein supplement (protein < 25% of energy) tends to influence pregnancy outcome favorably, while a very high protein supply may also be harmful.[7] It is therefore recommended that protein supplements are not required to meet this additional requirement during pregnancy. To achieve high quality protein content in an Indian diet, the foods can be varied, selecting foods with high protein content. For instance, pulses or legumes which have an individual protein efficiency ratio (PE) of 28% can be added as a cup of lentils or whole gram at meal time, or even between meals. Similarly a greater use of milk or milk based products (with a PE ratio of 15%), or non-vegetarian foods like eggs (PE ratio of 30%) or flesh food can further increase protein intake. All these food groups also add high quality protein to diet.[6]

Gestational Weight Gain

Fetal growth is reflected by gestational weight gain. A low weight gain is a risk indicator of intra-uterine growth retardation and perinatal mortality. On the other hand a higher gain is a risk indicator for maternal diabetes, macrosomia, delivery problems, birth trauma and asphyxia. It is now well known that intrauterine growth retardation and macrosomia may program obesity and metabolic syndrome later in life. The recommended total weight gain ranges for pregnancy are highlighted in Table 4.1.[8]

TABLE 4.1: Weight gain recommended for pregnancy

Prepregnancy weight category	Recommended total gain (kg)
BMI < 19.8	12.5–18.0
19.8–26	11.5–16.0
> 26.0–29.0	7.0–11.5

Source: Institute of Medicine. Nutrition during pregnancy, 1990.

Essential Fatty Acids

Some data exists in support of supplementation of essential fatty acids (EFA) like fish oil during pregnancy showing improved birth weight,[9] but random controlled trials have failed to elicit any such co-relation.[10]

MICRONUTRIENTS IN PREGNANCY

Vitamins

Fat Soluble Vitamins

Requirement of vitamin D increases twice the normal during pregnancy, therefore besides consuming rich dietary source of vitamin D, exposure to sunlight increased the vitamin production in the skin. An average well nourished woman would be having adequate reserves of the vitamin to sustain through the pregnancy period. Therefore the extra supplement of vitamin A may not be required. Good dietary sources include milk and milk products, green leafy vegetables, fruits like mangoes, papaya, vegetables like carrot, jaggery (source of β carotene, a precursor of vitamin A). Vitamin E requirement also increases during the last 8–10 weeks of pregnancy. The role of this vitamin is to prevent oxidation of the total fat reserves which are stored for providing for the growing fetus. Good sources of vitamin E are oily fish, flax seeds and green leafy vegetables.

Iron

As well known, iron requirements increase dramatically during pregnancy. The absorption of iron is directly proportionate to the level of iron stores in the body. When dietary iron stores are inadequate for the increased demands of iron, the maternal stores are depleted. By the first trimester, the iron stores are low or absent in women. However, during pregnancy, the iron status of the fetus is maintained near normal, even if depletion of iron stores and subsequently anemia occurs in the mother. Iron deficiency during pregnancy can produce anemia, fatigue and irritability in the mother and may impair growth of the fetus. Iron supplements should be taken with food to enhance iron absorption (meat, fish and fruits and vegetables rich in vitamin C).

Zinc

Low zinc intake during pregnancy increases the risk of delivering a low birth weight baby and may increase risk of birth defects.[11] Zinc requirements are about 50% higher during pregnancy.

Magnesium

Deficiency of magnesium can cause fatigue and muscle cramps and increase risk of premature birth and maternal hypertension. An intake of 400 mg/d is recommended. In a cross sectional study, birth weight has been shown to be positively co-related to magnesium intakes in early pregnancy.[12]

Calcium

During pregnancy about 30–40 g of calcium are transferred to the fetus during pregnancy, most of it during the third trimester.[8] The absorption of maternal calcium increases rapidly during pregnancy. An intake of about 1000–1200 mg of calcium throughout pregnancy reduces bone loss, since during late pregnancy, the calcium must be withdrawn from maternal bone and transferred to the fetus. Keeping in view the importance of most micronutrients, the deficiency of any of these can have adverse effects during pregnancy, both for the mother and the baby as shown in Table 4.2.[13]

Dietary and Environmental Hazards During Pregnancy

Alcohol

Consumption of alcohol during pregnancy is potentially hazardous due to the devastating effects on the outcome, termed as fetal alcohol syndrome (FAS).[14] It is characterized by abnormal facial

TABLE 4.2: Effects of micronutrient deficiencies during pregnancy

Nutrient	Effect on mother	Effect on fetus/ placenta
Vitamin D	Reduced bone density, may increase risk of osteoporosis	Impaired skeletal and tooth development, hypoglycemia, rickets
Vitamin A	Anemia	Low birth weight, premature birth
Vitamin E		Birth defects, spontaneous abortion
Folate	Anemia	Low birth weight, birth defects, miscarriage
Thiamine		Infant beriberi (severe B_{12} deficiency producing heart failure)
Iodine	Hypothyroidism	Severely impaired mental and motor development
Calcium	Increased risk of hypertension and eclampsia, decreased bone density may increase risk of osteoporosis	Impaired skeletal and tooth development, rickets
Magnesium	Increased risk of hypertension and eclampsia	Premature birth
Zinc		Birth defects, premature birth and low birth weight
Iron	Anemia	Low birth weight, premature birth, increased infant mortality

Source: Keen CL, et al. (eds), Maternal nutrition and pregnancy outcome. Ann NY Acad Sci:1993;678.

structure and impairment in growth and intellectual development. The mechanism involves the crossing over of alcohol and its metabolites through the placenta. The fetus does not have the enzymes to breakdown these toxic products including alcohol, which remain in the fetal circulation over prolonged period, thus exposing the fetus to high concentrations of alcohol for a long duration.

Caffeine

In pregnancy, the metabolism of caffeine is known to slow down, taking 2–3 times longer to metabolize. Intake of > 300 mg caffeine per day (equivalent to > 3 cups of caffeine/d) can be devastating due to its causing impaired growth and development and increasing risk of miscarriage.[15] Caffeine tends to constrict the blood vessels in the placenta which can result in reducing the supply of oxygen and nutrients to fetus.[16] It is recommended that pregnant women should best avoid coffee, black tea, chocolates and colas.

Food Additives

Additives like non sweeteners, i.e. saccharine, cyclamate and aspartame should be avoided by pregnant women due to the fact that these pass through the placenta and could be carcinogenic, especially when exposure begins *in utero* and continues through adult life.

Heavy Metals

Exposure of toxic metals like mercury, lead, cadmium and nickel can be harmful for the pregnant women, including the industrialized and agricultural chemicals due to their risk of being transported to fetus through the placenta. Even low levels of lead passing through the placenta increase the risk of premature birth, irreversibly impairing intellectual and motor development throughout childhood and lowering IQ.[13]

Hypervitaminosis A

Excess intake of vitamin A above the recommended levels during pregnancy (> 25000IU) has been linked to birth defects, including malformations of the skull, heart and the central nervous system.[17] It is interesting to note that deficiency of choline and vitamin E enhance the toxicity of high doses of vitamin A during pregnancy.

Tobacco

Children of mothers with history of smoking may have long-term impairments in physical growth and intellectual performance. The adverse effects are dose dependent and directly proportionate to the number of cigarettes smoked during pregnancy. The adverse effect is due to the reduced blood flow through the placenta and restricted oxygen and nutrient flow to the fetus. Smoking can deplete maternal stores of zinc, vitamin C, vitamin B_6, folate and vitamin B_{12}.[17]

Special Considerations During Pregnancy

Heartburn, Nausea, Constipation: A woman may encounter certain problems like heartburn, nausea and constipation during the entire period or specific periods of pregnancy. This is due to the changes in the hormonal levels during this period. The progesterone levels are raised which cause the muscle tone to relax and slow down the digestive process especially the peristalsis.[17] As a result there is a reflux of the gastric juices, at the lower esophagus, causing irritation and discomfort which is termed as heartburn. This can be minimized by eating smaller meals and avoiding taking meals immediately prior to physical activity or exercise. However, the relaxing of the muscle tone is otherwise beneficial as it helps to slow the transit time allowing increased nutrient absorption along with the gastro intestinal tract (GIT). The problem of reflux can also be alleviated by avoiding lying down immediately after meals (3–4 hours) and even when doing so to keep the head ended elevated. Another common problem of nausea can be tackled by having small frequent meals and not with meals which can be of help too.[17] Nausea may also be controlled by supplemental vitamin B_6 (25–75 mg/d) and magnesium (200–500 mg/d).[18]

Many women experience severe constipation and hemorrhoids during pregnancy which is due to increased water absorption from the stools which transits slowly along the GIT. Therefore liberal fluids and high fiber diet is recommended to ease the problem. Lots of fresh fruit and green vegetables and whole grain cereals can help the stool motility. Extra-vitamin C and regular moderate exercise can be helpful.

Hypoglycemia

Pregnant women are prone to develop hypoglycemia due to increased utilization of glucose by the fetus from the mother. This is particularly so at the early hours in the morning or if the woman has skipped a meal or is on a long fast. Skipping meals tend to produce more ketone bodies which can adversely affect the fetal development. Frequent small consumption of snacks and meals is recommended for these women to avoid hypoglycemic attacks.

Gestational Diabetes

About 5% of pregnant women may develop reduced ability to secrete insulin and control blood sugars resulting in gestational diabetes.[19] Hyperglycemia during pregnancy has an adverse effect on the fetus and the mother producing complications later on. Therefore dietary modifications with moderate exercise can help maintain normoglycemia and thus prevent complications. Supplemental zinc and chromium are known to enhance the action of insulin.[20]

Hypertension and Toxemia of Pregnancy

Extreme increase in the blood pressure during pregnancy can cause toxemia characterized by protein loss in the urine and fluid retention. This can prove fatal for both mother and the fetus.[21] These complications can be prevented by suitable dietary modifications. Too much restriction of salt can also increase the risk; therefore undue salt restriction should be avoided. Low calcium or zinc is known to increase the risk of toxemia. Calcium supplementation (2 g/d) during pregnancy can be beneficial. Supplemental B_6 (25–50 mg/d) may also be helpful in prevention and treatment of this disorder.[22]

Lactation Period

Nutritional Needs During Lactation

Breast milk is Mother Nature's unique gift bestowed upon the child through the mother. Milk production in the first 6 months of lactation averages about 750 ml/d, but women can vary in their output which can far exceed this volume being up to 2000 ml/d.

The composition of breast milk is unique due to the fact that it contains over 200 recognized components like:

- All nutrients (energy, protein, essential fatty acids, vitamins and minerals) needed by the new born for optimum growth and development.
- Enzymes to help the newborn digest and absorb nutrients.
- Immune factors to protect the infant from infection.
- Hormones and growth factors that influence infant growth.

All of the above components, though remain same in all mothers, the concentration of each of these are dependent upon her diet. Therefore during the period of lactation it is very important that the diet of the mother for the first 6 months is optimum which can in turn optimize the breast milk formation. Breastfeeding mothers need significantly more energy, proteins and micronutrients during lactation to support milk formation. For an exclusively breastfeeding mother, who would produce an additional amount of milk for the first 6 months, would require 600 kcals, and for partially breast feeding during 7–12 months, it would be 517 kcals or approximately 520 kcals.[6] The NIN (2010) recommendations have been computed by adopting the factorial requirement during lactation. This has been computed on the basis of secretion of 9.4 g/d of protein in milk during 0–6 months and 6.6 g during 6–24 months. Therefore the additional mean and safe protein intake at different months of lactation have been rounded off to 19 g/d for safe allowance for a lactating woman during 1–6 months and 13 g from 6–12 months. As for pregnancy, has protein requirements can be met from a balanced diet with a PE ratio between 12–13%.[6]

The requirements of most vitamins and minerals go up by 50%–100% compared to the pregnancy period. The quality of the breast milk can be influenced by the quality of the food consumed while breast feeding. The type of fat consumed during breast feeding influences the fat content of the breast milk. Vegetarians produce more milk with greater amounts of fatty acids present in plant foods. This is important since essential fatty acids (omega 3 fatty acids and EPA and DHA) are essential for the development of the nervous system of the new born.[23]

Vitamins like vitamin D are essential in the maternal diet since deficiency of this can lead to low levels in the infant too. Infants fed breast milk low in vitamin D may develop skeletal abnormalities and rickets.[24] There are other major minerals like calcium and magnesium which continue to be secreted in the milk despite low concentrations of the same in the maternal diet, draining from maternal reserves. Therefore if maternal stores of calcium are continuously low, these can be totally depleted leading to osteoporosis later in their lifespan.[21] Calcium supplements along with vitamin D during lactation and during the weaning period are important to maintain calcium balance and maternal skeletal health.[25]

REFERENCES

1. Plagemann A. Perinatal programming and functional teratogenesi: impact of body weight regulation and obesity. Physiol Behav. 2005;86:661-68.
2. Rasmussen KM. The influence of maternal nutrition on lactation Annual Review of Nutr. 1992;12:103-17.
3. Williamson CS. Nutrition in pregnancy. British Nutr Foundation. 2006;31:28-59.
4. Barasi EM. Human Nutrition-A health perspective, London: Arnold Publishing. 2003.
5. Prentice A, Goldberg GR. Energy adaptations in human pregnancy: limits and long term consequences. Am J Clin Nutr. 2000:S1226-S32.
6. ICMR, Nutrient Requirements and Recommended Dietary Allowances for Indians, A Report of the Expert Group of the Indian Council of Medical Research. 2010.
7. Otten JJ, Pitzi Hellwig J, Meyers LD (eds). Dietary Reference Intake (DRI) Washington, Institute of Medicine, National Academic Press. 2006.
8. Kramer MS, Kakuma R. Energy and protein intake in pregnancy. Cochrane Database Syst Rev. 2003;4.
9. Institute of Medicine (IOM). Nutrition during pregnancy: Report of the Committee on Nutrition during Pregnancy and lactation. Washington: National Academy Press. 1990.
10. De OnisM, Viller J, Gulmezoglu M. Nutritional interventions or prevent intrauterine growth retardation: evidence from randomised controlled trials. Eur J Clin Nutr. 1998;52:S83-93.
11. Ramakrishnan U, Manjerkar R, Rivera J, et al. Micronutrients and pregneacy outcome: a review of the literature. Nutr Res. 1999;19:103-59.

12. King JC. Determinants of maternal zinc status during pregnancy. Am J Clin Nutr. 2000;71:1334S.
13. Doyle W, Crafford MA, Wyan AH, et al. Maternal magnesium intake and pregnancy-outcome. Magnesium Res. 1989;20:205-10.
14. Keen CL Adrianne Bendich, Calvin C. Willhite (eds). Maternal nutrition and pregnancy outcome. Ann NY Acd Sci. 1993;678.
15. Beattie JO. Alcohol exposure and the fetus. Eur J Clin Nutr. 1992;46:S7.
16. Hinds TS. The effect of caffeine on pregnancy outcome variables. Nutr Rev. 1996;54:203.
17. Azais-Braesco V, Pascal G. Vitamin A in pregnancy: requirements and safety limits. Am J Clin Nutr. 2000;71:1325S.
18. Baron TH, Ramirez B, Richter JE. Gastrointestinal motility disorders during pregnancy. Ann Int Med. 1993;118:366.
19. Sahakian V, et al. Vitamin B_6 is effective therapy for nausea and vomiting of pregnancy: A randomized controlled study. Obster Gynecol. 1991;78:33.
20. Jovanovic-Peterson L, Peterson LM. Vitamin and mineral deficiencies which may predispose to glucose intolerance of pregnancy. J Am Coll Nutr. 1996;15:14.
21. Ritchie LD, King JC. Dietary calcium and pregnancy induced hypertension: Is there a co-relation? Am J Clin Nutr. 2000;71:1371S.
22. Institute of Medicine. Nutrition during lactation. Washington DC: National Academy Press. 1991.
23. Crawford MA. The role of essential fatty acids in neural development: Implications for perinatal nutrition. Am J Clin Nutr. 1993;57:S703.
24. Greer FR, Marshall S. Bone mineral content, serum vitamin D supplements. J Pediatr. 1989;114:204.
25. Kalwarf HJ, et al. The effect of calcium supplementation on bone density during lactation and weaning. N Eng J Med. 1997;337:523.

5 Nutrition for Premature Infants

Infants are termed as premature when they are born before 37 weeks of gestation, as compared with full term infants born from 38–42 weeks.[1] These infants usually weigh less than 2.5 kg and constitute about 10% of all births. Infant mortality rises from 5 times normal at 37 weeks of gestational age to 45 times normal at 32 weeks of gestational age.[2]

Some of the common terms associated with prematurity in infants are as presented in Table 5.1.

Most of the problems associated with premature births occur in infants with birth weights of 1,500 g or less, usually in those born at < 32 weeks of gestational age. These children are at increased potential risk of developing many problems due to their physiological immaturity (Table 5.2).

Premature infants with associated problems are also at increased risk of developing nutritional deficiencies due to:

Decreased nutrient intake: This is due to low stores of glycogen, fat, protein, fat soluble vitamins, calcium, phosphorous, magnesium and trace elements, caused by low deposition during pregnancy, since they are born earlier than normal anticipated term.

Increased growth rate: For premature infants to reach the expected weight by 1 year of age, they would need to increase their weight tenfold, considering that full term babies almost triple their weight age by 1 year of life. Therefore for such rapid growth, increased energy and nutrients are required.

Immature physiological systems: The ability for digestion and absorption are decreased due to:

- Low concentrations of lactase, pancreatic lipase and bile salts.
- The stomach capacity is decreased thereby reducing the gastrointestinal (GI) motility and gastritis.
- A coordinated suck and swallow action is not developed until 32–34 weeks of gestation

TABLE 5.1: Terms related to prematurity

Premature Infant	Infant born before 37 weeks of estimated age
Low birth weight	Birth weight < 2,500 g
Very low birth weight	Birth weight < 1,500 g
Very very low birth weight	Birth weight < 1000 g
Chronologic or birth age	Time since birth
Gestational age	Estimated time since conception
Corrected age	Age corrected for prematurity

Refer. 1

TABLE 5.2: Potential risks of premature infants

Undernutrition	**Osteopenia**
Anemia	Respiratory distress syndrome
Poor temperature control	Uncordinated suck and swallow
Apnea	Hypoglycemia
Retinopathy of prematurity	Infection
Necrotising enterocolitis	Limited renal function
Decreased gastric motility	Fat malabsorption
Asphyxia	Hypotension
Intraventricular	Hyperbilirubinemia
Bronchopulmonary dysplasia	

Refer. 2

- Hepatic enzymes are increased which make specific amino acids, conditionally essential (cysteine) or toxic (phenylalanine), due to the inability of the body to synthesize or degrade.
- Renal concentration ability is reduced.

Illness: Any of the following associated illnesses also would increase the energy requirements:

- Respiratory distress syndrome may delay the introduction of enteral feeding due to increased risk of aspiration. GI mobility too is decreased and feedings may not be tolerated.
- Patent ductus arteriosus may require fluid restriction which further hinders optimum calorie intake. In such conditions, the babies are generally kept nil per orally.
- The infant becomes at risk of developing necrotizing enterocolitis (NEC), in which case parenteral nutrition (PN) has to be administered, since the bowels have to be kept at rest. When refeeding, an elemental formula is indicated. There may develop complications of short gut syndrome and hence may require nutritional management for malabsorption.
- Hyperbilirubinemia may increase the insensible water loss and fluid requirement. In case exchange transfusion is required, enteral feeds.
  May have to be delayed. Thus NEC becomes a complication of exchange transfusion.
- Sepsis and suspected sepsis requires with holding of all enteral fluids till the infant becomes stable.

MANAGEMENT OF THE PREMATURE INFANT

Goal

The goal of management of the premature infant is:

- To provide optimal growth and development without metabolic complications.
- To match the fetal growth of full term infant.[3]

Within 24 hours of life, the infant should be administered PN to promote energy intake and homeostasis, to establish nitrogen (N) balance and to prevent essential fatty acid deficiency.[4] PN guidelines of specific nutrients are shown in Tables 5.3[1,5] and 5.4.[1,6] If fluids are not restricted, adequate nutrients can be provided by PN, provided by a peripheral intravenous line.

TABLE 5.3: Parenteral nutrition guidelines for macronutrients and minerals per day

Nutrients	Unit/kg
Energy (kcals)	80–90
Glucose (mg/kg/min)	6–12
Fat (g)	0.5–3.0
Protein (g)	2.7–3.8
Sodium (mEq)	2–4
Potassium (mEq)	2–3
Chloride (mEq)	2–3
Calcium (mg)	60–100
Phosphorus (mg)	43–70
Magnesium (mg)	3.0–7.2
Zinc (µg)	400
Copper (µg)	20
Chromium (µg)	0.05–0.2
Manganese (µg)	1
Selenium (µg)	1.5–2
Molybdenum (µg)	0.25
Iodine (µg)	1.0

Refer. 1, 5

TABLE 5.4: Parenteral guidelines per day for the preterm

VITAMINS	Dose/kg	Maximum dose/day
Vitamin A (µg)	280	700
Vitamin E (mg)	2.8	7
Vitamin K (µg)	80	200
Vitamin D (µ)	4	10
Vitamin C (mg)	32	80
Thiamine (mg)	0.48	1.2
Riboflavin (mg)	0.56	1.4
Niacin (mg)	6.8	17
Vitamin B_6 (mg)	0.4	1
Folate (µg)	56	140
Vitamin B_{12} (µg)	0.4	1
Biotin (µg)	8	20
Pantothenic acid (µg)	2	5

Refer. 1, 6

In preterm infants, fluids need to be so adjusted so as to avoid fluid overload, to prevent risks of developing NEC, bronchopulmonary dysplasia, PDA and intraventricular hemorrhage.[7] Pre-term infants have a limited ability to hydrolyze triglycerides; therefore higher levels of these are more often encountered with decreasing gestational age, infection, surgical stress malnutrition and with the SGA infant.

Enteral Nutrition

Weaning from parenteral to enteral nutrition is done when the baby is clinically stable. The transition needs to be done gradually to facilitate feeding tolerance and to prevent the development of NEC. The feeds are gradually increased in volume and strength as parenteral fluids are gradually decreased. This transition is done within a period of 3 days. The feeds are started as trophic feeds, i.e. small volume feeds given to nourish the gut. The feeds are increased gradually with improvement in the condition of the infant. For VLBW babies, the feeding is limited to 20 ml/kg/d or less to prevent NEC. Some of the risks and benefits of starting EN are presented in Table 5.5.[1,8,9,10]

Contraindication for Feeding the Premature Infant

Enteral feeding should not be initiated under the following conditions:

- Is receiving indomethacin or has received it within the previous 48 hours.
- Has a hemodynamically significant patent ductus arteriosus.
- Has an umbilical arterial or venous catheter. Feeding should be initiated until after > 8 hours.
- Is polycythemic
- Has respiratory instability or there is impending endotracheal intubation.
- Has hemodynamic instability as evident by sepsis, hypotension or is on vasopressin drugs.
- Has received an exchange transfusion within the past 48 hours.
- Has abdominal distension or other signs of GI dysfunction.
- Has had an episode of severe asphyxia in the previous 72 hours.

Table 5.5: Risks and benefits of introducing enteral feeding

Risks	Benefits
Necrotising enterocolitis	Shortens physiologic jaundice
Aspiration	Prevents cholestasis
Feeding Intolerance	Stimulates GI development
Intestinal perforation with transpyloric feeding	Allows full volume feeds earlier
	Increases weight gain
	Lowers alkaline phosphatase activity levels

Refer. 1, 8, 9, 10

Feeding Protocol

Feeding a premature baby can be done by any one of the methods as listed in Table 5.6.[11]

Since these infants have not yet developed co-ordinated sucking and swallowing, they must be fed by gavage, if breast feeding is not possible. Orogastric tubes are generally used to avoid the risk of occlusion of the nasal passage with a naso-

Table 5.6: Methods of feeding a premature infant

Breast/bottle	Most physiological methods
	Infant at least 32–48 weeks of gestation
	Infant medically stable
	Infant's respiratory rate < 60 breaths/min
Gavage	Supplement to breast or bottle feeding
	Suggested for infants < 32 weeks of gestation
	Recommended when resp. rate < 80 breaths/min
	Used for intubated babies
	Used for neurologically impaired neonate
Transpyloric	Used when gavage feedings not tolerated
	Used when infant is at risk of aspiration
	Employed when infant intubated
	Used for infant with decreased motility
	Must wait for passage of stool to begin feedings
	Requires radiographic assessment to check placement
	Complications include dumping syndrome, altered intestinal
	Microflora, nutrient malabsorption, perforation of intestine
Gastrostomy	Used for gastrointestinal malformation
	Used for neurologically impaired infant

Refer. 11

gastric tube. Secondly, repeated insertion of a naso gastric tube can cause inflammation of the nose with subsequent obstruction. As the infant matures, nipple feeding can be considered.

The feeding guidelines for the premature infant are as listed in Table 5.7.[11]

Breastfeeding

Breast milk where available can be offered. It may be required to be expressed (EBM), since the baby might be too weak or too small to breast feed. Moreover, the mother may not be available 24 hours during the period of prolonged hospitalization. Family support for the mother can help them enable to establish successful breast feeding. Kangaroo care (skin to skin contact between mother and infant) will facilitate parent infant bonding and has been linked with longer period of lactation by the mother who delivers prematurely.[12]

The mother's own preterm milk (PTM) has been found to be superior to other sources of preterm formula milk and is an important source of nutrients to the preterm baby. It differs from term milk with a higher concentration of total N, protein (up to 2.2 g%), sodium, chloride, magnesium, iron, copper, zinc, IgA, etc. (Table 5.8), thus making it 'baby specific'. The high protein content reduces to 1.3 g by 6 weeks.[13]

Other milk sources used are banked milk, expressed breast milk (EBM), milk fortified with human milk protein (HMF) and other ordinary and special formula milk powders which are commercially available. HMF is used when ordinary milk powder is used to supplement various nutrients like energy, protein, sodium, calcium, medium chain triglycerides. The amount used is 2 sachets per 100 ml of EBM or formula milk. The energy and protein content of one sachet of HMF are 6.5 and 0.2 g respectively, with carbohydrate being 1.2 g and fats 0.1g.[13]

Enteral Feeds

In case of enteral feeding, the type of formula selected depends upon various factors. The important factor to consider is that it should provide appropriate amounts of energy protein and other nutrients as laid down by the European Society of Pediatric Gastroenterology, Hepatology and Nutrition and the North American Society of Pediatric Gastroenterology, Hepatology and Nutrition in 2010 as shown in Table 5.9.[14] Ranges

TABLE 5.7: Suggested feeding guidelines for the premature

Weight	Feeding Interval	Initial volume (cc/kg/d)	Feeding increments (cc/kg/d)	Days to full feeding†
< 1,000	q 2 hrly	10	10	16
1000–1,500	q 2–3 hrly	10–20	15–20	10–7
1,501–1,800 sick‡	q 3 hrly	10–20	20–30	7–5
1,500–1,800 healthy‡	q 3 hrly	20–40	30–50	5–3
> 1,800 sick‡	q 3 hrly	20–40	30–75	5–2

Refer. 11

†Full feedings are defined as 120 kals/kg

‡Sick refers to infants with symptoms of any medical or surgical condition, other than uncomplicated prematurity. Healthy refers to term or preterm infants without any medical or surgical condition.

TABLE 5.8: Composition of term and preterm milk per 100 ml

Nutrient	Term	PTM 1st week	PTM 2nd week	PTM 3rd week	PTM 4th week	PTM 5th week	PTM 6th week
Energy	67	64	67	67	67	67	67
Protein (g)	1.1	2.3	1.9	1.6	1.5	1.4	1.3
Sodium (mmols)	0.6	1.7	1.3	1.2	0.9	0.8	0.8
Potassium (mmols)	1.5	1.7	1.5	1.3	1.3	1.2	1.2
Calcium (mmols)	0.8	0.7	0.7	0.7	0.7	0.7	0.7
Phosphorus (mmols)	0.5	0.5	0.5	0.5	0.5	0.5	0.5

Refer. 13

of advisable nutrient intakes are expressed both per kilogram body weight per day and per 100 kcal (Table 5.9). Calculation of the latter values was based on the minimum energy intake of 110 kcal/kg/d that are recommended. Thereby, the ranges of nutrient intake per 100 kcal will ensure that the infant receives the minimum or maximum of each specific nutrient at an intake of 110 kcal/kg/d. One should be aware that at higher energy intakes, the individual nutrient should not exceed an acceptable maximum level of intake.

The vitamin needs of the infant are met by use of fortified human milk, without addition of supplementation.[1]

For the infant receiving human milk iron supplementation can be initiated at 2–4 mg/kg/d, once full volume of feeds has been initiated. The infant receiving a combination of breast and formula can be given 2 mg/kg/d.

Adequate levels of calcium and phosphorous are essential to prevent osteopenia which is commonly reported in premature infants. Besides, the poor nutrient stores at birth, excessive losses of these minerals contribute to low levels of these infants. Prolonged PN, chronic diuretic therapy or diets of unfortified human milk are added risk factors for deficiency of calcium and phosphorus in these babies.

Premature infants are at risk of trace element deficiency due to poor nutrient stores at birth, rapid growth and dependence on adequate intake. Use of PN solutions however, minimize these deficiencies. Zinc deficiency in these infants has been reported when mother's milk is inadequate in this trace mineral, or where the infant is given oral copper and or iron supplements, which may compete with zinc for absorption.[15]

Intolerance to Feeding

At times premature infants may not tolerate feeds and may have episodes, which may require withholding of feeds or a delay in advancing feeds. Any signs of feeding intolerance should be considered seriously in view of the increased risk of developing NEC among these infants. The signs which can alert or indicate possible intolerance to feeding could be:

- Gastric residuals or emesis
- Blood in stool

TABLE 5.9: Recommended intakes for macro-and micronutrients for preterm babies

Nutrients (Min-Max)	Per/kg/d	Per 100 cals
Fluids	135–200	
Energy	100–135	
Proteins (g) <1 kg b wt	4.0–4.5.0	3.6–4.1
<1.8 kg b wt	3.5–4.0	3.2–3.6
Lipids (g)	4.8–6.6	4.4–6.0
Carbohydrate (g)	11.6–13.2	10.5–12
Sodium (mg)	69–115	63–105
Potassium (mg)	66–132	60–120
Chloride (mg)	105–177	95–161
Calcium salt (mg)	122–140	110–130
Phosphate (mg)	60–90	55–80
Magnesium (mg)	8–15	7.5–13.6
Iron (mg)	2–3	1.8–2.7
Zinc (mg)	1.1–2.0	1.0–1.8
Copper (μg)	100–132	90–120
Selenium (μg)	5–10	4.5–9.0
Manganese (μg)	8–15	7.5–13.6
Fluoride (μg)	1.5–60	1.4–55
Iodine (μ)	11–55	10–50
Chromium (mg)	30–11230	27–1120
Molybdenum (μg)	0.3–5	0.27–4.5
Thiamine (μg)	140–300	125–275
Riboflavin (μ)	200–400	180–365
Niacin (μg)	380–550	345–5000
Pantothenic acid mg	0.33–2.1	0.3–1.9
Pyridoxine (μg)	45–300	41–273
Cobalamin (μg)	0.1–0.77	0.08–0.7
Folic acid (μg)	35–100	32–90
Ascorbic acid (mg)	11–46	10–42
Biotin (μg)	1.7–16.5	1.5–15
Vitamin A (μg)	400–1000	360–740
Vitamin E (mg)	2.2–11	2–10
Vitamin K (μg)	4.4–28	4–25
Choline (mg)	8–55	7–50
Inositol (mg)	4.4–53	4–48

Refer. 13

- Metabolic acidosis
- Onset of apneic episodes
- Abdominal distension
- Diarrhea
- Hyperglycemia
- Temperature instability.

NUTRITIONAL ASSESSMENT

It is important to assess or determine the daily intake of the infant for adequacy, strength of formula or feeding method. The intake is evaluated against standard nutritional guidelines. Moreover, with passage of time the feeding techniques need to be advanced to the most physiological method possible for the infant. Breast or bottle feeds are introduced as the coordination of sucking and swallowing and breathing is developed at 32–34 weeks of gestation.[1] The time of feeding can be limited to about 20 minutes per feeding period to prevent fatigue or excessive energy expenditure.

ANTHROPOMETRIC MEASUREMENTS

Assessing weights on hospitalized premature infants can be difficult due to the interference of the medical equipment. The infant is also prone to cold stress during such procedures, which diverts energy from growth to heat production.

Weights when taken should be done at the same time each day to avoid diurnal variations. Initial weight loss reflects the loss of extracellular fluid which ranges from 10%–20% of birth weight during the first week of life.[11]

After regaining birth weight, the weight gain goal is 10–20 g/kg/d or 15–30 g/d. When the infant weighs 2.5 kg, a weight gain of 20–30 g/d is appropriate.[16]

Head circumference should be measured weekly. Alterations may occur from birth to 1 week of life due to head molding or edema. The goal is 0.5–0.8 cm/week. Length measurements may not be easy to obtain, which should increase by 1 cm/wk.

Skinfold and mid arm circumference are not very helpful for assessing diet changes, nor do they change rapidly, hence not required for routine medical care.

If there is inadequate weight gain in these infants over a period of time, it is worth looking into the causative factors so that appropriate measures can be taken to correct it. Some of the common causes of inadequate weight gain are presented in Table 5.10.[16]

Table 5.10: Common causes of inadequate weight gain

- Nutrient calculations are incorrect
- Infant is not receiving planned diet due to
  - Intravenous fluid administration interrupted to give blood or drugs
  - Infant unable to consume as planned orally and no gavage supplements provided
  - Feeding with held as the infant's respiratory rate increased or body temperature unstable
- Infant does not tolerate formula
- Infant is cold stressed
- Infant has outgrown previous diet plan
- Nutrition solution was incorrectly prepared
- Incorrect formula/feed provided to the infant

Assessing Feed Intolerance

Feeding intolerance is commonly encountered amongst premature babies, so continuous monitoring should be done to ascertain any signs indicating the same. This is important to prevent sepsis or NEC.[17]

Based on the assessment, feedings may need to be with held in conditions of signs of illness, including persistent apnea and bradycardia or temperature instability. Gastric residuals may also be an indicator to with hold feeds. With bolus feeding, a residual of up to 50% of the feeding volume or the hourly rate for continuous feeding is often accepted. Mucus residuals are not a concern, which are present in an infant recovering from lung disease. Undigested formula is an indicator of a large volume of feed offered, which means either the infant is not tolerating the formula or has poor GI motility, or there is intestinal obstruction or even NEC. In transpyloric feeds bile residuals are common.

Abdominal distension can occur due to air swallowing, feeding intolerance, infrequent stooling or NEC. An increase of 1.5 to 2.0 cm is considered significant, indicating with holding of feeds.[17]

A workup of sepsis and NEC should be considered when any one of the above signs is noted. Blood in stool is also a matter of concern and should be evaluated, as it could be a sign of illness, feeding tube irritation of the intestine, anal fissure or blood swallowed during delivery.

DISCHARGE OF THE PREMATURE INFANT

The premature is considered fit for discharge when body temperature is maintained, breast feeding is established or bottle/spoon feeding is enabled which is adequate to support growth and cardiorespiratory function is mature and stable.[18]

The care taker should also be prepared for discharge of the high risk infant. 24 hour visitation should be allowed for the parent to become active in caring for the infants. Rooming in with the infant facilitates care and gives confidence to the parent. Most infants can be discharged home on breast feeds or standard infant formula. The breast fed baby should receive a multivitamin with iron supplement, while for the infant on formula feed, iron may not be required, since most formulae are enriched with iron.[11]

The catch up growth in a preterm is about 10 times for the age or up to 5 times for the length, where as for the term baby it is about 200 g/week after the first 10 days of life. Initially there is a slight loss in weight, but it is regained by 10 days.[13]

REFERENCES

1. American Academy of Pediatrics and American College of Obstetricians and Gynecologists. Guidelines for Perinatal Care. 4th edn. Elk Grove. IL: American Academy of Pediatrics. 1992.
2. Wilcox AJ, Skjaervan R. Birth weight and perinatal mortality: the effect of gestational age. Am J Publ Health. 1992;82:378-82.
3. American Academy of Pediatrics Committee on Nutrition. Nutritional needs of preterm infants. In: Kleinman RE eds. Pediatric Nutrition Handbook 4th edn, Elk Grove Village, IL: American Academy of Pediatrics. 1998;55-88.
4. Riveria A, Bell EF, Brier DM. Effect of intravenous amino acids on metabolism of preterm infants during the first 3 days of life. Pediatr Res. 1993;33:106-11.
5. Hansen JW. Consensus Recommendations. In: Tsang RC, Lucas A, Uauy R, Zlotkin S, eds. Nutritional Needs of the Preterm Infant. Baltimore: Williams and Wilkins. 1993:288-89.
6. Greene HL, Hambidge KM, Schanler R, et al. Guidelines for the use of vitamins, trace elements and phosphorous ininfants and children receiving total pareneteral nutritio: Report of the Sub-Committee on Cliical Practice Issues of the American Society for Clinical Nutrition. Am J Clin Nutr. 1998;48:1324-42.
7. Aspen Board of Directors. Guidelines for the use of parenteral and enetral nutrition in adults and pediatric patients. Section VII. Nutrition support for low birth weight infants, JPEN. 1993;17(Suppl):1SA-52SA.
8. Berseth CL. Minimal enteral feedings. Clin Perinatiol. 1995;22:195-206.
9. Dunn L, Hulman S, Weiner J, et al. Beneficial effects of early hypocaloric enteral feeding on neonatal gastrointestinal function: preliminary report of a randomized trial. J Pediatr. 1988;112:622-29.
10. Meetze WH, Valentine C, McGuigan JE, et al. Gastrointestinal priming prior to full enteral nutrition in very low birth weight infants. J Pediatr Gastrointest Nutr. 1992;15:163-170.
11. Anderson DM. Nutrition for Premature Infants, In: Handbook of Pediatric Nutrition. 2nd edn. Samour PQ, Heln KK, Lang CE, eds. Jones and Bartlett Publishers, Massachussetts. 2004.
12. Hurst NM, valentine CJ, Renfro L, et al. Skin to skin holding in the neonatal intensive care unit influences maternal milk volume. J Perinatol. 1997;17:213-17.
13. Elizabeth KE. Low Birth Weight Babies. In: Nutrition and Child Development, 3rd edn. Paras Medical Publisher New Delhi. 2004;40-53.
14. Agostini C, Buonocore G, Carnielli VP, et al. Enteral Nutrient Supply for Preterm Infants: Commentary from the European Society of Pedaitric Gastroenterology, Hepatology and Nutrition Committee on Nutrition. J Ped Gastroenterol Nutr . 2010;50:1-9.
15. Atkinson SA, Zlotkin S. Recognizing the deficiencies and excesses of zinc, copper and other trace elements. In: Nutrition during infancy: Principles and Practice, eds. Tsang RC, Zlotkin SH, Nicholas BL, Hansen JW, 2nd edn. Cincinnati, OH: Digital Educational Publishing. 1997:209-32.
16. Schanler RJ. The low birth weight infant. In: Walker WA, Watkins JB eds. Nutrition in Pediatrics. 6th edn. Maldin MA: BC Decker, Inc; 1997:392-412, Saunders Company. 1998:337-46.
17. Robinson AF, Bhatia J. Feeding premature infants. Clin Pediatr. 1993;32:36-44.
18. American Academy of Pediatrics Committee on Fetus and Newborn. Hospital discharge of the high risk neonate- proposed guidelines. Pediatr. 1998;102: 411-7.

6 Feeding of Infants (0–6 Months)

The first consideration that comes to mind when we talk of feeding infants is the new born child, and feeding a new born obviously takes us to the most natural God given gift to the mother, that of breast-milk. As soon as the child is born, nature prepares both, the mother and the baby to make the best of this natural gift. Soon after birth the mother starts secreting milk and it requires an effort on the part of the baby to suck so that secretion is further enhanced. In our country from generations this gift of nature is well accepted and justified because the thought of feeding her child comes naturally to the mother and she is mentally geared to do so. The baby also responds spontaneously to the mother's love and the natural instinct of suckling is smoothly initiated. But, unfortunately, in our own country over the years this spontaneous practice of making the best of 'Nature's Gift' is slowly eroding with the result that both mother and child face a lot of problems. Therefore to bring our attention to this problem and help the mother revert to the dying practice of utilizing Nature's gift, WHO has dedicated one week (1–7 the August) every year as 'Breastfeeding Week'.

To begin with we shall first discuss why breast-feeding is important and the various factors associated with failure to feed or 'nurse'.

ADVANTAGES OF BREASTFEEDING

The main advantages of breast feeding are:

- It is a complete food by itself for the baby till 6 months of life in all respects. The proportion of all macro-and micronutrients are such that it is tailor made for the new born. It is rich in fats, especially the essential fatty acids and the protein quality is just right for the baby. It is unique that it is rich in lipase an enzyme which is poor in other sources of milk.
- It has water content which is adequate to meet the total requirement of the baby in the driest of summers. There is no need to feed water as long as the baby is exclusively breast fed. Offering water to a baby on breastfeeds can actually cause a reverse effect of reducing the mother's milk output by suppressing her prolactin concentration in the plasma. This fact has been well demonstrated by studies from Brazil by WHO.[1] It was shown that introduction of water or tea even if continuing breast feeds were twice as likely to stop breast-feeding before 3 months compared to those who were fed exclusively for 6 months.
- It is rich in antibodies in the form of immuno-globulins and leukocytes, which help the baby fight against any infections. A bacterium called lactobacillus bifidus present in breast milk prevents the baby from possible infections. The breast milk protein consists of whey protein (80%) in the form of lactalbumin, thus making it superior to cow's milk.[1] Table 6.1 gives a comparison between human milk and cow's milk.[10]
- The Ca:P ratio is ideal in breast milk as compared to other milk source.
- Though low in iron, the bioavailability is high due to presence of lactoferrin which prevents the baby from being anemic.

TABLE 6.1: Comparison between human milk vs. cow's milk

Characteristics	Human milk	Cow's milk
Energy (kcal/100 ml)	70	67
Protein (g/100 ml)	0.9	3.5
Whey: Casein ratio	80/20	20/80
Carbohydrate (g/100 ml)	7.0	5.0
Carbohydrate source	lactose	lactose
Fat (g/100 ml)	2.7–4.5	3.5
Linoleic acid (%)	10–15	4.0
Calcium (mg/lt)	340	1,200
Phosphorus (9 mg/lt)	150	955
Ca:P ratio	2.3	1.3
Iron (mg/lt)	1.0	0.5
Sodium (mEq/lt)	7.0	25.0
Potassium (mEq/lt)	14.0	35.0
Renal solute load	80.0	220.0
Oral solute load	250.0	263.0

Refer. 10

- Breast milk is available at just the right temperature for the baby avoiding the need to cool or heat it as required appropriate for consumption.
- The mother is free to move around anywhere with the baby without the hassle of organizing to carry formula milk or in premixed from or reheating it or carrying sterilized bottles along with.
- It is very economical as it saves the family from spending on expensive formula available in the market.
- It is sterile with minimum chances of contamination. The enzyme lactoferrin is bacteriostatic thereby inhibiting *E. coli* by rendering iron unavailable to it. An exclusively breast fed infant is about 14 times less likely to die from diarrhea, nearly 4 times less likely to die from respiratory diseases and almost 3 times less likely to die from other infections than a non-breast fed infant.[2]
- Breast milk ensures stability by emotional bonding of mother and child. It also gives a feeling of security to the child.
- It ensures certain maternal benefits also by decreasing postpartum bleeding.
- It burns off extra fat deposited during pregnancy besides possibly decreasing the risk of ovarian cancers in mothers at a later stage.
- Exclusive breast feeding up to 6 months also helps spacing between two pregnancies. As per WHO/UNICEF estimates, contraceptive prevalence would have to increase by 11% in order to compensate for 25% decline in breast feeding.[3]
- Contrary to the general myth among young mothers of the present generation, breast feeding helps her to lose the extra weight she had gained during the course of her pregnancy and helps regain her figure.

COLOSTRUM

This is the first viscous yellowish milk which is secreted soon after delivery. Unfortunately, most often this 'early' secretion is discarded by most mothers in certain communities, with the explanation that it is toxic for the baby. On the contrary colostrum is the richest source of proteins and immunoglobulins and the fat soluble vitamins like A and E. It is rich in secretory IgA, which prevents the baby from any gastrointestinal infections. However, it is lower in fats and carbohydrates as compared to mature milk. This secretion may not be in large volume and lasts for only about 2–3 days, but is very crucial for the baby as it helps in stimulation of mature milk by 2–10 days after birth. It also helps in stimulating peristalsis and acts as a lubricating protective effect on the mother's nipples.

FACTORS CAUSING LACTATIONAL FAILURE

As mentioned earlier, breast feeding is such a natural phenomenon which should be a spontaneous function, but still we find the incidence of successful breast feeding practice gradually declining. There can be a number of factors leading to lactation failure. We shall discuss in detail and see what steps can be taken to prevent this problem.

- **Initiation of breast feeding:** Breastfeeding should be initiated within half to one hour after delivery in the case of normal delivery and at least 4–6 hours after a cesarean section delivery. At birth, the baby is completely ready and alert to begin sucking. In an ideal environment, the onus lies on the part of the family members or the immediate care givers present around to put the baby to the mother's breast so that the sucking reflex is initiated. It should be impressed upon the mother that that the initiation of lactation is influenced greatly by the sucking reflex and if she on her part fails to make an effort at that time, lactation failure is bound to set in. Mature milk starts from the third to fourth day and the volume increases gradually from about 100 ml on the second day, rapidly increasing to 500 ml by the second week and going onto about 700–800 ml by 5–6 months. The mechanism involved is that sucking stimulates the production of prolactin (milk production) and oxytocin (milk ejection) so that lactation is maintained. Oxytocin reflex is also known as the 'let down reflex' due to its role in 'letting down' milk production. (Fig. 6.1)

- **Family support:** The role of the female family elders is very crucial in influencing good or poor lactation. If the mother, mother in law or any one closely associated with caring for the new mother encourages her to feed by reenforcing its importance, the mother is bound to follow their advice and be 'mentally geared' to feed her baby. On the other hand, if these same people give their own remarks about the baby not 'getting satiated by the mother's milk or that her 'milk is not adequate', or that the mother is 'too weak to feed', the mother is psychologically discouraged and begins to lose confidence in her own ability to satisfy her baby with her own feed. The lack of confidence is enough to inhibit the 'let down' reflex and gradually the milk production also dwindles. Added to this, is the fact that because of this reason, the mother herself or the family members begin to offer formula milk or cow's milk in their attempt to be over concerned. It may be noted that the milk production is inversely proportionate to the 'artificial' or 'top milk' fed to the baby, i.e. the more the baby is fed by the bottle; the lesser will become the breastmilk output. Therefore, a 'positive attitude' needs to be instilled in the mother and the care givers to maintain successful breastfeeding. Artificial feeds include water also which should not be offered before 6 months due to the fact that the water content in breastmilk is adequate enough for the baby's requirement as mentioned earlier. It is noteworthy

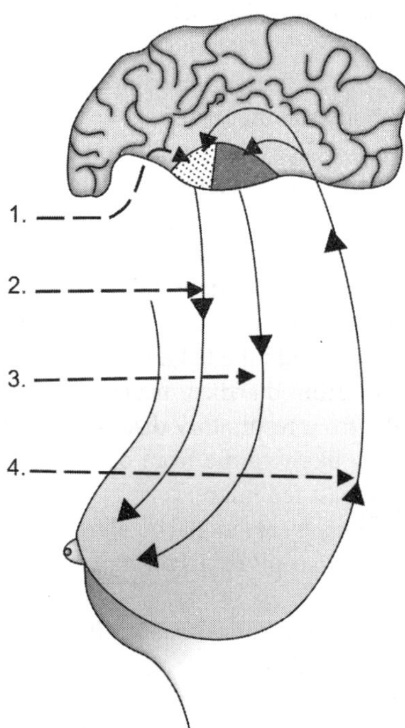

FIGURE 6.1: Diagram of physiology of lactation

to point out here that just supplementing water also along with breast-milk is enough to suppress the 'let down' reflex and lead to diminished milk output. Besides these factors, it is important that the mother be totally stress free, with no anxiety of any sort and comfortable since the let down reflex is greatly influenced by these factors.

- **Lack of privacy/rooming in:** We live in a society and hence social interaction is an integral nature of all humans. As per our traditions and social obligations, when a new born arrives, there is a row of visitors making a bee line to bless the mother and the child or, at other times, in families with limited space, the mother the mother does not get a chance to be on her own or have any privacy to be able to nurse the child in peace. This can often lead to distraction of her focus from the baby which itself can be a causative factor in lactation failure. Moreover, the mother is seen feeding her baby amidst other members of the family where there is some discussion going on or her attention is focused on the television or she may be attending any visitors too. This distraction from the baby can reduce the let down reflex further leading to decreased lactation. Therefore it is very important that some 'rooming in' be allowed to the mother and the child so that she can focus completely on her baby. This allows 'one to one' contact eye contact with the child and may be some verbal communication between the two which helps 'bonding' between the mother and child.

EARLY INTRODUCTION OF TOP FEEDS

Ideally breastfeeding should be done 'exclusively' for 6 months as recommended by WHO. But at times mothers in their zeal to feed their babies adequately end up 'overfeeding' them by resorting to artificial feeds. They feel that breastfeeds are not adequate or he remains 'hungry', or is not growing adequately. As a result they initiate top feeds in the form of formula, milk substitutes and even semi-solids much before 4–6 months. This results in decreased output of breastmilk by mothers and again to make up for this deficit, they further resort add more solids. This vicious cycle ultimately results in further decreased output and lactation failure. On the contrary, if the mother continues to breast fed at frequent intervals, the milk output is maintained and may normalize eventually. Approximately 700 to 800 ml milk is secreted per day in a healthy normal lactating women and this is sufficient till 5–6 months.

Mother's Employment

In our grandmother's age, lactation failure was unheard of as mothers mostly were housewives and their total energy and commitment was focused on the family and their needs. In the process with the arrival of the new born, the attention of the mother is totally focused on her baby and its care. Nursing comes naturally to her which she can continue without ever having the fear of discontinuing it. But in the present scenario, where majority of the mothers are working, there is a latent fear in their minds that sooner or later they will have to leave the baby at the hands of her mother in law, or the care taker or in the crèche. In such a condition she will have to resort to artificial feeding. So, in order to allow the baby to' acclimatize' to the top feeds, the mother tends to introduce these much earlier. As a result, her own feeds gradually decrease and the baby is deprived of the several benefits of her own feeds. This is particularly true of working mothers who have maternity leave and unable to continue nursing their child once they go back to their jobs. Therefore the fear that the baby may to accept the bottle later on, drives her to initiate the child to this technique, so that it is easier for the care giver or baby sitter to feed the child. This in a way also helps her to overcome her own guilt complex of not being able to feed her child herself. Besides, it is easier for the care giver to put the bottle to the baby's mouth rather than make an effort to feed him/her with a cup and spoon.

Mother's Problem of the Breast

A very common problem encountered my some mothers which can contribute to lactation failure is related to engorgement of breasts, mastitis or obstructed ducts or sore nipples. But it may be stressed here that these problems are rather a result of inadequate or improper feeding and the cure lies in more or proper feeding technique rather than discontinuing nursing.

Engorgement

This is a result of inadequate milk removal, poor ejection or failure to 'let down' or insufficient or in frequent nursing. Treatment comprises frequent nursing, warmth, massage or use of breast pumps.

Duct Obstruction

This can be due to tight fitting clothes exerting local pressure which can be which can be relieved by frequent nursing, moist heat and massage.

Mastitis

This problem is a result of prolonged engorgement or duct blockage if not tackled promptly. There can be development of abscess also, which may require antibiotic treatment. Management again involves counseling of proper nursing technique or removal of milk from blocked ducts. Analgesics can help mitigate the pain to the mother.

Sore Nipples

This is also due to improper feeding or holding the baby to the breast. When there is improper latching onto the breast, the baby is not able to suck adequately, at the same time hurting the mother's nipples leading to cracks and soreness. Correct positioning of the baby to the mother's breast and the mother's own posture while feeding can help avoid this problem. As seen from Figure 6.2, the baby is 'latched on' in the right position when the baby's chin is close to the breast, rather than only at the nipple. More of the alveolar is visible above the baby's mouth, unlike in the wrong position post of the alveolar area is visible and the baby's mouth is not wide open. In the right position, the mouth is wide open. Moreover, if not attached properly, breast feeding becomes painful for the mother unlike, 'as' in the right attachment the baby sucks deeply with slow, regular movements of the tongue. Feeding should not be discontinued due to this problem since correct positioning and 'latching on' to the breast will gradually heal the affected area. In a good attachment, the baby's chin is close to the breast while in the improper latching, the chin is away from the breasts. More of the areolar is visible above the baby's mouth than below it and the mouth is wide open with lower lip turned outwards. Nursing is not painful for the mother and the baby sucks slowly. In the wrong attachment, mouth is not wide open and much of the areolar is outside the baby's mouth. Breastfeeding is painful for the mother if the latching on is in correct.

Certain basic precautions if taken heed of can help avoid problems related to soreness of the nipples or blocked ducts, etc.

- Frequent expression of milk both manually or by use of breast pump can stimulate the 'let down' reflex and help in adequate lactation.
- Frequent short feeding, e.g. every 2 hourly for 5–10 minutes after the 'let down'. The mother can offer from one side first and after feeding for about 5–8 minutes, the child is satisfied, she can feed from the other side the next time she feeds. This will ensure uniform flow from both breasts. With increase in its requirement with age, it might become necessary to feed from both sides.

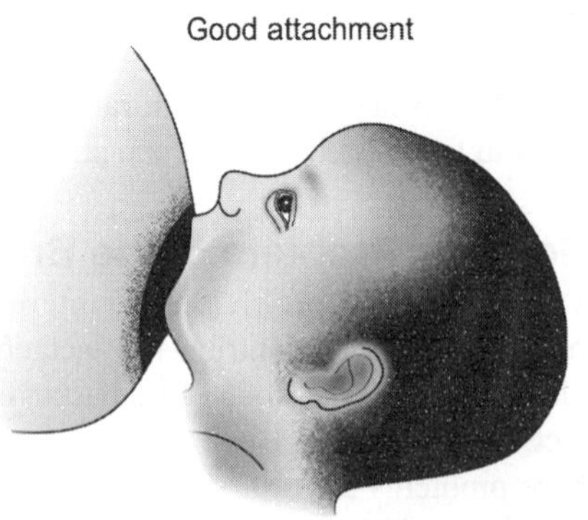

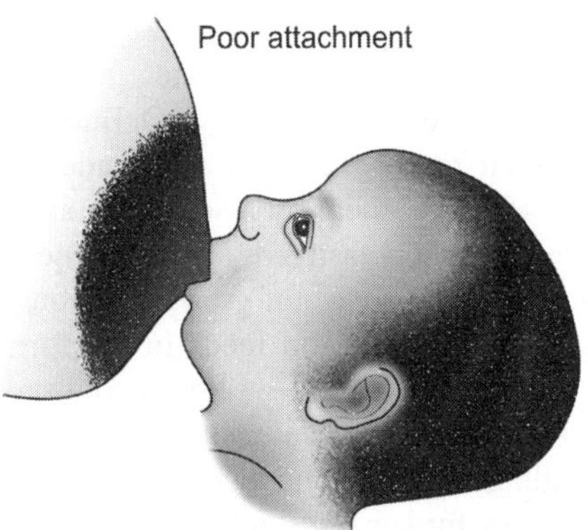

FIGURE 6.2: Feeding position adapted from KE Elizabeth[1]

- Proper 'latching on' of the infant to the breast.
- After the baby is satisfied, the mother should try to dislodge the baby from the breast gently by inserting her finger into the corner of the infant's mouth.
- The nipple should be washed only with plain water without using soap or any disinfectant solution.
- The nipple should be allowed to dry before covering. In case of severe pain or soreness, the mother can express manually rather than allowing the baby to suck, to avoid further pain.
- If soreness is very severe and painful, it would be wise to stop nursing at that nipple and express manually from the other side for 24–48 hours.
- A mild analgesic can help reduce pain to some extent.

To summarize, to encourage the mother to breast feed successfully and optimally for the first 6 months, care should be taken to keep her relaxed, help her build confidence in her ability to feed and give her adequate space for rooming in. She should be encouraged to maintain her own diet adequately without any food fads and have plenty of fluids especially water through out the day. Having a glassful of water just before nursing the child can also help the let down reflex. It is advisable that, rather than the elders or others in the family handling the baby, the mother must be allowed and encouraged to do herself, which helps in 'bonding' between the two and also gives a sense of security and satiety to the child.

ROLE OF PRELACTEALS

In most communities it is customary for elders in the family to offer prelacteals to the new born. These can be indifferent forms in different communities like, honey, 'janam ghutti' goat's milk or 'saunf' water, etc. This practice is not healthy due to the risk of any infections being passed on to the baby. Honey which is commonly offered as the first food in many communities can actually be responsible for passing any fungal infections. 'Janam ghutti' is usually given as pacifier and considered good for digestion. Bloating of abdomen due to aerophagia is very common due to which the baby cries. Mothers then resort to such practices which can indirectly harm the baby's system. Even plain water, either as such or boiled with saunf, etc. is not required. Such practices can adversely affect the sucking reflex which in turn suppresses milk output. There can be a risk of aspiration also into the air passages or lungs and secondly highly prone to infections if proper hygiene is not maintained. Therefore, the baby should be put on the mother's breast within half an hour of birth to stimulate the let down reflex by inducing the oxytocin.

Frequency and Duration of Exclusive Breastfeeding

The baby is the best judge in self regulating its timing of feeding. There should not be any fixed schedule of feeding. Demand feeding is the norm advised. Each baby differs from the other in getting satisfied and may have varying stomach capacities. Some may be satisfied earlier but may demand more frequently. Others may continue to be quiet for longer periods, but at a time may feed well from both breasts. Generally 5–8 minutes on each breast is sufficient to satisfy the baby and give a feeling of fullness. A 'crying' baby generally is taken as a signal of a 'hungry baby' by the mother and feeding him generally satisfies him. But crying may not always indicate hunger. At times a wet baby might cry too or he may be ill or experiencing some sort of discomfort in any form. 'Teething' can also be painful or irritable for a child and he may express that by crying. The mother with experience learns to assess the need of her baby and will know whether the child is really hungry or not. Usually babies themselves set their own schedule of about 3–4 hours depending upon how optimally they are able to suck at one given time.

The mother can be assured of her feed being adequate for the baby, by maintaining a record of his weight gain and the frequency of urination. If there is an upward trend in weight gain and if the baby passes urine about 5–6 times per day, she can rest assured that her milk is adequate for the baby and need not resort to formula feeds.

Artificial/Formula Feeding

Mothers with the fear of their babies being left underfed, generally resort to formula feeds right from early infancy. In our country formula feeding is generally discouraged due to the high risk of infections, and bottle contamination. There is also risk of over dilution leading to failure to thrive. Under exceptional conditions where either the mother has expired or the baby is adopted from unknown parents, or there are twins and the mother is not able to breast feed adequately, formula feed may be resorted to. Ideally cow's milk or the regular dairy milk can be used in undiluted form. The common myth that whole undiluted milk can not be tolerated by the infant should be dispelled off by proper counseling. Even it is whole buffalo milk, the excess cream formed after keeping for a few hours may be skimmed off in the early few weeks only, gradually shifting to whole milk. The main draw back of dairy milk or the locally available milk is that it is devoid of iron and therefore, iron supplementation may have to be given to prevent anemia setting in. Multivitamin drops too can be given along with. To counter the effect of higher sodium content and osmotic level in dairy milk, it is a good idea to feed plain water two to three times a day. Formula fed infants may not require iron or water supplements, since most commercial milk substitutes are all well fortified. The only drawback of formula milk, if used by the lower socioeconomic group, is that the dilution may be in excess of the instructions provided on the packaging, thereby leading to inadequate weight gain and if the water used for reconstituting is not sterile or hygienic, there can be added risk of gastrointestinal infections. In situations where the mother has to join back to work before 6 months, it would be a wise decision for her to express her milk (expressed breastmilk or EBM) and leave it behind with the care taker to be used with the other milk substitute being used. This EBM should be given with a clean spoon and cup. It can be safely kept for 4–6 hours without being contaminated. Refrigerating the EBM can keep it for almost 24 hours. Heating it may curdle it so it can be given as such. At times wet nurse is available who can nurse the baby, thus providing the benefits of human milk to the baby.

Adverse Affects of Bottle Feeding

Although bottle feeding is widely practiced and accepted in the western world, in the developing countries this practice should not be encouraged due to the associated risks of infections and contamination of the feeds. As mentioned earlier in this chapter, the introduction of the bottle in early infancy also can lead to nipple confusion and the maternal milk output begins to decrease prematurely. The various reasons to avoid the bottle in our country are:

- There is increased risk of gastrointestinal infections due to inadequate maintenance of the bottle hygiene. Even the mothers belonging to lower socioeconomic status tend to introduce the bottle due to the ease with which it can be put in the baby's mouth and the effort and time spared for attending to their household chores.
- The baby is confused between the bottle nipple and mother's nipple and finds it easier to latch on to the bottle than to the breast.
- Introduction of the bottle in early infancy also suppresses the mother's own milk output, thus depriving the baby of the essential nutrients which can be provided by breastmilk.
- The baby gets addicted to the bottle and develops a dependency on it, probably seeking security. This addiction prevents him to wean onto the cereal based semi-solids in the second half of the first year, gradually leading to getting anemic, as milk is a very poor source of iron.
- Many children who are hooked on to the bottle continue to use it for prolonged duration and even prefer to take other sweetened beverages/drinks from the bottle only, thereby compromising on their appetite.
- As the baby might tend to overfeed with the bottle, there can be a risk of these babies getting over weight also due to excessive milk intake, sometimes going up to 1–1.5 litres per day. The milk used also may be full cream, which can be a contributory factor for increased fat cells in the body from childhood itself. These fat cells once formed can not be reduced later in life and these children would continue to be 'chubby babies' growing ultimately into 'obese adults'.

On the other hand, there is another extreme spectrum of bottle fed babies-those with 'failure to thrive'. This happens in the lower socioeconomic group of mothers who tend to dilute the milk in order to stretch the limited available resources with them. This satisfies the baby for a short while but is deprived of the essential nutrients required for his optimum growth and development. Again, since it is easier and convenient for the mother to feed with the bottle (sparing her the precious time available for other house hold chores) and equally comforting for the baby to suck from the bottle, he will not accept any solid food offered to him. The cereal pulse based solid feed has to be chewed and this requires an effort on the part of both the mother and the child to feed, chew and swallow it. This makes it easier for both to give into the temptation of using the bottle for feeding mother and the child to feed, chew and swallow it.

Burping after Feeding

This is a very important step to be followed each time the baby is fed. Along with ingesting milk, babies take in a lot of air also, and if it is not expelled, the baby will cry soon after he is allowed to lie down. This is due to the abdominal distension caused by aerophagia. To relieve this problem, it is advisable to allow the baby to burp after each feed, by holding him upright with his head on the mother's shoulder and gently patting on the back till the baby burps out extra-air. It is advisable to make the baby lie on the right lateral side after feeding to prevent any aspiration or choking.

Duration of Breastfeeding

Exclusive breastfeeding should be done for 6 months as per WHO guidelines and continued along with cereal supplements till 2 years of age. However, most often it is observed that many mothers come with problems of the child not accepting any semi-solid food despite their best efforts. On further probing it is found that mothers continue to exclusively breast-feed well beyond 6 months without encouraging much of semi-solids with the result that the baby sort of gets addicted to the breast and refuses to accept anything else. Besides, prolonged breastfeeding gradually leads to anemia which in turn results in loss of appetite. Therefore, if the child is gradually weaned over to semisolids after 6 months, he gets acclimatized to a variety of foods and develops a taste for a variety of foods. But, yes breastfeeding should continue for as long as possible in addition to cereal supplements. In specific conditions, when the child is not accepting solids at all because of prolonged breastfeeding, the mother can be asked to stop breastfeeding, so that the child gets to accept solids.

Breastfeeding During Illness

There are very few indications when the mother is advised against breastfeeding her child. By and large a mother should continue to breastfeed her child even if she is ill like in viral infections, even tuberculosis, hepatitis or any other infectious diseases. In mastitis or breast abscess the mother can express her milk and feed the child. In case of the mother suffering from tuberculosis, she should be under constant supervision of a clinician for appropriate treatment for her own self as well as monitoring of the baby too for transmission of infection. In conditions where mother may be HIV positive, it is generally advised to continue breastfeeding keeping in mind the overall advantages of it as compared to the risk of transmission. If the baby is also positive, then there is no benefit in discontinuing breastfeeding in any case, but even if the baby is not positive, breast-feeding should be continued to be encouraged, as it can prevent further likely recurrent infections. As per the recommendations of WHO, breastfeeding should be promoted in HIV positive mothers in view of its role in providing immunity against other HIV related complications in already infected infants.[4] Perinatal transmission of the disease is known to be around 30%. Moreover, in situations where there is lack of adequate support for children of such mothers it is considered justified for the mother to continue breastfeeding (See chapter 39 also). The few conditions where the mother is advised against breastfeeding are when she is on certain drugs like in conditions of malignancy, thyroid or some psychotic problems. Drugs like laxatives also can affect the baby's gastrointestinal system temporarily.

In case of a child being ill also, except when indicated otherwise, like in situations where there may be risk of aspiration, etc,[5] there is no indication of withholding breastfeeds. In fact breast feeding should be continued since the child may not accept solids easily; in which case at least breast feed can help tide over that brief period of low intake. In

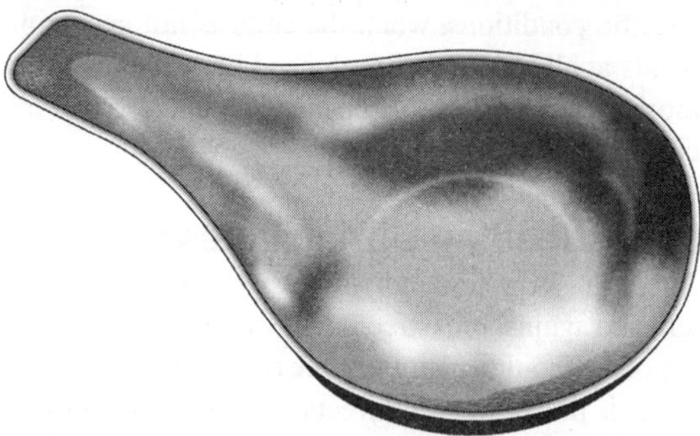

FIGURE 6.3: The traditional feeding spoon (palada)

conditions of viral or diarrheal illness which are very common in infants, breastfeeding should be encouraged to prevent them from dehydration and negative energy balance. It should be explained to the mothers that passage of stool after every feed in an exclusively breast fed baby does not indicate diarrhea and no medication should be offered. Over treating such babies with antibiotics can actually lead to drug induced diarrhea which can worsen the situation. It is a perfectly normal phenomenon for a breast fed baby to pass stool after every feed. Only after solid feeds have been introduced, do the stools begin to be slightly formed and decrease in frequency.

A baby born with cleft palate might encounter some difficulty in breastfeeding, if the palates involved. In such conditions, he can be fed expressed breast milk by spoon and cup or if required there are specially designed spoons available termed 'pallada' in local terminology (Fig. 6.3).

These have a long teat like design which can go easily into the baby's mouth for feeding milk. Care should be taken to avoid choking by maintaining an upright position of the baby while feeding.

Breastfeeding Promotion Network of India (BPNI)

A national network has been formed for the cause of promotion of breast feeding in our country known as the breastfeeding promotion network of India (BPNI). A global agency exists for the same cause known as World Alliance for Breastfeeding action. In 1992, UNICEF organized a global program of Baby Friendly Hospital Initiative (BFHI), which was adopted by India in 1993. Many hospitals today have been certified as 'BFHI' for which certain policies have been laid down:

- Hospitals need to have an official policy to protect, promote and support breastfeeding.
- All staff involved in maternity and child care hospitals/centers are trained in skills of promoting breastfeeding.
- To assist mothers in early initiation of breast feeding within half hour of birth for normal deliveries and within 4–6 hours of a cesarean section.
- All mothers are taught the right technique of breastfeeding and to maintain lactation.
- To ensure no food or drink or any other mill substitute other than breastmilk be offered to the baby and are strictly prohibited in the hospital.
- Mothers should be encouraged to breastfeed on demand.
- Any use of artificial teats, pacifiers, soothers and feeding bottles are strictly prohibited in the hospital.
- Maximum follow up support and assistance for exclusive breastfeeding up to 6 months be made available to all mothers.

The Infant Milk Substitute Act (IMS Act)

Around the same year in 1993, another Act known as Infant Milk Substitute Act (IMS Act) was passed, relating to regulation, production, supply and distribution of all types of milk substitutes including feeing bottles and infant foods. The World Health adopted an international code for marketing of breastmilk substitute way back in 1981. This code was subsequently adopted by the Government of India in 1993 and passed as an Act (Central Act 41 of 1992). This Act calls for strict prohibition of free samples of infant formula and other gifts, posters and advertisements and any financial inducements to health personnel. The Indian Academy of Pediatrics (IAP) has also adopted this code strictly.

Summary of Provision of the Code

- No direct promotion to the public by way of advertisement or distribution of discount coupons, free samples (Article 5.1 and 5.3)

- No promotion of products in healthcare facilities (Article 6.2 and 6.3)
- No free samples or gifts to mothers (Article 5.2 and 5.4)
- No contact with mothers by company sales personnel (Articles 5.5 and 6.4)
- No promotional samples or gifts to health workers (Article 7.3).

Information provided by manufacturers and distributors regarding products should be restricted to scientific and factual matter and should not convey the belief that bottle feeding is equivalent or superior to breastfeeding.

REFERENCES

1. Elizabeth KE, Feeding of infants and children. In: Nutrition and Child Development; 3rd edn. Paras Medical Publisher Hyderabad. 2002;pp1-28.
2. Victoria CG, Smith P, Vaughan JP, et al. Evidence for protection by breast feeding against infant deaths from infectious diseases in Brazil. Lancet. 1987;2:319-22.
3. WHO/UNICEF. Breast Feeding in the 1990's: Review and Implications for a Global strategy based on the Technical Meeting, Geneva, 25-28 June. 1990.
4. Akre J. Health Factors which may interfere with breast feeding. In: Infant Feeding: The Physiological Basis. Bull WHO. 1989;67(Suppl):41-54.
5. Gosh S. Infant Feeding, Food and Nutrition Board, Department of Women and Child development, Ministry of Human Resource Development, Government of India. 1993.

7 Nutrition for Older Children

"Tell me what you eat and I will tell you what you are"

Anthelme Brillat Savarin (1825)

A child having completed his second year of life will gradually begin to show many changes which are a part of his normal growth and development. His association with food assumes a varied spectrum, right from a language of communication to a show of emotions, to the extent of acceptance or rejection or selection of food.[1] But the fact remains that 'food' or more precisely 'good nutrition' continues to remain fundamental to the child's physical and mental growth and development.

Growth and development is a continuous process whereby each year builds upon the preceding one[1] It is here that the role of building good food habits assumes significance. Good food habits can not be acquired overnight or for one particular period. They have to be built over the years and these years begin right from one's childhood. At this point, parents, health workers and to some extent teachers can play a crucial role to help the child.

Unlike in the past when a child used to enter school not before the age of five, today, due to changing times, a child is exposed to the outside world as early as 2.5–3 years. It is here that the process of food becoming a social event begins, when the packed tiffins which are sent with him (to the Nursery or prepreparatory school or crèches), becomes a medium of another school activity. This participation inculcates certain habits such as sharing, widening circles of human relationship and also becoming a sociocultural activity.

BUILDING GOOD FOOD HABITS

Certain considerations towards building good food habits should be:

1. Maintaining regular meal timings in a pleasant environment.
2. Offering small in between snacks of a nutritious variety.
3. Avoiding monotony in various meals. Change is usually welcome and will help develop new tastes.
4. Food items should be such that the child is able to handle himself without messing or difficulty. Where and when required, adult help would be appreciated.
5. Avoiding use to tinned products or instant ready to mix preparations. A child fed on such feeds will not accept the simpler home based family diet later.
6. Whenever possible, one meal of the day should be a 'family affair' where all the family members sit together and enjoy food rather than considering it as just another routine affair.
7. Undue anxiety over food should be avoided as it can rebound as a reaction of food becoming a weapon by the child to win his point.

Diet for the Preschool Child (2–5 Years)

Growth and development although have a set pattern at various stages, need not necessarily be a uniform process for all children. Therefore, no two children should be assessed on a comparative basis but as an individual by himself. The velocity of growth tends to keep changing at various stages. During the second year of life there is a further deceleration of the growth rate. An average child gains 2.5 kg and 12 cm during this year. The decrease in appetite which had generally started by about 1 year extends well into the second year. This causes loss of some subcutaneous tissue, which had reached its peak by about 10 months of life.[2] As a result the 'plump look' baby gradually begins to change to a lean and muscular child. According to Beal, healthy well nourished girls reduced their milk intake as early as six months and returned to higher intakes at 2–3 years of age. Boys showed a reduction in their intake around nine months, but increased their intake by the end of two years. Pattern of appetite was seen to vary from child to child. In Beal's study, appetite of some children improved by five years or earlier, while other continued to eat poorly well into their school years.[3]

During the third to fifth year of life, weight and height gains are relatively steady. It is generally about 2 kg and about 6–8 cm gain in weight and height respectively.[2] Besides, dentition begins to appear by about 2½–3 years resulting in changes in food habits and likes and dislikes of specific food items. A study conducted by the National Nutrition Survey in its first phase was directed towards areas of low income in ten states. This study revealed an alarming amount of malnutrition which included every type of deficiency seen in under developed countries. However, cases of severe deficiency states like kwashiorkor, rickets and goiter were few, but still occurred. The incidence of failure to gain weight at a satisfactory rate was high among pre-school children. Anemia was widely seen in this age group and dental decay was found to be practically universal.[4] This study was in total contrast to the others where nutritional status of most children in USA was good, due to the fact that the latter studies were limited to children from middle income groups where such problems are uncommon.[3,5] Beal and her associates, in a longitudinal study, confirmed that at a given age set up, the individual patterns of growth varied widely just as their intakes of nutrients varied.[3] More recent observations made in the pediatric out patient department of PGI, Chandigarh also revealed similar trends. The intakes and nutritional status of children 0–2 years were found to be proportionate to the socioeconomic and literacy levels of the mothers. The better the socioeconomic status and literacy level, more satisfactory was the food intakes and consequently nutritional status of the children.[6]

RECOMMENDED NUTRIENTS AND FOOD GROUPS

Considering the RDA for various nutrients (Chapter 2, Tables 2.1 and 2.2) and those for various Food Groups (Chapter 2, Table 2.3), it may be appreciated that it is not very difficult to provide the recommended foods. These are basically the common day to day food stuffs prepared by every household. The concept of extra milk or fruit requirement does not hold any weight, because as observed from the RDA, it is the common cereal-pulse-vegetable combinations commonly prepared at home, that requires emphasis rather than milk, fruit or eggs meat, etc. Even small helpings of vegetables can be adequate to meet the requirements. Moreover making use of Mother Nature's gift to man- 'seasonal crop' can best serve the purpose. Carrots and most green leafy vegetables available in abundance during the winter season can fulfill our daily needs of Vitamin A, iron and calcium, in fact, also store for the lean period. Similarly the practice of consuming jaggery or 'gur' in winters and also groundnuts can provide adequate iron and proteins to us. In fact when ever available these should be consumed throughout the year. Fruits, if made use of seasonal gifts can also be easily accessible. Mangoes in summers are in abundance which can take care of the vitamin A requirements and perhaps even in building the store. Similarly, amla and guava—the cheaper fruits are in fact precious enough in terms of their high vitamin C content. This way a judicious selection of foods available, and formation of healthy good habits can easily provide the required nutrients for any individual for any given day. It is not necessary to be able to spend more' to 'provide more'. Rather overspending also leads to 'over nutrition' or wrong nutrition, which, if unbalanced can prove detrimental to the health of the children. Some easy to prepare low cost nutritious recipes are given (the Annexure).

Diet for School Children (6–12 Years)

Growth rate of children between 6–12 years of age continues to remain steady more or less ending in a preadolescent growth spurt by about 10 years in girls and 12 years in boys. The average weight gain during these years is about 3.0–3.5 kg per year and about 6 cm in height correspondingly.[2] This period of life is full of vigor and activity with increased physical out put. Appetite of these children also tends to show an increase and correspondingly they tend to show good gain in weight and height. Normally, the fat in the subcutaneous tissue which had decreased between ages 1–6 years in both sexes begins to redeposit as early as 8 years in girls and 10 years in boys with normal nutrition. They again tend to become chubby and look full and rounder just before the increased, velocity of growth at pre-adolescent stage of 12 years.[2] During this period girls and boys become conscious of their growth spurt and other changer of physical development. It is quite common to see uneven distribution of fat in them which during adolescence tends to spread our uniformly.

During these years, environmental stress and strains are not uncommon and most often children fall prey to all kinds to infections, some minor like virals, etc. to the more severe forms like tuberculosis or recurrent diarrheas. In such conditions, appetite is the first to suffer and their intakes decrease drastically, added to the lost in appetite are various fancies of children for particular goods which may not necessarily be nutritious. These result in failure to gain weight, and complaints of easy fatigability, decreased alertness in school and irritability are some common associated problems.

WHAT ARE FOOD FADS

Besides poor appetite consequent to infections, certain other factors are a major contributor to the poor or faulty dietary patterns among children. Old blind beliefs and wrong food fads of 'hot', 'cold', 'light' and 'heavy' foods are most commonly seen among the Indian population including the so-called educated class. Restriction of specific foods not suitable during a specific illness or being a cause of certain diseases adds to the problem of poor intake or faulty food habits, e.g. restricting banana during an episode of cold and coughs or it causes phlegm, or curd during fever due to its' cold' effect, of rice causing joint aches and cold; fats, jaggery and ground nuts are considered hot and heavy and hence avoided during summers. Treating most diarrheas and fevers with tea spiced with certain herbal leaves is another very common practice which can adversely affect the child's appetite besides compromising on their nutrition. On the contrary, banana being a good source of calories and potassium can provide enough nutrition during any illness. Rice based simple soft foods can equally be good with some added fat to increase the calories besides making it palatable in an otherwise anorexic condition. Jaggery and ground nuts commonly blamed for being hot and difficult to digest are on the contrary very good sources of vitamin A, and iron and proteins and calories respectively. These should be consumed not only during winters but through out the years when ever available. Sweets made from jaggery and addition of 1–2 tsps of groundnut powder can make an excellent source of calories, protein, vitamin A and iron.

HOW TO MEET THE REQUIREMENTS (RIGHT SELECTION)

As observed from the RDA (Chapter 2, Table 2.3) with increase in age, the stress is more upon cereals and pulses, the other groups like milk, fats and sugars remain more of less consistent. This requires a proper selection of foods. This means a child aged 7–10 years should be having approximately 10–12 chappatis or its equivalent in terms of rice, dalia, bread, etc. Pulses also should form an essential part of a meal, because the requirement of 60–70 g can only be met, if had as at least one serving (approximately 1 medium katori, i.e. 100 g cooked) twice a day. The same may otherwise be incorporated in the form of mixed flour as 'missi roti' bread sandwiches, 'khichdi' or even mixed dalia.

In between small feedings or snacks in the form of besan pura or pancakes of cornflour or bread pakoras with paneer on potato stuffings can be excellent cereal/pulse based nutritious combinations. Besan ladoos or groundnut and jaggery based sweets can also serve as good in between snacks to meet the day's requirements. Milk, however remains the same is in the early years (approx 200–300 ml). Seasonal fruits and vegetables in moderate amounts can easily meet the requirements of most vitamins and minerals besides providing adequate fiber. Here in lies the importance of proper selection of foods and building good food habits. As mentioned earlier in this chapter, good food habits can only be built over the years. A child may be having adequate or even extra calories but through milk based sweets, chocolates or any such junk foods available readily in attractive displays. The media exposure to tempting eatables sold in attractive packets, e.g. of potato wafers or instant noodles or cream soups are a major contributory factor for inculcating wrong selection and food habits. All these items may be providing enough calories but without the much needed proteins, vitamins and minerals.

It becomes very essential therefore that some adult supervision for the right selection of foods is made so that a balance is maintained between the requirements and the likes and dislikes of the child.

To sum up the following dietary guidelines may be kept in mind while planning meal for children between ages 2–12 years:

- The energy requirements of the child should be adjusted to maintain ideal body weight.
- Calories from solid fats and sugary beverages should be consumed with caution.
- Portion sizes of in between snacks should be monitored.
- Child should be encouraged to eat home based food and dine out only occasionally.
- A variety of fruits and vegetables, whole grains and legumes besides milk and milk products should be a part of the daily menu.
- Milk and milk products should be of the low fat category.
- Breakfast should never be skipped and should comprise a serving or two of cereal along with milk.
- Water is crucial for body metabolism and hence should be consumed liberally—between 1–1.5 litres at least.
- Adequate exercise in the form of sports or other outdoor games for at least an hour, is a must for all children to maintain ideal body weight and good health.
- Watching television while eating should be strictly discouraged. The total time spent watching television or computer games should not exceed 1.5 hours per day in intervals.

ANNEXURE

Low Cost Nutritious Recipes

1. Nutritious ladoo

Wheat flour	1/2 cup
Besan	1/2 cup
Fat	1/2 cup
Jaggery powder	1 cup
Till	2–3 tsp.

1. Roast the till without oil.
2. Fry the wheat flour and besan in the oil till golden brown.
3. Mix jaggery powder to the above mixture along with till and form into ladoos.

2. Carrot/pumpkin barfi

Pumpkin/Carrot	250 g/4–5
Jaggery/Sugar	50 g
Oil	1 tsp.
Coconut gratings	if available.

1. Peel the carrots and grate finely.
2. Prepare sugar syrup till slightly thick.
3. Add coconut gratings and cook till the mixture. leaves the side of the pan.
4. Four the mixture into a greased plate and cut into squares on cooling.

3. Panjiri

Wheat flour	100 g
Besan	100 g
Groundnut powder	200 g
Oil	7–8 tsps
Till	50 g
Ground jaggery/sugar	200 g.

1. Roast groundnuts and after peeling grind into coarse powder.
2. Roast till without oil till reddish brown.
3. Roast both flours separately first and then together in oil.
4. Mix till, groundnut powder and jaggery powder or sugar and store in a jar on cooling.

4. Soak soyabeans

Soyabean	50 g
Rice	100 g
Onions	25 g[1]
Carrot	1/2–1
Peas	2–3 tsp
Cabbage/cauliflower	100 g
Tomatoes	2
Spinach	1–2 leaves
Oil	5–6 tsps
Salt/spices	to taste.

1. Soak soyabeans overnight. Remove skin in the morning and boil or pressure cook for 10 minutes.
2. Clean and soak rice for 10–15 minutes.
3. Peel and slice vegetables into moderate size pieces.
4. Heat oil in a vessel pressure pan. Fry sliced onions and other vegetables slightly.
5. Add the soaked rice with 1 tsp. salt and let boil or pressure cook.
6. Serve with curd.

5. Moong dal/black chana 'chaat'

Moong dal/Black chana	25 g
Roasted ground nut powder	2 tsps
Tomato	1/2 g
Patato	1 g (boiled)
Roasted chana dal	2 tsp
Oil	1–2 tsp
Salt	to taste.

1. Soak the pulse overnight.
2. Next day remove from water and tie in wet muslin cloth and leave for 12–24 hours till sprouts appear.
3. Pressure cook or boil the sprouted pulse for 5 minutes to soften it.
4. Fry the vegetables lightly and add boiled potatoes later.
5. Add the steamed pulse along with salt and spices.
6. Serve with line.

6. Missi Roti

Wheat flour	15 g
Gram flour (based)	15 g
Spinach/fenugreek leaves	3–4
Onion	1/2
Oil	1½ tsp
Salt	to taste.

1. Chop spinach/fenugreek leaves finely after washing.
2. Knead the flour with chopped leaves and onion adding salt to taste.
3. Make small balls and roll out to make medium size paranthas.
4. Fry on both sides with oil and serve hot.

7. Poha

Chidwa (rice flakes)	25 g
Ground nuts	10 g
Onion	1/2
Roasted gram dal	10 g
Potato	1/4–1/2
Carrot (sliced)	1/2
Salt	to taste
Oil	2 – 3 tsp.

1. Wash the chidwa and keen aside.
2. Slice potatoes, carrots and onions finely.
3. Heat oil and fry the above vegetables.
4. Add ground nuts and roasted dal to the above and fry till brownish.
5. Now add the wet chidwa along with some salt and turmeric powder and mix all the ingredients well.
6. If desired add finely chopped coriander leaves and green chilli mix again and serve.

8. Upma

Suji	1/2 cup
Groundnuts	10 g
Carrots sliced	1/2
Potato sliced	1/2
Tomato	1
Onion sliced	1
Salt	to taste.

Mustard seeds	1/4 tsp.
Oil	3–4 tsp.
Water	1½ cup.

1. Fry suji in oil till brown and keep aside.
2. In a karahi heat oil and fry mustard seeds till they sprout. Then add the vegetables and groundnuts.
3. Add to the above thrice the amount of water as suji and boil adding salt.
4. Once the mixture boils well add the fried suji gradually, stirring simultaneously till the whole mixture forms into a smooth 'halwa' like consistency.
5. Serve with any chutney, pickle or sauce.

REFERENCES

1. Robinson C H. Nutrition for Children and Teenagers, In: Normal and Therapeutic Nutrition, 14th edn. Oxford &IBH Publishing CO. 1972; pp321-36.
2. Behr man R E, Kliegman R M, Jenson H B. Growth and Development, In: Nelson Textbook of Pediatrics Part I, 16th edn. Harcourt Publishers International Co. 2000; pp23-65.
3. Beal VA "Dietary Intake of Individuals followed through and childhood, Am J Pub Health. 1961;51(8):1107-71.
4. Schaefer AE and Johnson OS "Are we well fed?" The search for the Answer, Nutr. Today, 1969;4(No.1): 2-11.
5. Morgan AF eds. Nutritional status, USA. Bull.769, California Agricultural Experiment station, Barkley. 1959.
6. Madhu Sharma BR Thapa Impact of Socio-economic and literacy level on nutritional status of children (un-published).

8 Nutrition for the Adolescents

"We are indeed much more than what we eat, but what we eat can nevertheless help us to be much more than what we are"

Adelle Davis

Adolescence is the period of transition from childhood to adult and any transitional phase involves some stress and strain. An adolescent some times finds himself in a peculiar circumstance of adjustment to a new environment and may experience the pain of setting in to the groove of the big world. It is also a period of rapid growth and maturity, both physiologically and psychologically.

In the past few years the adolescent group has become a focus of great interest for physicians, nutritionists, social worker and psychologists, due to the realization that this is the group that required a lot of support and right guidance in term of physical growth, sexual maturation, optimum nutrition and sound mental help.

Thirty five percent of adult weight and 11–18% of adult height is acquired during the adolescent age. Nutrition plays a key role to support this rapid growth and development. More than 80% of the adolescent population lives in the developed countries where growth in number and proportion of children and adolescents has far exceeded in any other age group.

According to studies from National Institute of Nutrition figures[1], the population projections for India indicate that the number of adolescent will increase from 200 million in 1996 to 215.3 million in 2016.

Adolescence has also been referred to as a window of opportunity to prepare for a healthy productive and reproductive life, and prevent the on set of nutrition related chronic diseases in adult life. At the same time this is the last chance to address adolescent specific nutrition issues and possibly, also correction of some nutritional problems originating in the past.

This is the period when they get conscious of their looks, figure and personality. Eating behavior during this period is greatly influenced by school pressures, peer pressures, media influence and parental support.

Anemia and chronic under nutrition, are the two major problems encountered during this phase. This picture of malnutrition is mainly the result of exposure to media and easy access to junk foods through more available money on hand. It would not be an overstatement, as endorsed by authors that under nutrition in the early teens is directly linked to life style related diseases of adult hood like diabetes, hypertension and cardiovascular disease.[2]

These life style and eating behaviors, along with psychosocial factors are particularly important threats to adequate nutrition. Therefore this period of adolescence can be considered a timely period to shape and consolidate healthy eating and life style behaviors, there by preventing or postponing the onset of nutrition related chronic diseases in adulthood.

Certain nutrition issues are adolescent specific and need to be targeted with specific strategies and approaches. These include:

- Increased nutritional needs
- Growth assessment
- Adolescent eating patterns and life style
- Nutrition related to early pregnancy.

Increased nutritional needs: The period of adolescence has also been termed as the period of 'youth'. This is that time of life which begins at puberty. For girls, puberty typically occurs between 12 and 13 years of age, while for boys it occurs between ages 14 and 15 years, and the velocity or spurt of growth is the fastest during this period. The nutritional needs proportionately increase during this phase.

Calories: The increased rate of growth and activity during this period puts an additional demand for energy which varies as per the body size, level of activity and sex. The RDA for micronutrients and minerals, calcium and iron are as shown in Table 8.1.[3]

As seen from the table, the caloric needs of boys from preadolescent (10–12 years) begin from around 2200 calories, increases to almost 2600 by the time they are 18 years. Similarly for girls, the range begins from approximately 2000 calories at about 10–12 years and increases to about 2100 calories. This is a significant increase from childhood phase. The peak increase for boys is around 16 years while for girls it is around 12 years. The recommendation for distribution of these calories from carbohydrates, fats and proteins is 55–60%, less than 10% saturated fats and abut 30% respectively. Various studies from Indian groups indicate a poor nutritional status of adolescents, especially in terms of energy intakes.

Proteins: Adequate intake of proteins is also very important for growth and maintenance of muscle mass. The average requirements for all age groups range from about 55–70 g, except for the boys between 16–18 years, whose requirement peaks to about 80 g per day. In the North Indian communities like Punjab, Haryana and even Delhi, these requirements are not very difficult to achieve, given the consumption of milk and milk products and non-vegetarian foods which are predominant in their dietary habits. However in the fast growing culture of media friendly youth, involved in a string of fashion competition, the fear of gaining extra kilos and preserving the ideal figure, may deter them from adequate and right type of dietary habits.

Fats: The recommendations for dietary fats for Indians have been revised by the Expert Group of ICMR, 2010.[3] For the adolescent girl and boy the total fat intake of less than 25% of energy is considered to affect growth. For this a minimum level of visible fats should range between 35%–50% of energy. However, fat intake of more than 35% of energy may increase the risk of diet related noncommunicable diseases and should be avoided. An average figure between 20%–30% of energy is considered safe for this group of children.

Calcium: The skeletal account for at least 99% of body stores of calcium and the gains in skeletal weight is most rapid during adolescent growth. About 45% of the adult skeletal mass is formed during adolescent growth. The largest gains are made in early adolescence between 10–14 years in girls and 12–16 years in boys. During peak adolescent growth, calcium retention is on an average about 200 g/d in girls and 300 g/d in boys. The efficiency of calcium absorption is only about 30%. Therefore it is important that to reduce the risk of osteoporosis in later adult life, adequate calcium is provided in the diets of adolescents. Activities like cycling, gymnastics skating, dancing and supervised weight training for at least 30–60 minutes a day three to four times a week can help build bone mass and density. In the well to do middle class houses where milk consumption is an essential component of a day's

TABLE 8.1: Recommended dietary allowances for adolescents

Age group (years)	Sex	Wheat (kg)	Calories/ day	Protein g/d	Fat (visible) g/d	Calcium mg/d	Iron mg/d
10–12	Boys	35.4	2190	54	35	600	34
	Girls	31.5	1970	57	35	600	19
13–15	Boys	47.8	2450	70	45	600	41
	Girls	46.7	2060	65	40	600	28
16–17	Boys	57.1	2640	78	50	500	50
	Girls	49.9	2060	63	35	500	30

Source: (ICMR 2010)[3]

meal, especially in the North Indian Community, deficiency is not very common. Of course, as mentioned earlier, with today's youth focused on more weight management, deficiency of calcium can pose a major risk.

Iron: Iron deficiency anemia is very common in adolescence, in view of their increased blood volume and muscle mass during growth and development. The increased lean body mass (LBM) composed mainly of muscle is more important in adolescent boys than in girls. In the preadolescent period, LBM is about the same for both sexes. With the onset of adolescence, boys undergo a very rapid accumulation of LBM for each additional kilogram of body weight gained during growth ending up with a final LBM maximum value, double that of girls. In girls increased body mass and onset of menarche also account for increased requirements. It has been observed widely among the youth, that their meal pattern is such that adequate tissue replacement cannot be met with. Good iron sources are whole grains, pulses, green leafy vegetables, jaggery and nonvegetarian foods like egg yolk, organ meats like liver. Iron from nonvegetarian sources like lean meats and fish (known as haem iron) is better absorbed than iron from non haem iron. But even in nonvegetarian families, these foods do not form a regular feature in majority of them. Therefore, left with the vegetarian sources, the adolescent of today's generation is quite averse to include whole cereals or leafy vegetables in their diet. Most of the refined or processed foods available at the super market, which they mainly rely on, are all devoid of iron which can be a significant contributory factor for anemia. Nutritional anemia it self is a major national nutritional problem and can be responsible for a host of eating and behavioral problems like anorexia, irritability and lethargy. Iron supplements can be given to those who tend to be anemic.

Growth assessment: Anthropometry is the one most important criterion to monitor growth assessment. The report of the WHO expert committee for anthropometric methods and reference data[4] includes specific recommendations for appropriate use of anthropometry in all age groups including adolescents, for screening or program response evaluation at the individual or population level. Reference data tables are provided, as well as calculations to convert weight and heights into BMI values. Anthropometric data may help identify stunting underweight, overweight and obesity. Stunting or short height for age may reflect malnutrition in the past irrespective of the current problem. The assessment of obesity and adiposity level is more difficult in adolescents than in adults due to rapid changes in body composition. The velocity of growth values at different stages of life, are greater during the first five years of life, then slows down, and again reaches its peak during the adolescent years. During puberty, boys gain about 20–38 cm in height, while girls about 16–25 cm. Similarly weight gain is about 20 kg in boys and 16 kg in girls by the time of puberty.

Growth pattern of adolescent Indian boys and girls (10–19 years) as per the National Nutrition Monitoring Bureau (NNMB) data is shown in Figures 8.1 and 8.2.[5]

The WHO recommended standard reference growth charts is the NCHS standard, validated in 1963–1975 and updated in 2000 on more than 20,000 well nourished healthy US population from birth to 18 years. The 50th centile of the normal distribution curve is the median and is considered as standard value or 100% of the expected. The International Obesity Task Force (IOTF) has defined BMI > 18.5 as normal; > 25 corresponding to 90th centile as overweight and > 30 corresponding to 97th centile as obesity. Studies on Indian children[6] have reported that 79% of the poor rural girls from Rajasthan below 13 years have a BMI below 18.5, which is otherwise considered as normal. Therefore it was suggested that values < 15 be indicative of underweight or chronic energy deficit (CED) and < 13 as severely underweight. The upper cut off of 22 for overweight and 25 for obesity in young adolescents during the growth period seems appropriate and in accordance with IOTF standards (Refer also Chapter 3 for BMI).

In addition to weight, height and BMI, upper segment to lower segment ratio is also considered. An upper segment to lower segment ratio of 0.9–1.0 is expected among adolescents and in adults it is 1.1. Higher U/L segment ratio is characteristic of short limb dwarfism and bone disorders like rickets.

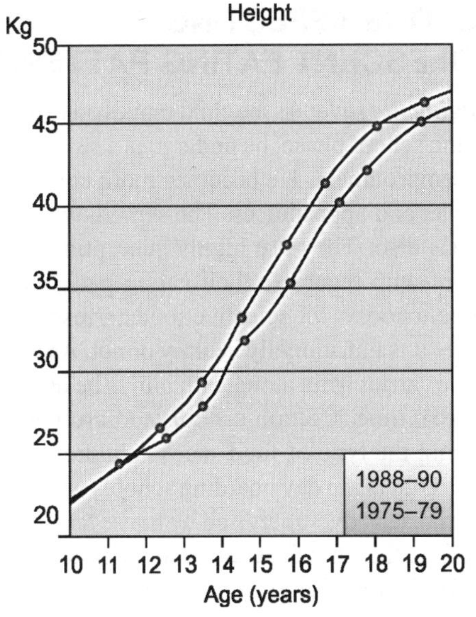

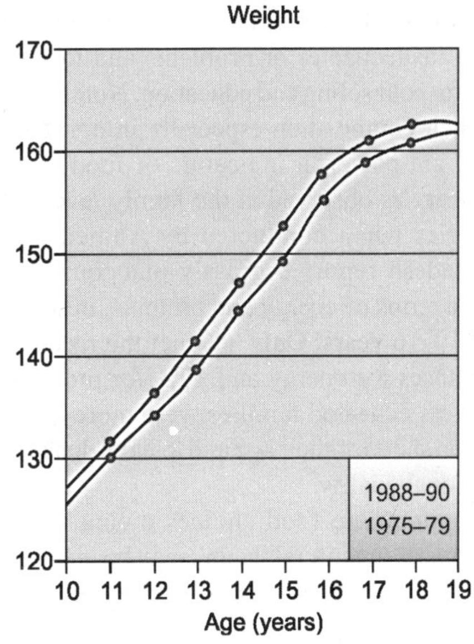

Figure 8.1: Growth pattern of adolescent boys
(*Source:* NNMB, NIN, Hyderabad 1975–1990)

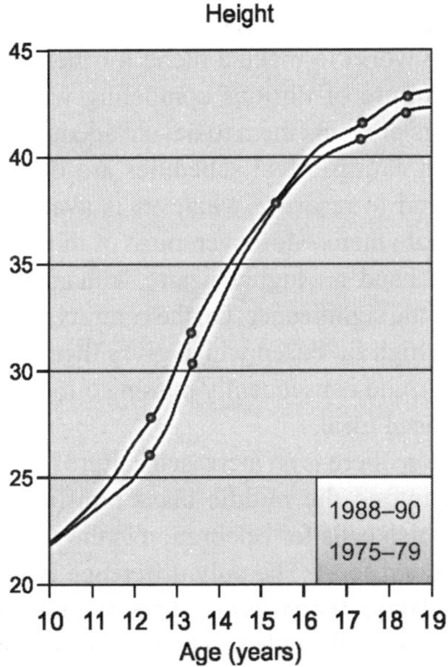

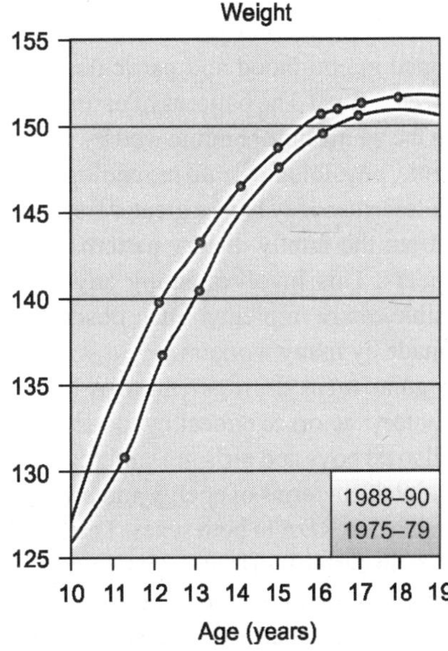

FIGURE 8.2: Growth pattern of adolescent girls
(*Source*: NNMB, NIN, Hyderabad 1975–1990)

BMI measurements of adolescents are recommended wherever and whenever feasible, irrespective of the type of nutrition problems to be expected. Whether too high or too low, inappropriate BMI in adolescents should trigger an appropriate response from health care providers.

Dietary assessment: Diet assessment involves enquiring about the dietary intake pattern of individuals. This is intended to provide clues of eating inadequacies or problems and to serve as a basis for counseling and education. Number of meals and their composition especially in nonstaple food items, are powerful indicators of food security or insecurity as observed at the family level.[7] Dietary enquiries when conducted by Ahmed, et al.[8] in Bangladesh reported grossly inadequate intakes, both in terms of energy and proteins, in school girls aged 10–16 years. Only 8% met the recommended allowances for energy and 17% for proteins. Girls from less educated families were more likely to be thin and short for their age and to have diets of poorer nutritional quality.

Inappropriate food choices owing to personal preferences or cultural factors may be identified with too little or too much of certain type of foods. Finally, the enquiry may reveal a risk of eating disorders, and for this, questions on body image and dieting are in order.

Adolescent eating pattern and life styles: Dietary habits that affect food preferences are generally developed in childhood and particularly during the adolescent years.[9] The patterns of eating vary widely among the youth and are influenced by various social, economic, physiological and psychological factors.[10]

Adolescents today have a greater freedom to break away from the family dietary patterns and eat with their peers. This involves eating any type of food accessible easily in plenty. Such observations have been made by many workers.[11]

Irregular meal timings can also be one of the contributory factors to unhealthy food habits. A study on well to do boys and girls in Delhi revealed that the dietary intake in terms of energy and protein was less as compared to RDA in both sexes. The calorie deficit was 27% in case of girls and 25% in case of boys,[12] observations from a study on adolescents from Chandigarh, revealed that the calorie distribution from macronutrients was highly skewed.[13] In the diets of these adolescents, the carbohydrates contributed about 50–64% of the total calorie, but that contributed by proteins was only around 11% against a desired level of 15%. On the other hand, as high as 29% of the calories came from fats against the RDA of 20–25%.

FACTORS AFFECTING ADOLESCENT EATING PATTERN

Changing life style: As the child moves on to his teens from the school phase, he undergoes a sea of change in his environment. He becomes more conscious of his looks and appearances. The same holds true for the girls also. They are highly susceptible to peer pressure with regard to their eating patterns. They become 'choosy' for selective foods, irrespective of whether it is nutritionally healthy or not. As a school child he carries tiffin along with him to be had during the break time. Certain schools too are particular regarding the type of food/snacks children bring to school. Others are day boarding schools where lunch is a social activity, supervised by house teachers. But as soon as they finish school and enter college life, the tiffin boxes disappear and they rely on college canteens for eating. They are very susceptible to peer influenced eating styles. Cold drinks, sweetened beverages, pizzas, samosas, burgers, noodles, etc. are a routine affair and replace meals. Besides, they enter into the big world to make a niche for themselves. The new culture of tuitions competing with their meal timings prevents them to devote adequate time to spend on eating. Meal schedules are disturbed and they tend to resort to whatever is available at hand to satiate them. Moreover, most of these foods available 'at hand' are highly bizarre, with nutritional content of little significance. On the contrary, they are high sugar, high fat based which gives them instant gratification, and consequently missing out on home based balanced meal.

In addition, there is an increased culture of dining out, even among the middle class families. Any occasion which calls for celebration in the family, is focused around food. The only difference is that in the good old days, food was organized at home under the supervision of the elders, while today, it is much easier and convenient to hire caterers or even organize in big restaurants. Here again, the menu is vast and highly energy dense thanks to the liberal fat and carbohydrate contents of such recipes. Adolescents tend to get hooked on to these types of foods and develop a taste for them, as a result of which they begin to dislike home based food.

Increased consumption of junk foods: They tend to rely heavily on junk foods like potato chips or fries, burgers, pizzas, etc. Cold drinks like colas, aerated sweetened beverages and bakery products are consumed while on the move. Most of the foods may not feel very 'heavy', but being energy dense due to their high fat content, they are devoid of important minerals like calcium and iron, which make the adolescent highly 'at risk' for developing anemia and osteoporosis at a much younger age. The emergence of multinational fast food joints are patronized by a large number of adolescents and youngsters.[14] A study from Ludhiana on teenager's eating behavior observed that fast foods were mostly consumed in between regular meals, some of the favorites being samosa, bread pakora, potatochips, noodles, pastry, patties and cola drinks.[15]

Missing meals: It has been reported that the number of meals missed or eaten away from home increases from early adolescence to late adolescence, reflecting their growing independence and more time spent away from home.[16] The meals omitted are generally compensated by snacks and other fast foods. The general trend is that the meal missed maximum is the breakfast, followed by lunch. Very often mothers seem to be satisfied if their teenager has a glassful of milk in the name of breakfast. This is because due to the pressure of competition and matching up to the expectations of their parents/ teachers, they do not have adequate time to take a wholesome cereal based breakfast. Lunch is often skipped due to the long working hours and again lack of time to be home for a good lunch. In the bargain they end up snacking on what ever is conveniently available. Observations made on the dietary pattern of adolescents in Chandigarh revealed that the snacks/ junk foods comprised about 25% of the day's calories while percent calories from breakfast was 19% and lunch and dinner combined comprised 41% of the day's intake.[13] A study from Spain, showed that high energy breakfasts were associated with higher intakes of minerals and vitamins, lower serum cholesterol levels and improved biochemical indices of nutritional status.[17]

Prolonged television viewing: Adolescents are easy prey to the television culture and this practice has led to an increased percentage of couch potatoes. It has been reported that television viewing is commonly associated with eating habits of teenagers amongst both under nourished and obese groups. In a study from Indore, 44% of underweight and 53% of the obese children associated television viewing along with meal timings.[18]

Nibbling: This is another very common habit, rather a time pass activity among most adolescent groups. It was found to occur in almost 54%–70% of the children irrespective of normal or over weight children.[18] This incidence of nibbling could be also attributed to the fact that they feel hungry or 'munchy' more often, as most of them can not or do not adhere to a regular three meal pattern with two in between snacks time. This makes them more vulnerable to lay their hands on whatever tit bits are available around. Secondly, most adolescents who 'are' concerned about their over weight status, resort to this practice, by skipping a whole meal to reduce calories and end up munching here and there to satisfy their hunger. They do this under the false concept that these foods tend to be 'light', where as actually they are energy dense (either high fat or sugar). They ultimately end up ingesting more calories than they would have done by a regular meal which would be balanced in all nutrients. Many authors have made similar observations from time to time at different periods.[19,20]

Meal timings: An ideal meal pattern for a child or adolescent age group is a three meal pattern with two in between snacks. These include breakfast, lunch and dinner. This pattern helps to meet the increasing energy and other nutrient requirements of these children. But in practice this concept has literally disappeared from the schedule of our youth. As mentioned earlier in this chapter, breakfast mostly is skipped (if at all they do so, it comprises nothing more than a glass of milk per force). Lunch timings may not be fixed due to their varied schedule or due to 'snacking' during the in between period. The last meal, dinner, may be a heavy one, if they are hungry or again it may be skipped, if in the name of dinner or supper, some snacks are consumed at some fast food joint along with their peers. As high as 41%–44% of children do not follow any fixed meal pattern.[18]

Adolescent Related Nutritional Disorders

Obesity

Obesity is emerging as a very common nutritional related disorder and if timely intervention is not done, it can lead to serious chronic disorders in adulthood. The changing life style of the present generation as discussed earlier, is the main contributory factor. Lack of physical activity and other outdoor games along with faulty eating habits takes a toll on their health. The major long-term health problems associated with adolescent obesity are its persistence in adult life and its association with cardiovascular disease risk in later life. Based on the Harvard Growth Study males who were over weight at age 13–18 years were found to be at increased risk of mortality five to six decades later compared to subjects who were lean during adolescence.[21]

In general longitudinal studies suggest that obesity tracks into adulthood, particularly if it is present in adolescence.[22] It is well established that the amount of body fat and its distribution affects metabolic disease risk. In a cross sectional study of Bogalusa, anthropometric measures of adiposity were found to be related to lipid and insulin concentrations, even before adulthood.[23] It is estimated that half of cardiovascular disease mortality is nutrition related, and 33%–50% of type 2 diabetes cases (WHO 1990).

Hypertension is another high risk disease among obese adolescents. Other nutrition related chronic diseases such as cardiovascular diseases, diabetes mellitus Type II, and cancer may only appear in adult life, but are associated with dietary and life style risk factors at adolescence, most of which are in association with obesity.

STUNTING AND MALNUTRITION

Stunting is commonly observed among adolescents in under nourished populations. Short stature in adolescents is usually caused by infection and inadequate dietary intake during the preschool years. Fetal mal formation may also be a contributory factor. In India, by and large the girls are found to be worse off than boys. This gender difference can perhaps be explained by the deeply rooted socio-cultural and economic practices that discriminate against females of all ages. Various studies have shown that most of the growth deficit in adolescents occurred during the first 3 years of life. The positive effects of energy and protein supplementation during the first 3 years of life indeed persisted at adolescence: height, weight and fat free mass were still higher in the supplemented than non-supplemented individuals.[24] The consequences of stunting and malnutrition are delay in maturation especially in girls, reduction of work capacity and ultimately high risk pregnancy.

IRON DEFICIENCY ANEMIA

Anemia may either be the cause of malnutrition among young adolescents, or malnutrition itself may be the cause of anemia. Prevalence of anemia is estimated to be about 27% in developing countries while only 6% in industrialized countries. According to the ICRW/USAID studies[25] anemia in adolescents was quite high in Nepal (42%) and in India (55%). The prevalence was as high in boys as in girls. The high prevalence of anemia itself can also be a cause for stunting due to failure to achieve their full growth potential. The consequences of anemia can also affect the outcome of pregnancy, especially if it is a teenage pregnancy. Besides it can also result in high risk of low birth weight, prematurity, still births and maternal mortality.

CALCIUM DEFICIENCY

It is well known that calcium requirements for skeletal development are greater during adolescent period, since maximum bone mass is acquired during adolescence. The amount of calcium reserves made during this period determines the risk of osteoporosis in adulthood. Deficiency of calcium also increases the risk of bone fractures even among adolescent period if at least 60% of the RDA is not met with. Calcium deficiency during adolescence has also been co-related with post-menopausal bone loss. Regular consumption of dairy products during this period is associated with lower levels of post-menopausal bone loss.

NUTRITION RELATED DENTAL DECAY

According to WHO, in developing countries, dental health may deteriorate rapidly as a consequence of dietary changes. Sucrose or the common table sugar is the main carcinogenic factor since it is generally in a form which sticks to the teeth. Starch or complex carbohydrates are not harmful, therefore diets high in starch but low in sugar have a very low caries producing potential. Also, partly hydrolyzed starch as found in highly processed foods and snacks items which are literally consumed by youngsters can be carcinogenic. Risk of tooth decay can increase with increased consumption of snack foods, processed or tinned products and other high sugar foods. Therefore, early malnutrition and dietary changes associated with adolescent life styles and socioeconomic development may lead to increasing prevalence of dental decay in adolescents and adults.

DIET AND VIOLENCE—A NEW DIMENSION

'We are what we eat' Our Vedas have long since dwelt at length on the effect of various types of foods we eat and how they can be responsible for the overall personality and behavioral temperament of an individual. The concept of 'cold' or 'hot' foods is deeply buried in the Indian psyche and any changes related to our physical, psychological and even sexual behavior have been attributed to the type of dietary life style of an individual. According to the ancient science, food has been categorized as 'satvic' or 'tamasic', meaning either producing soothing and healthy effects or having a negative influence like aggression, violence, etc. Though not scientifically proven, there might be some basis for this concept.

Today we can see this impact of dietary pattern on the personality and behavior of our young generation. Violence among children and adolescents is fast leading to a magnitude of epidemic. This trend has led many research workers to look into the depth of the etiology of this new problem, that of malnutrition as a cause of 'child violence'. This phenomenon is steadily spreading across the globe—the developed and the developing countries. Reports of kids killing their own peers over petty issues are increasingly being heard and seen. It is time now that this problem is tackled efficiently with the right approach. Several workers now have established this link between malnutrition and child violence. Malnutrition can involve either excess or deficiency of certain important nutrients during the growth of the child.

High Calorie (Junk) Malnutrition

The link between high calorie malnutrition and crime and senseless violence has been well documented.[26] High calorie malnutrition is defined as calorie excess with nutrient deficiencies, resulting in inadequate ability to utilize these calories efficiently. The possible hypothesis attributed is, the incomplete oxidation of some of the by products which are toxic and might interfere with the acid base balance of the body. Most of these high calories are contributed by a high consumption of junk foods. It was seen that these high calorie foods comprised too much sugar, refined foods and stimulants. Children thriving on such foods were the ones with violent behaviors and were found to be hyperactive. It is believed that hyperactivity and restlessness lead to impatience and a desire for instant gratification. These unfulfilled desires lead to frustration and anger, which may lead to violent behavior.

High calorie malnutrition can create 'irritable brainstem' since this tissue, (brain) demands highly efficient oxidative metabolism. This 'irritable brainstem' can 'turn up the volume' of the response and in the worst scenario create temporary insanity and take over the complete behavior of the individual. Triggering factors for such behaviors can be as trivial as being refused an expensive car or watch or being rebuked for not concentrating enough on one's studies.

Vitamin and Mineral Deficiencies

Besides excess calories, lack of certain vitamin deficiencies can also trigger violent behavior. Deficiency of vitamin B_1 (thiamine) is reported to result in irritability and poorly controlled behavior due to failure of cholinergenic behavior. Supplements of thiamine in the diets of such children for several months resulted in complacency of behavior, which initially were very aggressive and difficult. Other factors like medications (hormone therapy) can contribute to the mood swings and behavioral changes in women. Deficiency of vitamin B_{12} is also known to trigger violent behavior.[27] The role of other nutrients like iron, cobalt, zinc and iodine are also known to influence behavioral changes in children. A deficiency of iron, for instance is well known to impair mental performance.

Some foods commonly known to contribute to child violence are:

Sugar and white flour: These contribute to empty carbohydrates, leading to high calorie malnutrition by providing calories without vitamins and other supporting nutrients, to assimilate these calories.

Sugar drinks: High in phosphoric acid which causes calcium depletion. They are also high in sugar contributing to 'high calorie malnutrition'. Caffeine in soft drinks is likely to stimulate the adrenal glands leading to nutrient deficiencies.

Coffee and tea: Besides caffeine, these contain tannin which inhibits absorption of vitamin B_1.

MSG: Mono sodium glutamate an essential ingredient of all Chinese cuisine, are associated with violent behavior.

Trans fatty acids: These fats replace healthy animal fats that provide fat soluble activators needed for mineral absorption.

Liquid vegetable oils: Being very high in omega 6 fatty acids, these inhibit the proper utilization of omega 3 fatty acids, which are vital for brain function.

EATING DISORDERS

Eating disorders in children are becoming a matter of concern besides posing a great challenge to the dieticians and the pediatricians. These may range from a state of starvation to that of excessive feeding, both of which can pose serious problems for an adolescent. These disorders can start as early as 9 years of age or before puberty. Girls are more commonly affected but it has been observed that 5% of all cases are males.[28] It is estimated that about 5–10% of post-pubertal females are affected by these disorders. Girls are almost nine times more likely than boys to develop any sort of eating disorder. This has also been described as a 'wealthy persons' disease, implying that only families from the higher socioeconomic groups are susceptible.[29]

Anorexia nervosa, bulimia nervosa and binge eating disorders are complex, multidimensional disorders having psychological, medical, socio cultural and nutritional components.[30] These disorders are reported widely and alarming statistics support the need for serious interactive measures.

As per definition, diagnosis of eating disorders can be made when all features of the disorder are met.[31] These include:

- A fear of becoming fat and a drive to be thin.
- An obsession with food, weight, calories and dieting.
- The use and abuse of eating or not eating to cope with emotional discomfort, stressed life events and developmental challenges.
- An increased incidence of depression, obesity, substance abuse and eating disorders in the families of sufferers.
- A world view valuing external appearance over personal integrity.
- ***Anorexia Nervosa:*** Anorectics have an abnormal fear of gaining weight even if they appear very thin. They take pride in being thin and can go to the extent of remaining hungry and causing pain to themselves. They tend to regulate their intake by quantifying their food portions, rather than by depending upon their sensation for hunger. There are two types of anorectics:
- Those who keep themselves emaciated through strict dieting and food restriction (dieters).
- Those who are not able to lose the amount desired by dieting alone and hence resort to self induced vomiting and purging (vomiters and purgers).

These children often feel they are not good enough when compared to peers and also other family members and have a distorted image of their own selves. The clinical signs and symptoms of these patients include bradycardia, hypothermia, hypotension, constipation, insomnia, restlessness and depression. These features are known to revert upon refeeding and return to normal weight. Treatment of such patients involves:

- Nutritional Support

- Psychotherapy
- Family therapy.

For nutritional support, high calorie diets in liquid or solid form as per the condition and acceptance of the patient is advised. Education regarding food, weight, body composition and normal growth and development is encouraged. Nutritional intervention to relieve the affects of starvation is accepted as an essential prerequisite for desired results.

Specific principles for nutritional support include[32]

- A gradual weight gain is recommended since sudden weight gain can result in congestive heart failure, gastric dilation and malabsorption.
- Meals should consist of adequate amounts of carbohydrates, fats and proteins, being nutritionally balanced. The food preferences need to be considered too.
- Adequate dietary fiber from whole grain cereals is encouraged to avoid constipation.
- Small frequent feedings may be encouraged to avoid a feeling of bloating.
- Cold or room temperature foods can be advised to reduce satiety sensations.
- If caffeine intake is in excess, it should be reduced.

Bulimia nervosa: This disorder involves recurrent episodes of eating by rapidly consuming large amounts of food very fast. They seem to lose control on their eating behavior and may indulge in self induced vomiting, purging by use of laxatives and diuretics, vigorous exercise to control weight and even strict dieting. Such disorders generally develop after a distressing life event like death of some one dear, some major set back or disappointment, even perceived personal failure or memories of childhood abuse. The frequency of this disorder can occur on an average of at least 2 days a week for at least 6 months. Such patients tend to set unrealistic diet goals for themselves which may be quite rigid. They may lay undue stress on low fat foods like fruits, vegetables, nonfat yoghurt, etc. Their focus is primarily to serve caloric restriction.

Treatment in this disorder involves counseling, education about food, weight, etc. Counseling is a very important mode of intervention in these patients which includes psychotherapy blended with nutritional issues.

Summary of Recommendations in Eating Disorders

- Establish patient goals for 'normal' eating. Set calorie level for weight maintenance to ideal weight control and reduce risk of increased hunger.
- Ensuring at least three regular meals per day.
- Small frequent meals may be helpful.
- Food patterns can be maintained and eating patterns can be monitored.
- Develop exercise guidelines that support moderation and are practiced,
- Dispelling myths regarding diets, eliminating food rules.
- Gradual negotiation with them to add foods from their preconceived for bidden list of meal pattern.

High Risk Groups of Adolescents

Adolescent Pregnancy

Pregnancy in adolescence adds more risks and complications for pregnant teens compared to any other age group. They have higher rates of low birth weight infants, especially among those younger than 15 years old. The nutritional status of the pregnant adolescent is influenced by both physiologic and environmental/social factors. Since the pregnant teen is still growing, there occurs a maternal and fetal competition for nutrients, thus indicating increased nutrient needs in addition to pregnancy. Besides, there is also a risk of low pregnancy weight and minimal nutrient stores at the time of conception. Other factors affecting the nutritional status are lack of adequate antenatal care, limited resources for a good healthy diet, poor eating habits and emotional stress.

Energy needs can vary greatly, depending on pubertal maturation and physical activity. The RDA of protein is 60 grams, which is 14–16 grams more than for a nonpregnant teenager. Adequate energy intake will spare the protein to be used for growth. An iron supplement is routinely prescribed, besides vitamin B_6, C, folate and calcium.

Education and counseling are needed for the pregnant teen to accept the needed weight gain and avoid risks of possible complications.

TABLE 8.2: Recommended energy intakes for adolescent athletes

Age group (Years)	Sports group	Suggested energy intake (per day)	
		Girls	Boys
12–15	All Sports	2700 kcal (DIET A)	3200 kcal (DIET B)
15–18	All Sports	3100 kcal (DIET A)	3500 kcal (DIET B)
>18	Skilled games	3100 kcal (DIET A)	3500 kcal (DIET B)
>18	Endurance events and Team games	3500 kcal (DIET A)	4500 kcal (DIET D)
>18	Power games	4200 kcal (DIET C+ supplements*)	5200 kcal (DIET D+ supplements*)

*Supplements providing 600–700 kcal, as specified in the diet scale
(*Source*: SAI and NIN)[33]

TABLE 8.3: Diet scales for various sports groups

Food articles	Qunatity			
	Diet A	Diet B	Diet C	Diet D
1. Wheat soya flour	120 g	180 g	210 g	310 g
2. Other cereals	200 g	260 g	300 g	400 g
3. Pulses	30 g	30 g	40 g	60 g
4. Green leafy vegetable	100 g	100 g	100 g	100 g
5. Other vegetables	200 g	200 g	200 g	200 g
6. Roots and tubers	100 g	100 g	100 g	100 g
7. Fruits	150 g	150 g	200 g	200 g
8. Milk	750 g	750 g	750 g	750 g
9. Soya oil	25 g	25 g	30 g	40 g
10. Butter	15 g	15 g	15 g	25 g
11. Sugar	30 g	30 g	30 g	30 g
12. Meat/Fish/Poultry	100 g	100 g	100 g	100 g
13. Eggs	Two nos.	Two (no.)	Two (no).	Two (no.)
Energy	2775 kcal	3195 kcal	3528 kcal	4459 kcal
Protein	114 g (16.4%)	146 g (18.3%)	161 g (18.3%)	206 g (18.5%)
Fats	92 g (29.8%)	92 g (25.9%)	97 g (25.0%)	112 g (22.6%)
Carbohydrates	373 g (53.8%)	445 g (55.8%)	500 g (56.7%)	656 g (58.5%)

(*Source*: SAI and NIN)[33]

Supplements for power games:

S. No.	Food article	Quantity
1.	Eggs	Two
2.	Milk	500 ml
3.	Meat	100 g
4.	Fruit	100 g

Energy: 660 kcal
Protein: 44 g
Fats: 25 g
Carbohydrates: 65 g
(*Source*: SAI and NIN)[33]

Athletes

Adolescents involved in sports generally feel pressurized to maintain a certain weight or to perform at a certain level. In the bargain, some of them may be tempted to adopt unhealthy behaviors like crash dieting, taking supplements for muscle building, or to improve performance or eating unhealthy foods to fulfill their appetites (See Chapter 9 also).

There are certain guidelines to be followed to plan for a day's diet of an adolescent. These are based on their nutrient requirements, as recommended by Sports Authority of India training centers and National Institute of Nutrition, in 2002–03 during the training and competing phase. Ideally they should meet the daily calorie requirement as per the age and sex. Drastic changes in body weights should be avoided. A typical balanced diet for an athlete should comprise around 55% carbohydrates, 15% proteins and 35% fats. On an average an adolescent weighing around 50–70 kg may require about 3000-3600 calories per day, keeping in mind the sports activity that he/she may be involved (33). The suggested energy intakes for different age groups are as given in Table 8.2.

To meet these requirement, scales has been fixed for the various food groups as given in Table 8.3

REFERENCES

1. K Venkaiah, K Damayanthi, MU Nayak and K Vijayraghvan. Diet and Nutritional Status of rural adolescents' in India. Nutrition News, National Institute of Nutrition, Hyderabad, Oct. 2003; Vol. 24, No.4.
2. Rolland Cachera MF, Daheeger M Guillode, Batuileun Avons P, et al. Trekking the development of obesity from one month of age to adulthood. Ann Hum Biol. 1893;14:219-99.
3. ICMR. Nutrient Requirements and Recommended dietary allowances for Indians; A Report of the Expert Group of the Indian Council of Medical Research. 2010.
4. Mercedes de Onis and Monika Blossna. The WHO Global database on child growth and malnutrition: methodology and applications. Int J Epidemiol. 2003;32:518-26.
5. National Nutrition Monitoring Bureau, National Institute of Nutrition, Indian Council of Medical Research, Hyderabad. 1975-1999.
6. Chaturvedi S, Kapil U, Gnaneskaran N, et al. Nutrient Intake amongst adolescent girls belonging to poor socioeconomic group of rural area of Rajasthan. Indian Pediatr. 1996;33:197-201.
7. Ali M, Delisle HA. A participatory approach to assessing Malawi villagers' perception of their own food security. Ecol Food Nutr. 1999;38:101-2.
8. Ahmed F, Zareen M, Khan MR, et al. Dietary patterns, nutrient intake and growth of adolescent school girls in urban Bangladesh. Pub Health Nutr. 1998;1:83-92.
9. Cusatis DC, Sharma BM. Influences on adolescent eating behavior. J Adolesc Health. 1996;18(1):27.
10. Rees JM. The overall impact of recently developed foods on dietary habits of adolescents. J Adolesc Health. 1992;22(1):14.
11. Bull NL, Barbet SA. Food habits of 14–25 years old living accommodation and social class as factors affecting the diet. Health Visitor. 1985;58:9-10.
12. Kapil U, Minocha S, Bhasin S. Dietary intake amongst 'well to do' adolescent boys and girls in Delhi. Indian Pediatr. 1993;30:1017.
13. Sharma M, Ray M. Nutritional status of children visiting the adolescent clinic in a tertiary care centre at Chandigarh, 2005 (unpublished).
14. Truswell AS, Hill ID. Food habits of adolescents. Nutr Rev. 1981;39(2):73-88.
15. Sadana B, Khanna M, Mann SK. Consumption pattern of fast food among teenagers. Applied Nutrition, 1997; 22(1):14.
16. Guthrie HA. Nutrition from childhood through adulthood. In: Introductory Nutrition, 6th edn. Times Mirror/ Mosby. 1986.p.569.
17. Preziosi P, Galan P, Deheeger M, et al. Breakfast type, daily nutrient intakes and vitamin and mineral status of French children adolescents and adults. J Am Coll Nutr. 1999;18(2):171.
18. Kanchanwala R, Husain MH. Food habits of adolescents in relation to their body weight status and impact of diet counseling. Applied Nutr. 2003;28(1&2):33-9.
19. Bull NL. Studies of dietary habits, food consumption and nutrient intakes of adolescents and young adults. Wld Rev Nutr Diet. 1998;524-74.

20. Lawson M. Nutrition in childhood. Proceedings of a conference. London: Routledge. 1992.
21. Must A, Jacques PF, Dallal GE, et al. Long-term morbidity and mortality of over weight adolescents: a follow-up of the Harvard Growth Study of 1992-35. N Engl J Med. 1992;327:1350-55.
22. Serdula MK, Ivery D, Coates R J, et al. Do obese children become obese adults? A review of literature. Prev Med. 1993;22:167-77.
23. Freedman DS, Shear C L, Srinivasan SR, et al. Tracking of serum lipids and lipoproteins in children over an 8 year old period. The Bogalusa Heart Study. Prev Med. 1985;14:203-16.
24. Riveria JA, Martorell R, Ruel M, et al. Nutritional supplementation during the preschool years influences body size and composition of Guatemalan adolescents. J Nutr. 1985;125(Suppl 2):91-97.
25. Kurz KM, Johnson-Welch C. The nutrition and lives of adolescents in developing countries: Findings from the nutrition of adolescent girls research program. ICRW. 1994.
26. Lonsdale D. Crime and Violence: A hypothetical explanation of its relationship with high calorie malnutrition; J Adv Med Fall. 1994; 7(3):171-80.
27. Dommisse JV. Subtle vitamin B_{12} deficiency in Psychiatry: A largely unnoticed but devastating relationship? Medical Hypothesis. 1991;34:131-40.
28. Levine M. How schools can combat eating disorders: Anorexia nervosa and bulimia. Washington DC. National Education Association. 1987.
29. Berg F. Afraid to eat. Children and teens in weight crisis: Hettinger D; Healthy Weight Publishing Network. 1997:69.
30. Garner D, Garfinkel P. Handbook of Psychotherapy for anorexia nervosa and Bulimia Nervosa. New York's Guilford Press. 1985.
31. Levine M. How schools can combat students eating disorders; Anorexia nervosa and bulimia. Washington D C: National Education Association; 1987.
32. Rock CC, Yager J. Nutrition and eating disorders: a primer for clinicians. Int J Eating Disorder. 1987;6: 267-279.
33. Lal, PR. Evolution of Sports and Nutrition. An overview. J Traumatology and Allied Sports Sciences. 2003;Vol. 2.

9 Nutrition for the Athlete Child

It is well established that health and fitness of children is associated with the physical behaviors of parents,[1] thereby implying that family fitness should be encouraged. Physical involvement of children in their daily routine is well recognized by all sections of society, which is the reason why some time period is set aside for games and sports in most educational institutions. Inducting some form of activity for every child is considered very important in order to initiate lifetime habits of physical exercise.[2]

Taking part in recreational or competitive sports at a younger age helps developing skills, confidence, good health and fitness. Attitudes about physical activity and an active lifestyle are often formed in the first ten years of life.[3]

PHYSIOLOGICAL EFFECTS OF EXERCISE

Sports activity for a child has many physiological effects in children, especially cardiorespiratory, which is important for children and adolescents due to the following benefits:

- Improves strength and flexibility.
- Conditions the cardiorespiratory system.
- Increases endurance.
- Develops power, agility and speed.
- Aids in development of muscles.
- Exercises neuromuscular skills.
- Controls body fat percentage.
- Provides mental well being.

It is recommended that at least 20 minutes of exercise be performed, which should involve large muscles, produce mild perspiration and ensure heart beat to be at 60%–80% of maximum rate. Such an activity done at least 3–5 times a week can give the maximum benefits from cardiorespiratory work outs.[4,5]

Children preparing in sports activity should be assessed by physicians and health professionals to rule out any deleterious consequences of exercise activities undertaken by them. For participation and training in competitive sports by children, it is advisable to determine the match of maturation age with the sport, injury risk and general health status. This can be done prior to participation by a pediatrician or a physician trained in sports medicine.[6,7] Children preparing for sports activity also need to be imparted education on proper training, diet and injury prevention.[4]

NUTRITIONAL RECOMMENDATIONS

Good nutrition is crucial for appropriate growth, development and excellence in performing. Children participating in sports activities need to pay attention to their nutritional needs specific to their age and gender. The recommendations for such children are adequate supply of nutrients provided from a balanced, healthy diet as per the recommended dietary allowances (RDA). There is no indication that there are increased needs for any other nutrient beyond the RDA, although some teens may need more protein during periods of rapid growth.[8] In case of any individual deficiencies observed during the child's review, the specific nutrients can be supplemented and appropriate nutritional counseling session imparted. Arbitrary use of over the counter supplements however should be discouraged by the youth. Depending on the intensity of their activity and type of sport, the nutrient requirements may increase significantly which if not covered adequately can result in adverse effects of the growth and development of the children. Eating for sport activity should be an extension of healthy eating.

Principles of Healthy Diet for a Sports Child

The principles of a healthy diet for a child involved actively in sports should be:

- The child has a proper breakfast, comprising a cereal/bread, a drink like milk or fruit juice or a fruit.
- The child has two main meals—lunch and dinner apart from the morning breakfast, with a mid morning and an evening snack. These could be dairy products, cereals or fruit.
- The child has adequate fluids, preferably pure water or milk.

The Pregame Meal

Before an event or a practice session, the diet of the child should be:

- High in carbohydrates for energy, maintaining normal glycemic levels. Complex carbohydrates like rice, pasta, suji, potatoes are good choices.
- Moderate in protein (1–1.5 g/kg/d).
- Low in fat/fiber to reduce digestive stress.
- Low in salt.
- Preferred and familiar to the child's taste.
- Should have taken about 3–4 hours before any intense physical activity (Table 9.1) providing about 200–350 g of carbohydrates (4g/kg). This helps improve performance efficiency.
- Options of foods are low fiber cereal, with milk, fruit, milk shake or milk with an apple.
- The carbohydrate content of the food in the meal immediately preceding a meal should be reduced to avoid gastrointestinal distress.
- Prehydration with 120–250 ml water or fluid helps to maximise absorption of fluid without urination. After exercise begins, the kidney slows down urine production to compensate for water loss.

The Post Meal Diet/Refuelling

After an intense sports activity, the body needs to be 'refuelled' with the losses, preferably within 30 minutes of ending a sport activity. Delaying carbohydrate intake for too long after exercise reduces resynthesis of muscle glycogen. Resynthesis is most efficient when approximately 100 g of carbohydrates are consumed immediately or within 30 min of exercise.[15] The meal or snack should be a balance of carbohydrates and proteins depending upon the time of the day, whether it is meal time or a mid meal time of the day.

Energy

The base calorie requirement for the athlete is as per the recommended allowances. For the Indian athlete these recommendations are based on the guidelines recommended by Sports of Authority of India and National Institute of Nutrition, 2002–03[9] as given in Table 9.1.

To meet these requirements, scales have been fixed for the various food groups as given in Table 9.2.

Any increase in the calories for an activity will depend on the child's age, sex, present weight, desired weight, particular sport and level of involvement. Achieving the desired weight and maintaining the same will be the indicators of adequate calories. Because of the variance in the age of sexual development for children and the connection of body fat composition to development, body fat measurement should not be used as a qualification of weight status or goal, as in adults.[8,10] Frequent monitoring is recommended if weight change is desired to prevent too rapid loss or gain, which otherwise can affect the performance. It is therefore advisable to make the weight changes prior to the sports season.[11]

Carbohydrates

The carbohydrate content of the child involved in an intense sport activity or one who might be involved for long duration of practice may be increased in the diet to provide extraenergy.

TABLE 9.1: Recommended energy intakes for adolescent athletes

Age group (Years)	Sports group	Suggested energy intake (per day)	
		Girls	Boys
12–15	All Sports	2700 kcal (DIET A)	3200 kcal (DIET B)
15–18	All Sports	3100 kcal (DIET A)	3500 kcal (DIET B)
> 18	Skilled games	3100 kcal (DIET A)	3500 kcal (DIET B)
> 18	Endurance events and Team games	3500 kcal (DIET A)	4500 kcal (DIET D)
> 18	Power games	4200 kcal (DIET C+ supplements*)	5200 kcal (DIET D+ supplements*)

*Supplements providing 600–700 kcal, as specified in the diet scale
(*Source*: SAI and NIN)[9]

TABLE 9.2: Diet scales for various sports groups

Food articles	Qunatity			
	Diet A	Diet B	Diet C	Diet D
1. Wheat soya flour	120 g	180 g	210 g	310 g
2. Other cereals	200 g	260 g	300 g	400 g
3. Pulses	30 g	30 g	40 g	60 g
4. Green leafy vegetable	100 g	100 g	100 g	100 g
5. Other vegetables	200 g	200 g	200 g	200 g
6. Roots and tubers	100 g	100 g	100 g	100 g
7. Fruits	150 g	150 g	200 g	200 g
8. Milk	750 g	750 g	750 g	750 g
9. Soya oil	25 g	25 g	30 g	40 g
10. Butter	15 g	15 g	15 g	25 g
11. Sugar	30 g	30 g	30 g	30 g
12. Meat/Fish/Poultry	100 g	100 g	100 g	100 g
13. Eggs	Two nos.	Two (no.)	Two (no).	Two (no.)
Energy	2775 kcal	3195 kcal	3528 kcal	4459 kcal
Protein	114 g (16.4%)	146 g (18.3%)	161 g (18.3%)	206 g (18.5%)
Fats	92 g (29.8%)	92 g (25.9%)	97 g (25.0%)	112 g (22.6%)
Carbohydrates	373 g (53.8%)	445 g (55.8%)	500 g (56.7%)	656 g (58.5%)

It is worth considering that carbohydrate feeding does not prevent fatigue, but only delays it. The carbohydrate should be of the complex types which are digested and absorbed easily. They are also important to improve the performance level of the young athlete. This nutrient can efficiently fuel the body before, during and after sports events or competition. But the timing of carbohydrate is important.[12] Carbohydrates consumed during endurance exercise lasting longer than 1 hour ensures the availability of sufficient amounts of energy during the later stages of exercise and improves performance. The type of foods which can be consumed during the competitions and the timings when they can be best consumed are listed in Table 9.3. Easily digested foods high in carbohydrate, but low in protein and fat should be had. Allowing time for partial digestion and absorption provides a final addition to muscle glycogen, additional blood sugar and also relatively complete emptying of the stomach. Some good sources of complex carbohydrates are whole grain cereals, brown bread, rice, and liberal amounts of fruits and vegetables.

TABLE 9.3: Eating during competition

3–4 hours before (600–700 cals)	2–3 hours before (300–400 cals)	1–3 hours before (100 cals)	2–3 hours after
Fruit/vegetable juice	Fruit/vegetable juice	Fruit/vegetable juice	Bread, biscuits, muffins
Fresh fruit	Fresh fruit	Fresh fruit (low fiber, like plums, melons, peaches	Fruit yogurt
Bread, rusk	Bread, rusks, muffins	Sports drink	Large banana
Peanut butter, lean meat, low fat cheese	No butter or cream cheese		Fruit juice
Low fat yogurt			
Baked potato			
Cereal with low fat milk			

Refer. 9

Proteins

Protein is required for muscle building, therefore adequate amounts should be provided in the diet though vey high amounts are not recommended. This can be achieved by a balanced diet as per the RDA. Consuming greater protein than required is not advisable, because by consuming more than that required, the carbohydrate status may be compromised, thereby affecting the ability to train and compete at peak levels. High protein intake may also result in diuresis and potential dehydration.[15] Studies have shown that the need for protein in exercise depends more on the energy intake, since proteins will be used as energy source if calories are insufficient.

Foods like dairy products, nuts and legumes, fish, poultry, and soyabeans are good sources. It is worth keeping in mind that strong muscles come from regular training and exercise rather than excess of protein form the diet.

The traditional concept among athletes and body builders that they require high protein or amino acid supplements in the form of powders or pills is unfounded and should be discouraged. Large amounts of protein intake can cause dehydration, hypercalciuria, weight gain and stress on the kidney and liver. Moreover substituting amino acid supplements for food can also cause deficiencies of other micronutrients like iron, niacin and thiamine.

Fats

About 20–30% of the calories are provided by fats in a normal balanced diet for a young athlete. It is the most concentrated source of energy for fuel for light to moderate intensity exercise, besides providing the essential fatty acids. But severe fat restriction (<15% of energy) is also not advisable as it can limit performance by hindering intramuscular triglyceride storage, which is a significant source of energy at all intensities of exercise. Moderate to low fat meal is recommended for the premeal diet as high fat intake can interfere with performance and also cause gastrointestinal discomfort.

Vitamins and Minerals

Besides the macronutrients mentioned above, vitamins and minerals too are essential for a healthy body with good stamina. Of particular concern for the young athlete is calcium for healthy and strong bones and iron for stamina and endurance. Lack of calcium can lead to weak bones prone to stress fractures. Calcium rich foods are milk and milk products, while for iron, foods like meat, eggs, legumes especially soyabean and whole cereals are good sources. The iron from animal sources is the heme iron which is more easily and efficiently absorbed as compared to nonheme iron from vegetable sources like green leafy vegetables, cereals, legumes and dry fruits.

Fluids

An athlete child participating in a sport activity needs adequate hydration to prevent exhaustion and dehydration. Extra-fluids are needed to replace for losses through perspiration. Dehydration can lead to a feeling of overheating and exhaustion which can affect the child's performance level. The fluid needs include the amount required for normal hydration plus extra for training, participation and cool down activity.[11,13] Some common signs of dehydration should be explained to the athlete which are:

- Thirst
- Dizziness
- Fatigue
- Nausea
- Headache
- Chills
- Muscle cramps.

If not treated promptly severe dehydration can be very serious. It is therefore recommended to drink adequate water before, during and after the events. The athlete should be taught to recognize signs and symptoms of dehydration so that he/she an act promptly and consume adequate fluids. The color of the urine is an early sign to look for. Dark, scanty urine indicates dehydration, while a good amount, pale yellow urine indicates adequate hydration.[13] A guide to the fluid schedule is given in Table 9.4.[14]

It should be explained to the young athlete that certain fluids should be avoided as they can cause gastric disturbances and affect performance. These are:

- Carbonated drinks, regular fruit juice, fruit drinks, lemonade.
- Energy drinks containing lot of sugar or caffeine

It is recommended that a child of about 10 years of age or younger should drink until he or she does not feel thirsty and then should drink an additional half cup of water. Older children and adolescents should follow the same guidelines, but they should consume an additional cup of fluid.[15] It is a good idea to allow children to allow children to leave the playing field periodically to drink. It may not be easy for children to get to drink adequate fluids in the form of water. Providing them a sport drink that will tempt them to drink and rehydrate is the key to prevent active children from becoming dehydrated.

Sports drinks: These may be offered to a young athlete involved in active sports, but care must be taken that these should provide:

- Fluids to cool down the body and replace losses.
- Carbohydrates for quick energy—40 g–80 g/lt. from sources like glucose, fructose, sucrose or maltodextrin.
- Sodium and potassium lost in sweat—300–700 mg/lt. or at least 70 mg/250 ml.
- Should be noncarbonated and free from fizz.
- Should be free of amino acids, oxygen or herbal ingredients.

Exercise Recommendations in Specific Age Groups

Newborns—3 years

Unstructured safe play without special exercise equipment is good for the infant for healthy development.[16] Walkers and other baby equipment should be discouraged as they tend to hinder the muscle coordination of the child by restricting free movement.

TABLE 9.4: Fluid schedule before, during and after exercise

Time	Amount	Type of Beverage
4 hrs or less before exercise	>250–500 ml (1–2 cups)	Water—best choice
2 hrs or less before exercise	400–600 ml of fluid	Water—best choice
During exercise	Keep fluids with you when exercising; sip during work out–enough to replace losses through sweat (150–350 ml every 15–20 min advisable)	Water—best choice Sports drink—if exercising for >1 hour
Immediately after exercise	As per thirst if already had adequate during exercise (450–675 ml approx)	Water—best choice Other options—milk or chocolate milk, 100% fruit juice, sports drink

Reference: American Dietetics Association, Dieticians of Canada and the American College of Sports Medicine: Nutrition and athletic performance- Position Statement, J Am Diet Assoc 2000;100:1543.

Ages 3–8 years

Children tend to mimic parenteral activities, so the entire family should be involved in some physical activity so as to develop habit of participation by the children.[17] Activities in this age should be focused on participation and not on the aim of winning. However, it is important that children should not be imposed upon for ant activity due to over zealousness of the parents.[12]

Ages 8–12 years

Children by this age should be encouraged to perform cardiorespiratory exercised which can continue into adulthood. Those interested in perusing serious sports involvement and/or competitions, their maturation level should be assessed by a health professional.[6,13,17]

There can be vast differences in the maturation level of children of the same age group, and it is obvious that an early matured child will excel in a sport due to his/her maturity associated skill and muscular level. Children should be explained the physiological changes that occur during puberty so that they can prevent unsafe practices aimed at changing body composition for sport participation or appearances.[17]

Ages 13–18 years

At this age eating habits of teens usually are erratic, unhealthy (mainly snacking and reliance on fast foods, etc.). It is important to impart normal healthy nutrition education through class rooms or incorporated into their lifestyle to build good dietary habits. Exercise for them should be a continuous activity all the year round, rather than concentrating only during the practice or training sessions.

Ergogenic Aids

Ergogenic aids are popularly used and recommended by trainers for increasing the performance level in competitions, and readily available over the couter but it must be kept in mind that these have not been tested in pediatric subjects and should be discouraged.

Most athletes are prompted to use ergogenic aids to boost performance by many coaches and trainers. Supplements like β hydroxyl-β-methylbutyrate and creatine are commonly prescribed and made available to athletes. However, there is no evidence to prove any extra-benefits of such products on the performance levels, even though such claims are made by various advertisements. The safety of long-term use of creatine too is not established either, even though there are no scientific reports of any deleterious side effects of these supplements. However, anecdotal claims of having had muscle cramps or dehydration problems have been reported.[15] Caffeine is another common ergogenic aid used by athletes but is not suitable for children because of its side effects. Moreover it is also considered as illegal in International competitive sports.[18]

REFERENCES

1. Ross JG, Gilbert GG. A summary of findings. (The National Children and Youth Fitness Study). J Phys Educ Recreation Dance. 1995;56:1-48.
2. Healthy Children 2000, National Health Promotion and Disease Prevention. Objectives Related to Mother, Infants, Children, Adolescents and Youth. US Department of Health and Human Services, DHHS Publication No. HRSA-M-CH-91-2,1991.
3. Birrer RB, Levine R. Performance parameters in children and adolescent atheletes. Sports Med. 1987;4:211-27.
4. Sady SP. Cardiorespiratory exercise training in children. Clin Sports Med. 1986;5:493-514.
5. US Department of Health and Human Services. 1991: 11-12. Physical activity and fitness risk reduction objective 1.4. In: Healthy Children 2000. US Department of Health and Human Services.
6. Emery HM. Considerations in child and adolescent athletes. Rheum Dis Clin North Am. 1996;22(3):499-513.
7. Goldberg B, Saraniti A, Witman P, et al. Preparticipation sports assessment: An objective evaluation. Pediatrics. 1980;66:736-45.
8. American Dietetic Association. Timely Statement of the American Dietetic Association: nutrition guidance for adolescent athletes in organized sports. J Am Diet Assoc. 1996;6:611-61.

9. Lal PR. Nutritional Recommendations for Indian Sports Persons-A Review. J Indian Dietetic Association, 2006;31(1&2):1-19.
10. American Dietetic Association. Timely statement of the American Dietetic Association: nutrition guidance for child athletes in organized sports. J Am Diet Assoc. 1996;6:610-11.
11. Schoonen JC. Adolescence. In: Benardot D ed. Sports Nutrition. A Guide for the Professional Working with Active People. Chicago: The American Dietetic Association. 1993:113-21.
12. Jennings DS, Nelson S. Play Hard Eat Right. Minneapolis, MN: Chronimed Publishing. 1995.
13. Spear BA. Nutritional management of the child athlete. In: Williams CP ed., Pediatric Manual of Clinical Dietetics. Chicago: The American Dietetic Association; 1998:139-1448.
14. American Dietetics Association, Dieticians of Canada and the American College of Sports Medicine: Nutrition and athletic performance- Position Statement, J Am Diet Assoc. 2000;100:1543.
15. Berning JR. Nutrition for exercise and sports performance. In: Krause's Food &Nutrition Therapy. Mahan KL and Stump SE eds. Saunders Elsevier, Missouri. 2008.
16. Committee on Sports Medicine 1986-88. Infant exercise programs. Pediatrics. 1988;82(5):800.
17. Steen SN. Nutrition for the school age child athlete. In: Berning JR, Steen S, eds. Nutrition for Sports and Exercise 2nd ed. Gaithersburg, MD: Aspen Publishers. 1998:199.
18. Nancy L. Nevin Folino. Sports Nutrition for children and adolescents. In: Handbook of Pediatric Nutrition, eds. Samour PQ, Helm KK and Lang CE. 2nd edn. Jones and Bartlett Publishers Massachusetts. 2004.

10 Interaction of Nutrition and Infection in Children

INTRODUCTION

The fact that nutrition and infection act synergistically to worsen the clinical outcome of any disease, and conversely good nutrition status is essential for maintaining maximum resistance to infections and ability to recover from them, has been well established.[1] Infections have a deleterious effect on the nutritional status of the host through physiologic and anatomic changes. These changes become evident in such systemic reactions as fever, leukocytosis and stimulation of adrenal cortical activity. Local reactions include diarrhea, tissue inflammation and necrosis, increased mucus secretion, fatty liver and changes in skin and hair.

A well nourished child has greater ability to fight infections due to his/her greater resistance and recovers faster as compared to a child with poor nutritional status and impaired resistance. The nutritional status is determined by diet and factors that condition the requirement, absorption, assimilation and utilization of nutrients including activity levels and environmental factors in particular infection and stress.

The effects of repeated infections become cumulative if sufficient intervals do not pass between two episodes and adequate time is not allowed for the dietary intake to optimum levels. The effect of chronic infections will depend upon their nature and severity and the pre-existing nutritional status of the host.

The mechanisms of by which infection worsens nutritional status include:

- Reduced appetite
- Tendency of solid food to be discouraged
- Increased metabolic N losses
- Decreased N absorption especially in infections of the gastrointestinal tract.

Moderate to severe malnutrition can have serious consequences, especially in infants and children both short-term and long-term. In well nourished children, the body reserves normal dietary intake can avoid malnutrition unless they get prolonged infections. Malnutrition and infection can however become a vicious cycle (Fig. 10.1). An inadequate dietary intake leading to weight loss, lowered immunity, mucosal damage, invasion by pathogens finally result in impaired growth and development in children.

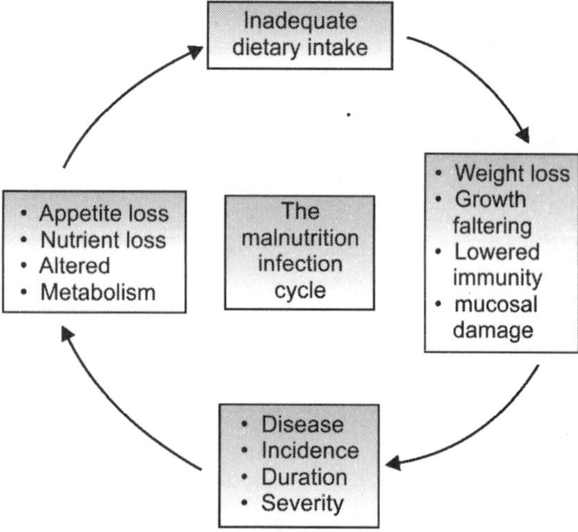

FIGURE 10.1: Spiral of malnutrition and infection

A sick child's nutrition is further aggravated by diarrheas, malabsorption, loss of appetite, diversion of nutrients for immune response and urinary N loss, all of which lead to nutrient losses and further damage to defense mechanisms. These in turn cause decreased intake. Added to this fever may further increase both energy and micronutrient requirements. Infections like malaria and influenza have mortality rates proportionate to the degree of malnutrition.[2]

The observed effect of infection on nutritional status varies with time, place and person. The age or the physiological state of the host often determines whether nutritional deficiency will `be manifest or clinically unapparent under a given circumstance. Growing children and pregnant and lactating women are particularly vulnerable. An added stress such as infection, often relatively innocuous by itself, may be sufficient to precipitate acute malnutrition.

SYNERGISM AND ANTAGONISM

Malnutrition is usually aggravated by infection, the consequences of which are bound to be more serious in a malnourished host than in a well nourished one. This effect of malnutrition being aggravated by infection leading to decreased immunity or infection aggravating malnutrition is termed as 'synergistic'. The simultaneous presence of malnutrition and infection resulting in an interaction is more serious for the host than would be expected from the combined effect of the two working independently. A state of vicious cycle is formed when an infection precipitates clinical malnutrition and which further becomes more and more sever in the malnourished host.

In a different situation when malnutrition is more likely to discourage multiplication of the agent than to affect the resistance mechanisms of the host, the action is termed as 'antagonistic', the combined effect being less than would have been expected.

Metabolism and Infection

Decreased Food Intake

In most infections some degree of anorexia is generally associated, and if this condition persists, it can account for a significant part of the adverse effect of infection on nutritional status especially in children. In addition to this, the normal dietary character is generally altered by either elders or care givers with a view to exert lesser load on digestion in an already compromised system. This results in with holding certain foods from the diet, e.g. solid foods and their substitutes which are offered may not always be energy dense, e.g. sweetened gruels or beverages like tea, etc. These factors finally contribute to the development of clinically evident nutritional diseases. It is therefore very important to ensure adequate feeding which is possible to be given orally in most cases and to refrain from discouraging or withdrawing of specific foods from the diet. Prolonged administration of grossly inadequate diets leading to severe nutritional deterioration of patients is commonly encountered even in hospitalised patients who assume a critical condition at times, besides prolonging the length of hospital stay and early recovery.

Decreased Nutrient Intake

There is a considerable decrease in nutrient utilization especially in conditions of acute diarrhea due to decreased absorption of nitrogen (N), fat and carbohydrates. Studies have confirmed that moderate diarrhea in a young child may result in an increased caloric loss, almost more than 500–600 cals/d.[3] Similar effects of malabsorption of other micronutrients like vitamin A, iron, folate too have been observed. This is due to increased transit time and the direct effect of toxins produced in the lumen, besides bacterial overgrowth into the small intestine and flattening of the intestine villi and microvilli.

Effect of Malnutrition on Infection

Nutrition and disease (infection) are interconnected: low nutritional status makes infections worse. A direct correlation has been observed between mortality from infections and nutrition for children, but not for breastfed infants. Malnutrition makes the host more susceptible to infectious diseases and when illness occurs, it is more severe, prolonged and carries increased risk of permanent damage or death. Malnutrition is also directly linked to the severity of the disease, e.g. diarrhea can become a life threatening disease due to dehydration. The duration of illness too is influenced by the state of nutrition resulting in longer duration and time taken for recovery.

Malnutrition directly affects all forms of immunity which may not be nutrient specific. Studies have shown that the defense mechanisms affected by nutritional status include interference with production of antibodies and bactericidal capacity of phagocytes, complement formation, number of T lymphocytes and T cells, subsets, the complement system and more.[4] Other factors apart from malnutrition influencing disease, are environmental, which coexist with malnutrition, leading to infection, e.g. over crowded housing, poor hygiene and sanitary arrangements which cause spreading of infection. Therefore along with adequate nutrition, environmental and socio-economic conditions need to be improved too.

Interaction between Malnutrition, Disease and Immunity

Nutrition deficiency affects immunity through specific mechanisms. Adequate nutrition is essential for adequate immune response, which is responsible for building resistance to infectious diseases in humans.[5] One effect of low nutritional status is reduced production of hydrochloric acid in the stomach, thus making the pH level higher than normal, allowing multiplication and passage into the small intestines of pathogens responsible for diarrheal disease. Deficiency of vitamins A, B and are also known to impair immunity seriously.[6]

Infection worsens the nutritional status and malnourished children are more easily affected by the synergistic effect of these further impairs immunity. The combination of infectious diseases, reduced food intake and altered metabolism is associated with hampering of growth and development in young children.[7] Infections like diarrhea are associated with decreased absorption of all major macro micronutrients: carbohydrates, fats and proteins besides affecting vitamins and trace elements. Intestinal transit time is reduced which allows for less absorption time and pathogen induced damage to the intestinal mucosa.[8]

Micronutrients and Immunity

Micronutrients are basic components of every cell in the body, serving as chemical messengers, building blocks and enzymes. For tissues to function efficiently, all of them need to be present in the right proportion. As these are not stored in the body in large amounts, regular daily intake is important to maintain tissue levels. An erratic or inadequate supply of these weakens the cells and forces them to 'limp along' thereby increasing vulnerability to disease. In the body both the humoral and cellular components of the immune system are dependent on nutrition. Marginal deficiencies of micronutrients like vitamin A, E, C, B_6, B_{12} and folate and minerals like zinc, manganese, magnesium, copper and selenium can impair production of new white cells and their activity against foreign substances and cells.

Vitamin A

Vitamin A maintains the integrity of the epithelium in the respiratory tract and gastrointestinal tract (GIT). The WHO estimates that worldwide 100–140 million children are vitamin A deficit, thereby increasing the risk of diarrhea, plasmodium falciparum malaria, measles and overall mortality.[9] As early as 1868, Scrimshaw had inferred that no nutritional deficiency is more consistently synergistic with infectious diseases than that of vitamin A.[1] In children concentration of vitamin A in the blood are appreciably reduced in pneumonia, rheumatoid arthritis, tonsillitis and rheumatic fever.[10]

Intestinal absorption of vitamin A is also impaired in the presence of giardia lamblia. In pathologic states, like obstructive jaundice, chronic nephritis and pneumonia, vitamin A is excreted in the urine. Children with meningitis, infantile diarrhea, chronic tuberculosis, measles, whooping cough and severe chicken pox frequently develop xerophthalmia,[1] thereby confirming that infection precipitates acute clinical avitaminosis A in children with latent deficiency. The deficiency of vitamin A in the form of xerophthalmia, keratomalacia and bitot's spots are still commonly found among malnourished infants in the developing countries. Vitamin deficiency and measles are closely interacted. Measles in a child is more likely to exacerbate any existing deficiency and children who are already deficient in vitamin A are at much greater risk of dying from measles. Post-measles diarrhea is often very prolonged and has a very high mortality.[11] Since measles depletes the body reserves of vitamin A, vaccination against measles often includes a high dose of vitamin A. Supplementation of vitamin A reduces the risk of developing respiratory tract infections, reduces mortality from diarrhea and enhances immunity.

Vitamin C

Studies have demonstrated an increased loss of vitamin C in the urine during the height of the primary reaction to vaccination against small pox and to vaccination with attenuated measles virus, as well as during the acute clinical stages of measles and chickenpox. Clinical manifestations of ascorbic acid deficiency and low urinary excretion of this vitamin were reported for school children of Madagascar Island having severe ascariasis or other intestinal parasitic disease.[1]

Iron

Infections influence iron metabolism directly through loss of blood and a resulting anemia. An inadequate dietary intake of iron compensates for a mild to moderate hookworm infestation, thereby preventing iron deficiency anemia. Chronic malaria is also known to produce anemia due to significant losses of iron. Chronic infections of bacterial or viral origin produce 'anemias of infection', a term coined due to the fact that it may interfere with iron binding capacity and erythrocyte life span. Some acute infections include hemolytic anemia.

Zinc

Zinc being a trace mineral, is required for activities of more than 300 enzymes, carbohydrate and energy metabolism, protein synthesis and degradation, nucleic acid production, heme biosynthesis and carbon dioxide transport. Deficiency of zinc can reduce nonspecific immunity, including neutrophil and natural killer cell function and complement activity; reduces numbers of T and B lymphocytes; and suppresses delayed activity, hypersensitivity, cytotoxic activity and antibody production.

Inadequate zinc prevents normal release of vitamin A from the liver and is associated with growth retardation, malabsorption, fetal loss, neonatal death and congenital abnormalities. Patients with Chron's disease, diarrheal illness and pneumonia have found to be having low concentrations of zinc. Supplementary zinc is associated with reduced duration of diarrheal diseases and pneumonia among children living in developing nations. Resistance to infection and improved appetite were found with continuous potassium and magnesium as well as zinc supplements.[12]

Effect of Infection on Malnutrition

Apart from malnutrition having an adverse effect on the severity or duration of infection, the opposite too can be equally contributory: infection also can have an adverse effect on the nutritional status, which further contributes to growth faltering in children. Loss of appetite during infection can directly result in decreased intake leading to poor growth and high mortality. It was shown that even with minor infections, the rate of protein breakdown increases at the same time as appetite decreases and protein and other nutrient deficiencies are accelerated. An infection increases the basal metabolic rate, which may double the energy requirement. Increased demand for glucose can deplete glucose stores in muscle fat. Carbohydrate and fat metabolism are also affected. The outcomes of an infection can be more serious for a malnourished child, since the body reserves are depleted even under ordinary circumstances.

Intestinal Parasites

Parasitic infections like that of helminths are highly prevalent and known to influence the nutritional status in children considerably. Giardia lambia in children is another very common parasite encountered among children and contributing to log standing chronic malnutrition.

Systemic Infections

Measles: Other systemic infections like measles and tuberculosis are the commonest cause of influencing the nutritional status among children. The myths associated with measles as a curse of the goddesses, prohibit adequate feeding of children which results in considerable deterioration of their nutritional status. This further leads to protein energy malnutrition, in which vitamin A and iron are commonly encountered in these post-measles children. A high mortality from measles in the developing countries is well known. This is attributable in part to the poor nutritional status of the children. Evidence from studies in Guatemala has shown that supplementary feeding alone can reduce fatalities significantly.[1] More complications were observed in malnourished than in well nourished children in India.[1]

Tuberculosis: Tuberculosis is a frequent cause of malnutrition and vice versa where a malnourished child is more susceptible to contact the disease, given their low immunological status. Malnutrition alters the clinical manifestation in children and also impairs prompt recovery. It has been shown to be an independent predictor of death in hospitalized patients diagnosed with tuberculosis. Children with multi-resistant tuberculosis are mostly severely malnourished due to inadequate dietary intake and prolonged inflammatory process and long courses of toxic drugs. Drugs used to treat tuberculosis are commonly associated with gastrointestinal side effects and vomiting and these further impair food intake. Optimizing nutritional status of such children is bound to confer some benefit on the host and course of recovery. Nutritional intervention like nasogastric feeding where oral intake is compromised can confer significant benefits by improving the nutritional status and prevent growth failure.

HIV infections: HIV infections cause considerable weight loss and protein depletion and play a significant role in morbidity and mortality. The development of malnutrition I HIV/AIDS is multifactorial and includes disorders of food intake, nutrient absorption and intermediary metabolism. Some common causes of decreased food intake in HIV infections are nausea, vomiting, taste alterations, dysphagia, anorexia, early satiety, depression, food access or preparation problems and voluntarily reduced intake to avoid diarrhea. Interventions like nutritional counseling, oral supplements and nasogastric feeding where indicated, are known to improve nutritional status and faster recovery, besides reduced complications.[13]

Gastrointestinal infections: A number of studies from the developing world have established that acute diarrheal disease and upper respiratory tract infections occur more frequently and last longer among malnourished than among well nourished children.[1] Intestinal parasites like hookworms and giardia may be associated with reduced intake, malabsorption, endogenous nutritional loss and anemia.[14] Parasitic infections are known to cause malnutrition, but the extent to which malnutrition can cause parasitic infections is not clear. Helminthic infection in school aged children is associated with cognitive deficits.[1] Children free of parasites have better nutritional status, grow faster, learn more and are freer of infections than are children with parasites.

Infection and Protein Nutrition Status

Bacterial infections of the GIT have an adverse effect on protein nutrition which is of major public health importance especially in the developing countries. In children during the weaning period, where inadequate diets lead to malnutrition, like in typhoid fever there has been found to be a two to three fold increase in nitrogen excretion together with a decrease in urinary creatinine due to loss of muscle mass. A decrease in serum albumin is characteristic of acute infections. Acute bacterial infections like pneumonia produce marked changes in all blood serum components, especially a decrease in albumin and an increase in alpha and beta globulins.

Similarly in tuberculosis, it has been observed that urinary nitrogen excretion was markedly increased. Several reports from various authors have confirmed that tuberculosis can precipitate kwashiorkor in children already suffering from chronic malnutrition, due to the strongly negative effect on nitrogen balance.[1]

Therefore it is clear that increased excretion of nitrogen and decreased intake of food associated with tuberculosis not only complicate clinical management, but also can pose an important public health problem in regions where protein energy malnutrition is prevalent.

Apart from the above mentioned infections almost all bacterial infections produce an increased urinary excretion of nitrogen. Generally they also result in some decrease in protein intake. Both these effects depend upon the severity of the disease with respect to urinary nitrogen, on the nutritional state of the host as well. Acute episodes can often delay the clinical recovery from the illness.

Infection and Growth and Development

Besides altering absorption, metabolism and excretion of specific nutrients, infections also reduce food intake by an action on appetite. Moreover, it is common to with hold solid food or modify diet during any episode of infection, thereby reducing nutrient intake. Purgatives or other drugs administered as part of therapy also tend to interfere with nutrient intake. As a result severe or prolonged illness has an adverse effect on growth and malnutrition, especially in an already nutritionally compromised child.

REFERENCES

1. Scrimshaw NS, Taylor CE, Gordon JE. Interaction of nutrition and infection. WHO Monograph Series No.57. WHO, Geneva. 1968.
2. Muller O, Garenna M, Kauyate B, et al. The association between protein energy and malnutrition, malaria morbidity and all cause mortality in West African children. Trop Med Int Health. 2003;8:507-11.
3. Rosenberg IH, Solomons NW, Scneider RE. Am J Clin Nutr. 1977;30:1248-53.
4. Scrimshaw NS, San Giovanni JP. Synergism of nutrition, infection and immunity: an overview. Am J Clin Nutr. 1977;66(2):464S-77S.
5. Chandra RK. Nutritional regulation of immunity and risk of illness. Ind J Pediatrics. 1989;56(5):607-11.
6. Pollard John H. 'Morbidity and longevity' in Ross, John A (ed), International Encyclopedia of population. The free press, Macmillan, New York. 1982;2:452-8.
7. Scrimshaw NS, Taylor CE, John E. Intractions of nutrition and infection. Monograph Ser No. 37, World Health Organisation, Geneva.
8. Lunn P. 'Nutrition, immunity and infection' in Schofield R, Reher D and Bideau A (eds). The Decline of mortality in Europe. Clarendon Press. pp. 131-45.
9. Shank RE, Coburn AF, Moore LV, et al. The level of vitamin A and carotene in plasma of rheumatic subjects. J Clin Invest. 1944;23:289-95.
10. Neidecker-Gonzales O, Nestel P, Bouis H. Estimating the global cost of vitamin A capsule supplementation: a review of the literature. Food Nutr Bull, 2007;28:307-16.
11. Tomkins A, Watson E. Malnutrition and infection-a review. Nutrition policy No.5,1989,http://www.unsystem.org/scn/archives/npp05/ch4.html. Accessed 31 March 2008.
12. Khanum S, Ashworth A, Hutley SRA. Controlled trial of 3 approaches to the treatment of severe malnutrition. Lancet. 1994;344:1728-37.
13. Heckler LM, Kotler DP. Malnutrition in patients with acquired immune deficiency syndrome. Nutr Rev. 1990;48:393-401.
14. Stolzfus RJ, Dreyfus ML, Chwaya HM. et al. Hookworm control as a strategy to prevent iron deficiency. Nutr Rev. 1997;55:223-32.

11 Vegetarianism in Children

The term 'vegetarian' is commonly defined as a person who excludes meat, sea food and poultry from his/her diet. However, this term may further be categorized as lacto-ovo vegetarian or lacto-vegetarian or strictly vegetarian, depending upon the type of foods that are excluded from one's diet (Table 11.1).

The most common type is the lacto-ovo-vegan who includes dairy products and eggs in their diets. On the other hand, vegans are strictly vegetarians in the literal sense, since they exclude all animal products and by products including honey and gelatin besides milk and eggs.

An increasing popularity of vegetarianism is being observed since a decade or more globally. In general, the most frequently cited reason for doing so is health benefits and disease prevention.[1]

For pregnant women and parents of vegetarian children, moral and religious considerations are more commonly given as reasons for doing so.[2]

The seventh day adventist religion strongly encourages a lacto-ovo-vegetarian diet, while other religions like the Jains, Muslims, Hindus, especially the Hare Krishna cult have prohibitions against eating some or all forms of animal foods.

ADEQUACY OF VEGETARIAN DIETS

The American Dietetic Association (ADA) and the American Academy of Pediatrics (AAP) have endorsed that well planned vegan and vegetarian diets can meet the nutritional need and promote normal growth of infants and children.[3,4]

In fact it has been observed that a vegetarian style of eating follows the dietary guidelines and meets the requirements of the recommended allowances for nutrients, if taken in a well balanced and planned way. A number of studies have shown that children and adolescents following a well designed vegetarian diet grow and develop normally.[5,6] Birth weights of infants born to well nourished vegetarian women

TABLE 11.1: Categories of vegetarian diets

Vegetarian type	Foods excluded	Protein source	Nutrient risk
Partial Vegetarian	Red meat	Poultry, fish, eggs milk, cheese, yoghurt, beans, lentils	Iron
Lacto-Ovo-Vegetarian	Red meat, fish, poultry	Milk, cheese, yoghurt, eggs, lentils, beans	Iron
Lacto Vegetarian	Red meat, fish, poultry, eggs	Milk, cheese, yoghurt, lentils, beans	Iron, vitamin D
Vegetarian	Red meat, fish, poultry, eggs, milk cheese, yoghurt	Beans, lentils, nuts	Proteins, energy, iron, fat soluble vitamins, B_{12}, Vitamin D, calcium, zinc

have been shown to be similar to birth weight norms and to birth weights of infants born to non-vegetarian mothers.[7]

The nutritional advantages of vegetarian diets have been well established and it has been indicated that the style of eating can lead to lifelong healthy eating habits when adopted at a younger age. Children and adolescents on vegetarian diets are known to have a lower intake of cholesterol, saturated fats and total fats and a higher intake of fruits, vegetables and fiber than their non-vegetarian counter parts.[8,9] Vegetarian children are also known to have decreased risk for several chronic diseases like diabetes mellitus, cardiovascular diseases, hypertension, obesity and some other types of cancer.[10] Vegetarian diets are mainly rich in carbohydrates, omega 6 fatty acids, dietary fiber, carotenoids, folic acid, vitamin C vitamin E, potassium and magnesium.[11,12]

It has been stated that lifestyle changes incorporating a low fat vegetarian or vegan diet could not only prevent various degenerative diseases like coronary artery disease, but even reverse them.[13,14]

NUTRITIONAL RISKS

A vegetarian diet if not well balanced or planned can have negative effects since they may be low in vitamin B_{12}, calcium, omega 3 fatty acids, vitamin D, iron, zinc, niacin and iodine. However, if adequately balanced, it can meet all the nutrients and can be appropriate for all stages of the life cycle including pregnancy, lactation, infancy, childhood and adolescence.[11] It is likely that vegans may be associated with malnutrition where as children eating lacto-ovo-vegetarian diet consume diets closer to the recommended allowances than children whose diets include animal foods.[14]

Vegetarian mothers who breast feed their infants need to be careful to provide adequate vitamin D, calcium and iron sources so as to produce nutritionally complete breast milk for at least the first 6 months of life. In case of vegan mothers it would be worth considering supplementing of the above nutrients to avoid deficiency, which could result in neurological damage in infancy, especially due to vitamins B_{12} and folate (progressive myelopathy and neural tube defect).

In infants beyond 6 months of life, semi solids should be introduced gradually which may include cereals and pulses. However due to the high fiber content they tend to be bulkier. To reduce this bulk, addition of fats and sugars can help to increase the density of foods. Cereals and pulses in their finer form can be prepared like washed dals or suji, dalia, etc. Full fat dairy milk may gradually be introduced along with fortified soy based foods.

The nutritional areas of concern for vegetarian children include:

- Providing sufficient energy and nutrients for normal growth.
- Providing an adequate iron intake to prevent iron deficiency anemia.
- Identifying adequate sources of vitamin B_{12} to prevent deficiency.
- Obtaining sufficient vitamin D and calcium to prevent rickets.
- Ensuring adequate provision of long chain (n-3) of acids from non-meat sources like seeds and nuts.
- Consuming food in appropriate form and combination to ensure nutrients can be digested and absorbed by the child.

Energy

Without adequate energy the child can gradually lead to failure to thrive. Vegetarian diets being high in bulk (fiber), concentrated sources of energy like oils can be used to increase the energy content of the foods. Foods like seeds, nuts and peanut butter when incorporated in the dishes planned for toddlers can provide concentrated source of calories along with minerals and proteins.

Proteins

Vegetable and pulse proteins have a lower concentration and range of essential amino acids than those from animal or fish sources. The protein needs therefore may be slightly higher than the recommended allowances due to the lower biological value of some plant proteins. Vegetarian children can derive their required amount of protein if offered a variety, including pulses and grains and the frequency of feeding. Dairy products in lacto-ovo-vegetarian children or even those who are lacto-vegetarian, can provide ample amount of proteins in their diets.

Calcium

Milk and milk products are a natural source of calcium for infants and children for both vegetarian and non-vegetarian children. Vegans will need to derive their calcium from fortified sources like soya milk, tofu or other soya products. If consumed recommended amounts for specific age groups, the calcium requirement can be met easily.[15] It must be kept in mind that since toddlers need an adequate fat diet too for proper growth and development, the use of whole fat milk can be beneficial at least till the age of 2 years. Breast feeding during the second year of life too can provide adequate fat. It is worth considering also that the same product from different manufacturers can differ by more than 100% of any nutrient per serving, e.g. chocolate milk or yoghurt from two different manufacturers can vary in their nutrient content considerably.[15,16] The absorption rate ranges from 50% of the calcium in fortified orange juice to about 30% from other sources.[15]

Among the vegetarian sources green leafy vegetables like spinach, though containing a good amount of calcium, is rendered as poor source due to it being bound to the high oxalate content present in it, thus inhibiting its absorption. Similarly peanuts though a good source of calcium, are high in oxalates which make it a poor source for this nutrient. Foods like broccoli, cauliflower, sesame seeds and figs are also good sources of calcium for vegetarian children. Nuts like walnuts and almonds are also very rich in calcium (Table 11.2).

TABLE 11.2: Some good vegetarian sources of calcium[17]

Food sources	Calcium (mg%)
Milk (cow's)	120
Milk (buffalo)	210
Curd (cow's)	149
Skimmed milk powder	1370
Soybeans	240
Rajma	260
Black channa (Horse gram)	287
Bengal gram, whole	202
Ragi	344
Beans, cluster	130
Beans, field	210
Lotus stem, dry	408
Fenugreek	395
Curry leaves	830
Mint	200
Mustard leaves	155
Spinach	73
Bathu	150
Walnuts	100
Almonds	230
Coconut, dry	400
Groundnuts	90
Figs	80
Lemon	70
Phalsa	129
Raisins	87
Apricot, dry	110
Dates, dried	120

Source: Gopalan C, Rama Sastri, SC Balasubramanian. Nutritive value of Indian Foods, NIN, ICMR, Hyderabad. 2000.

Vitamin D

Vitamin D is found in liquid milk although not in all other milk products. Exposure to sunlight too is a good source of this vitamin for children who may expose their hands and feet for 20–30 minutes at least thrice a week.[18] As per literature available[19] specific age groups require a vitamin D supplement like.

- infants who are exclusively breast fed.
- infants consuming < 500 ml of vitamin D fortified milk per day.
- children and adolescents who do not receive adequate sunlight exposure.
- children who are not on any multivitamin containing at least 200 IU of vitamin D.

An important factor to be kept in mind is the calcium balance bioavailability. Optimal calcium balance can be facilitated by adjusting other factors in the diet like sodium, oxalates, iron and proteins. Protein and sodium both increase urinary calcium loss. Since vegetarian diets are moderate in proteins, calcium absorption can be increased by powering the oxalates and phytate content of the diet.[15]

Iron

Iron is one micronutrient which needs careful consideration in a vegetarian or a vegan diet, since plant sources have lower iron content as compared to animal sources and even the bioavailability of iron from vegetarian sources is lower than as compared to the nonvegetarian sources. A number of studies have shown that vegans and other nonvegetarians were not found to suffer from iron deficiency any more than nonvegetarian children.[20,21] However while one study agreed that iron deficiency anemia is not more common among vegetarians, they found 'vegetarian' children had reduced levels of hemoglobin and iron compared to 'omnivores' due to 'the absence of animal iron sources with high utilisability'.[22] Studies from India have confirmed that 'strict vegetarian' mothers as well as their new borns have a greater risk and incidence of anemia and iron deficiency.[23] Keeping in view the bioavailability of iron from vegetable sources, it is recommended that iron intake of vegetarian children be 1.8 times that of nonvegetarians.[11,22] Foods like cereals, nuts, seeds, legumes especially soy based are significant sources of iron (Table 11.3), so a well planned vegetarian diet including these foods should not lead to iron deficiency anemia. However, fruits and raw foods should be avoided for infants and children.[11] An important point to be borne in mind while planning a diet with iron sources, is that, inhibitors and enhancers play an important role in the bioavailability of iron. For instance, ascorbic acid can enhance the bioavailability of iron while phytates like tannin in tea, wine or legumes can also inhibit iron absorption.[11]

Iron being an integral part of many proteins and enzymes which help in cell growth and differentiation and is involved in transporting of oxygen to the red blood cells, care should be taken to so plan a diet for vegetarian and vegan children, that it provides a good amount of bioavailable iron too.

TABLE 11.3: Vegetable food sources of iron

Foods	Iron (mg%)
Bajra	8.0
Ragi	3.9
Wheat Flour	4.9
Bengal gram flour	4.9
Bengal gram dal	5.3
Bengal gram roasted	9.5
Soybean	10.4
Horse gram, whole	6.7
Amaranth	18.4
Cauliflower greens	40.0
Colcasia leaves	10.0
Mint	10.2
Mustard leaves	16.3
Dates, dried	7.3
Custard apple	4.31

Source: Gopalan C, Rama Sastri, SC Balasubramanian. Nutritive value of Indian Foods, NIN, ICMR, Hyderabad. 2000.

Zinc

Overt deficiency of zinc in vegetarians has not been found to be greater than in nonvegetarians.[24] Phytates have been the main factor in inhibiting the availability of zinc from food.[11] High fiber foods, processed foods like sprouted beans and leavening bread have also known to lower the phytate content of the diet. Therefore some vegetarians may require a higher intake of zinc than the dietary reference intake for their specific age. Major plant sources of zinc include cooked dietary beans, sea vegetables, fortified cereals, soy foods nuts, peas and seeds, legumes and cheese.

Cobalamin (B_{12})

B_{12} is an important vitamin belonging to the B complex vitamin group. It is necessary for cell division and blood formation. Lacto-ovo-vegetarians can obtain their requirement of B_{12} from eggs and dairy products. Vegetable sources of this vitamin include cereals, bread, nuts and some fortified soy products.

It is important for vegan breastfeeding mothers to supplement vitamin B_{12} or include sources which are rich in this nutrient, since a deficiency of this vitamin may lead to certain neurological disturbances that could occur in their baby.[25,26] Another factor causing B_{12} deficiency may not be due to lack of the dietary source but due to limited absorption like that in those following a macrobiotic diet.[27]

Meal Planning for a Vegetarian Child

All infants begin life as vegetarians, since they are mainly breastfed for the first part of the year and even later are weaned on to formula milk or cereal based semisolids. The milk produced by vegetarian mothers is nutritionally adequate and so the infants of such mothers also grow and develop normally.[27] But babies who have not received breastfeeds should receive appropriate cow's milk or soy based formula to support normal growth.

Solid foods are added to the diet gradually as per the normal infant feeding guidelines (See Chapter 6). A vegetarian diet planned as per the dietary recommendations can meet the nutritional needs of toddlers and preschoolers and can aid in healthy growth and development.

In India the problem of vegetarianism is not a 'grave' concern, since it is largely a lacto-vegetarian population followed by a significant number being lacto-ovo-vegetarians. Even among the nonvegetarian population, the consumption of nonvegetarian sources is not a daily routine followed in all meals and yet in most well to do families the vegetarian sources of foods are consumed in adequate amounts which take care of the nutritional requirements of the older population. However, in case of children, nutritional anemia is a very common feature observed in very well to do families. This is because of faulty feeding habits, mainly being prolonged breastfeeding with inadequate solid foods or excess consumption of milk or milk products which are low in iron. It is therefore very important that children of vegetarian families take special care to incorporate all those foods which can provide all the micronutrients besides adequate macronutrients. A healthy eating style of the vegetarian family as a whole can go a long way in inculcating good and healthy eating pattern in children too.

REFERENCES

1. Yankelovick, Clancy, Shulman. Survey of adult Americans, Time Magazine and CNN. April 1992.
2. Finley DA, Dewey KG, Lonnerday B, et al. Food calories of vegetarian and nonvegetarians during pregnancy and lactation. J Am Diet Assoc. 1985:678-85.
3. American Academy of Pediatrics Committee on Nutrition.1998. Soy protein based formulas: Recommendations for use in infant feeding. Pediatrics. 1998;101:148-53.
4. Messina VK, Burke KI. Position of the American Dietetic Association: vegetarian diets. J Am Dietet Assoc. 1997;97:1317-21.
5. Nathan I, Hackett AF, Kriby S. A longitudional study of the growth of matched pairs of vegetable and omnivorous children, aged 7-11 years in the north west of England. Europ J Clin Nutr. 1997;51:20-25.
6. Sanders TAB, Reddy S. Vegetarian diets and children. Am J Clin Nutr. 1994;1176S-81S.
7. O'Connel JM, Dibley MJ, Sierra J, et al. Growth of vegetarian children. The Farm Study. Pediatrics. 1989;84:475-81.
8. Novy MA. Are strict vegetarians at risk of vitamin B_{12} deficiency? Cleveland Clinic J Med. 2000;67:87-88.
9. Sanders TAB and Manning J. The growth and development of vegan children. J Human Nutr Dietet. 1992;5:11-21.
10. Rajaram S, Sabate J. Health benefits of a vegetarian diet. Nutrition. 2000;16:531-33.
11. "Position of the American Dietetics Asociation and Dietitians of Canada: Vegetarian diets" http://www.adajournal'org/article J Am Dietet Assoc. 2003;06
12. Key TJ, Appleby PN, Rosell MS. Health effects of vegetarian and vegan diets. Proceedings of Nutr Soc. 2006;65:34-41.
13. Ôrnish D, Brown SE, Sckerwitz LW, et al. Can lifestyle canges reverse coronary heart disease? The Lifestyle Heart Trial: Lancet. 1990;336;8708:129-33.
14. Alder M, Specher B. Atypical diets in infancy and early childhood. Pediatrics Annals. 2001;30(11):673-80.
15. Weaver CM, Plawecki KL. Dietary calcium: adequacy of a vegetarian diet. Am J Clin Nutr. 1994;(5S):1238S-41S.

16. Coughlin CM. Vegetarianism in children. In: Handbook of Pediatric Nutrition, eds. Samour PQ, Helm KK and Lang CE. Jones and Bartlett Publishers, Inc Massachusetts. 2004;1133-48
17. Gopalan C, Rama Sastri, SC Balasubramanian. Nutritive value of Indian Foods, NIN, ICMR, Hyderabad. 2000.
18. Mangels A, Messina V. Considerations in planning vegan diets: Infants. J Am Diet Assoc. 2001;101:670-77.
19. Gartner LM, Green FR. Prevention of rickets and vitamin D deficiency: new guidelines for vitamin D intake. Pediatrics. 2003;111:908-10.
20. Larsson CL, Johansson GK. Dietary intake and nutritional status of young vegans and omnivores in Sweden. Am J Clin Nutr. 2002;76:100-06.
21. Ball MJ, Bartlett MA. Dietary intake and iron status of Australian vegetarian women. Am J Clin Nutr. 1999;70:353-58.
22. Krajcoviova – Kudlackova M, Simoncic R, Bederova A, et al. Influence of vegetarian and mixed nutrition on selected hematological and biochemical parameters in children. 1997, http://www.adajournal.
23. Sharma DC, Kiran R, Ramnath V, et al. Ind J Clin Biochem. 1994;9(2):100-02.
24. Freeland- Graves JH, Bodyz PW, Epright MA. Zinc status of vegetarians. J Am Diet assoc. 1980;(77):655-61.
25. Graham SM, Arvela OM, Wise GA. Long-term neurological consequences of nutritional vitamin B_{12} deficiency in infants. J Pediatr. 1992,121(Pt 1):710-14.
26. Johnson PRJ, Roloff JS. Vitamin B_{12} deficiency in infant strictly breast fed by a mother with late pernicious anemia. J Pediatr. 1982;100:917-19.
27. Messina M, Messina V. The Dietitians guide to vegetarian diets. Issues and Applications, Gaithersburg, MD: Aspen Publishers. 1996.

12 Food Allergies and Intolerances

"What is food for one, is to others bitter poison"

Lucretius

Food allergy is an immune system response to a food that the body mistakenly believes is harmful. Once the immune system decides that a particular food is harmful, it creates specific antibodies to it. The next time one eats that food, the immune system releases massive amounts of chemicals, including histamine, in order to protect the body. These chemicals trigger a cascade of allergic symptoms that can affect the respiratory system, gastrointestinal tract (GIT), skin or cardiovascular system.

Symptoms range from a tingling sensation in the mouth, swelling of the tongue, or throat, difficulty in breathing, vomiting, abdominal cramps, diarrhea, hypotension and also loss of consciousness to death. Symptoms typically appear within minutes to 2 hours after consumption of food which is allergenic to the individual.

Food allergies are usually mediated by IgE antibody directed to specific food proteins. However, other immunological mechanisms can also play a role. Foods most commonly causing these reactions in children are milk, egg, peanuts, soya and fish.

Adverse reactions to food may be toxic or non toxic:

1. Toxic reactions are not related to individual sensitivity but occur in anyone who ingests a sufficient quantity of tainted food. e.g. reactions to histamine in scombroid fish poisoning. On the other hand, nontoxic adverse reactions to food depend on individual susceptibility and are either nonimmune mediated, i.e. food intolerance[1] as shown in Table 12.1, or immune mediated, i.e. food allergy.

PATHOGENESIS

Allergic reactions to food are either IgE mediated or non-IgE mediated[2] as given in Table 12.2. The role of IgE mediated reactions in food allergy is well established. Persons who are genetically prone to atopy produce specific IgE antibodies to certain proteins to which they are exposed.

TABLE 12.1: Some conditions related to food intolerance

- Gastrointestinal disorder
- Structural abnormalities, hiatal hernia, pyloric stenosis, Hirschsprung's disease, tracheoesophageal fistulas
- Disaccharide deficiencies – lactose, sucrase, iso-maltose complex, glucose galactose complex
- Pancreatic insufficiency, cystic fibrosis
- Gallbladder disease
- Peptic ulcer disease
- Malignancy
- Galactosemia
- Phenylketonuria
- Jitteriness (caffeine)
- Pruritis (histamine)
- Headache (tyramine)
- Disorientation (alcohol)
- Psychologic disorder
- Neurologic disorder
- Auriculotemporal syndrome (facial flush from tart food)

Refer. 1

TABLE 12.2: Food allergy; target organs and disorders

Target organs	IgE mediated disorder	Non-IgE mediated disorder
Skin	Urticaria and angioedema atopic dermatitis	Atopic dermatitis Dermatitis herpetiforms
GIT	Oral allergy syndrome Gastrointestinal "Anaphylaxis" Allergic eosinophilic gastroenteritis	Proctocolitis Enterocolitis Allergic eosinophil Gastroenteritis Enteropathy syndrome Celiac disease
Respiratory tract	Asthma Allergic rhinitis	Heiner syndrome
Multisystem	Food induced anaphylaxis, food association exercise induced anaphylaxis	

Refer. 2

The symptoms of IgE mediated reactions typically involve the skin, respiratory system and GIT.[3]

A schematic picture of the pathogenesis is depicted in Fig. 12.1.[4] As mentioned above, when the food enters the GIT and undergoes protein digestion, the antigen (Ag) processing begins. As the antigen presenting cells present Ag to the T cells, specific cytokines are produced. In the allergic individual, the T-cells will secrete increased amounts of IL-4, IL-5 and IL-13, among the mediators and reduced amounts of IFN-α and TNF-α when compared to that in an individual who is not allergic. The T-cell in turn regulates eventual specific IgE production by B cells. This specific IgE is attached to mast cells with mediator release at the mucosal site. Thus the clinical symptoms follow.

The usual protective mechanisms-gastric pH, digestive enzymes, mucosal glycoproteins and peristalsis prevent this transmission to a certain extent. But the gut may not be able to effectively exclude intact antigens because of immaturity (infants), injury, malabsorption or infection. Agents causing increased intestinal permeability like alcohol, tobacco or aspirin and exercise immediately after food intake may hasten the process.

During the first year of life, the infant diet is the most powerful determinant of the growth and development of the child and food allergy is the most common health problem. It is well established that the feeding of solids is best delayed up to 6 months to reduce the risk of allergy.

In infancy, food allergy is expressed as crying colic, vomiting, diarrhea, rashes, eczema and cold like respiratory congestion. Some infants with food allergy can become seriously ill and fail to thrive unless their allergy is recognized and corrected.

Infants, who develop food allergy in their first year of life, may 'outgrow' the first effects but tend to grow into children with more pervasive health, behavior and learning problems unless their diet is properly managed.

COMMON FOOD ALLERGENS

Over 90% of IgE mediated food allergies in childhood are caused by eight foods: cow's milk, hen's egg, soy, peanuts, tree nuts (and seeds), wheat, fish and shellfish.[5] In children milk (casein, lactoglobulins and egg ovalbumin, conalbumin) is the common agent causing food allergy. Prevalence wise, most common food allergens at all ages in western countries are citrus fruits, tomato, egg, strawberry, soy, wheat and fish. Among Indians, common food allergens are cashew nut, coconut, wheat, fish (esp. shellfish), peanut, milk, egg, meat. Amongst spices, mustard and garlic are known to cause allergic reactions.

Skin Manifestations of Food Allergy

Skin is one of the most commonly targeted organs in food hypersensitivities. Clinical manifestations of food hypersensitivity range from symptoms of atopic dermatitis, to urticaria and angioedema and herpetiformis.

Dermatitis herpetiformis is typically associated with gluten sensitive enteropathy, which involves a chronic papulovesicular skin disorder. Almost all skin allergies provoking skin manifestations involve pruritis as a hallmark of the disease.[6]

Respiratory Manifestation of Food Allergy

Acute respiratory manifestation of food allergies involves either cutanous or GI symptoms. Egg, milk,

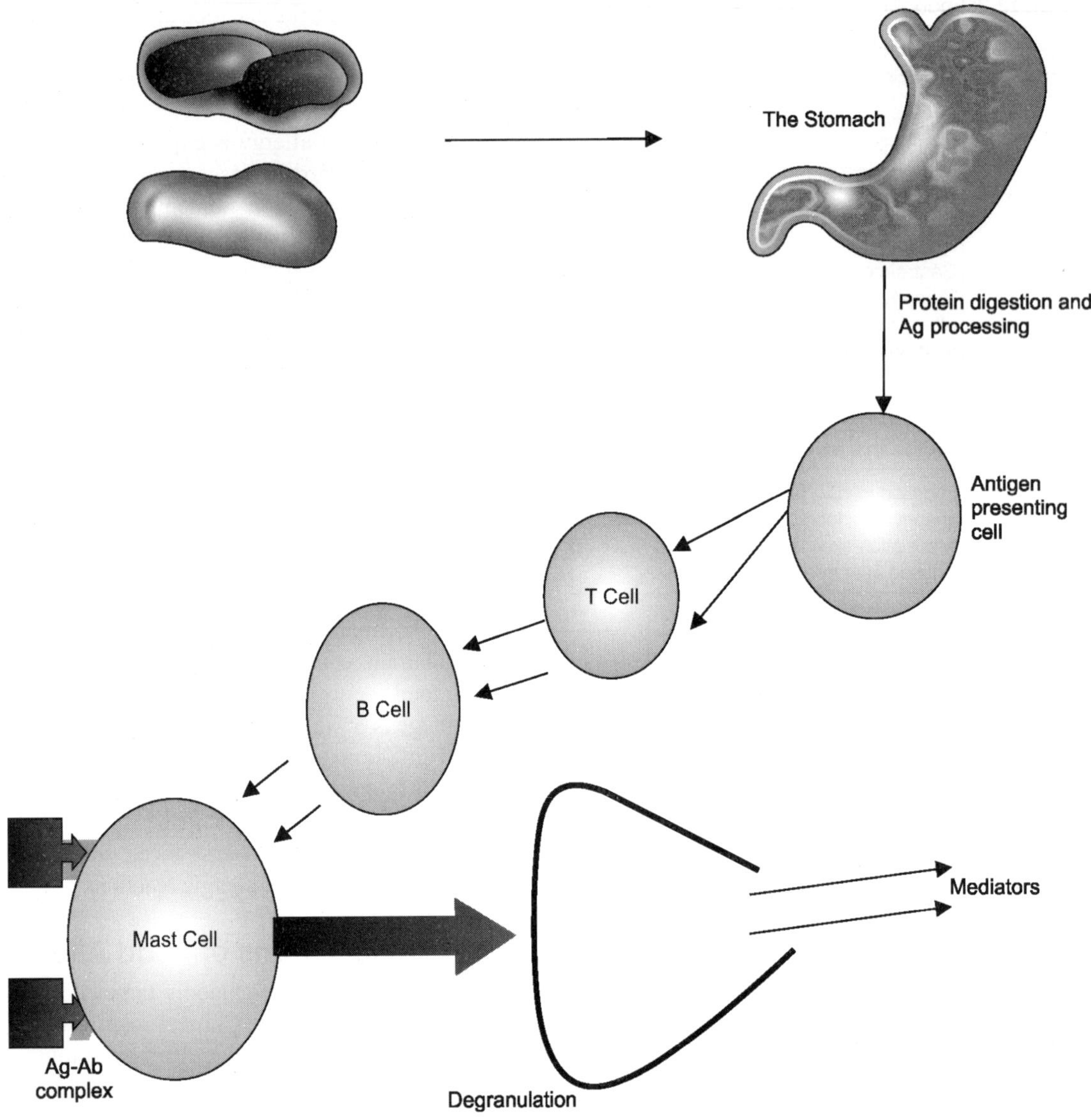

FIGURE 12.1: Pathogenesis of food allergy

Refer. 4

peanut, soy, fish, shellfish and tree nuts are the most common food allergens confirmed to elicit respiratory reactions.[7]

It is observed that food induced allergic reactions are more common in young pediatric patients than in older children and adults. Allergic sensitization or clinical reactions to foods in infancy predict the later development of respiratory allergies and asthma.

Food induced allergies may increase airway hyperresponsiveness in patients with moderate to severe asthma and may do so without inducing acute asthma symptoms.

Respiratory symptoms, especially asthmatic reaction, induced by food allergens are considered risk factors for fatal or near fatal reactions. Following features indicate the need for evaluation of food allergy in patients with asthma.

- Asthma triggered after ingestion of particular foods.
- Unexplained acute, severe asthma exacerbations.
- Patients with asthma that is accompanied by other manifestation of food allergy (e.g. anaphylaxis, moderate to severe atopic dermatitis).

Manifestations of GIT

The GIT is a very common target organ for IgE mediated reactions to foods. Symptoms of GI "anaphylaxis" occur shortly after ingestion of the offending food and include nausea, vomiting, abdominal pain and diarrhea.

Diagnosis of Food Allergy

Once food allergy is identified as a likely cause of symptoms, confirmation of diagnosis and identification of implicated food(s) needs to be done.

Diagnosis becomes easier when history implicates, a particular food like in patients with acute reactions e.g. urticaria or anaphylaxis. In patients with atopic dermatitis or asthma the causative factors are more difficult to pinpoint the causal foods.

MAINTENANCE OF FOOD DIARY

A regular maintenance of food diary indicating all the foods taken and occurrence of symptoms, the frequency of incidence or the severity can all help the physician come to definite conclusion.

Elimination Diet

Once there is suggestion of food related illness and tests for IgE antibody to food are positive, elimination of the particular food from the diet is the first step. Disappearance of symptoms on elimination can be highly indicative of that particular food as causative agents. Challenge with the same food once improvement is achieved, can justify the elimination of the food if symptom reoccur.

Oral Food Challenges

Double blind placebo-controlled food challenges are considered the gold standard for diagnosing food allergy.[3,8]

In this procedure, the patient avoids the suspected food for at least 2 weeks, antihistamine therapy is discontinued and doses of asthma medications are decreased as much as possible. After intravenous access is obtained, graded doses of either a challenge food or a placebo food are administered. The food is hidden either in another food or in opaque capsules. However this procedure is done under medical supervision strictly, so that any severe reactions if occur can be handled immediately.

PRICK PUNCTURE SKIN TESTING

This method involves determining the presence of specific IgE antibody, when the patient is not on antihistamines. The skin is punctured through glycerinated extract of a food. A local wheal and flare response indicates the presence of food specific IgE antibody, with a wheal diameter of more than 3 mm indicating a positive response.

The predictive value of this test is over 95% and hence of more value when they are negative. On the other hand the positive predictive value is only 50%, therefore this test cannot be considered in isolation. Intradermal allergy skin tests are not very reliable as they are highly false positive. Fresh extracts of fruits and vegetables are recommended for this test since the protein in commercial extracts of most fruits and vegetables are prone to degradation.[9]

In Vitro Testing (RAST)

This test Radio Allergosorbent (RAST) test is more practical than prick test for screening of food allergy in primary care office setting. As with skin tests this test too is highly sensitive for confirming negative result, i.e. ruling out an IgE mediated reaction. But when highly sensitive assays are used, the levels of food specific IgE antibody correlate with clinical reactivity to only certain foods (milk, egg, peanuts, and fish).

Tests are Positive

1. Eliminate food
2. If the patient has multiple sensitivities or an unclear history, perform open or single blind food challenges.
   a. If the challenge test is positive.

1. Eliminate foods (if only a few foods)
2. If multiple foods are implicated, consider double blind, placebo-controlled food challenges.
   a. If challenge is positive, eliminate food.
   b. If challenge is negative, reintroduce food.
3. Diagnosis established
   a. Educate patient about treatment and avoidance
   b. Re-evaluate at appropriate intervals if tolerance is likely.[10]

Oral Allergy Syndrome

As the name denotes, symptoms are limited to the oral cavity. They are characterized by pruritis and edema of the oral mucosa occurring after ingestion of certain fresh fruits and vegetables.[11]

The reaction occurs primarily in patients with allergic sensitivity to pollens and is caused by IgE antibodies directed toward cross reacting proteins found in pollens fruits and vegetables. A characteristic feature of this syndrome is that patients are usually not symptomatic to cooked foods since the causative allergens are heat labile.

CHINESE RESTAURANTS SYNDROME

As the name denotes, reaction occurs after ingestion of chinese food. The manifestations may be in the form of sensation of warmth and burning over head and shoulders, headache, stiffness and weakness of limbs. The culprit attributed is the monosodium glutamate (MSG) or ajinomoto, the essential ingredient of any Chinese cuisine.

SULPHITE SENSITIVITY

Sulphite based compounds containing sodium bisulphate which are present in wines, vinegar, beverages, dried fruits and even medicine and eye drops, TPN and dialysis fluids can also cause hypersensitivity. Asthma, anaphylaxis and cutanous reactions are common manifestation. Cross sensitivity can also occur with MSG and aspirin.

AURICULOTEMPORAL SYNDROME (FREY SYNDROME)

This syndrome is often misdiagnosed as a food allergy. It is manifested immediately as unilateral rarely bilateral flushing, sweating or both, localized to the distribution of the auriculotemporal nerve, in response to gustatory or tactile stimuli.[12]

In children the flushing usually begins within seconds after eating and subsides approximately 30–60 minutes later.

HEINER SYNDROME

This is a non-IgE mediated adverse pulmonary response to food. It is not a very common manifestation but can present in infants by an immune reaction to cows milk protein with precipitating antibody IgG, resulting in pulmonary infilterates, pulmonary hemosiderosis, anemia, recurrent pneumonia and failure to thrive.

ANAPHYLAXIS

This refers to a dramatic multiorgan reaction associated with IgE mediated hypersensitivity. Foods commonly associated with anaphylaxis are peanuts, tree nuts (walnuts, almonds, cashew, hazel-nuts) and shellfish. This is more common in patients with underlying asthma.[13]

Food associated, exercise and induced anaphylaxis occur in two forms. It may occur when exercise follows the ingestion of a particular food to which IgE mediated sensitivity is usually demonstrable (e.g. celery) or less commonly may occur after the ingestion of any food.

CELIAC DISEASE

This is actually an example of non-IgE mediated disease. In this the causative factor is the gliadin fraction of the protein gluten in wheat. It presents over a period of time, may be months or years with steatorrhea, flatulence and failure to thrive. The characteristic diagnostic feature is extensive flattening of villi of the jejunal mucosa.

ALLERGIC EOSINOPHILIC GASTROENTERITIS

This is an IgE mediated disease, but many patients do not exhibit specific IgE antibody to foods. Manifestations are severe reflux, postprandial abdominal pain, vomiting, early satiety and diarrhea. The diagnosis is suggested by presence of inflammation and significant eosinophilic infilteration of the oesophagus, stomach or small intestine.

INFANTILE PROCTOCOLITIS

This involves the lower GI tract and is of short duration. The ingestion of the responsible food (usually cow's milk protein or breast milk from mothers who are consuming cow's milk) causes diarrhea with blood in the stool.

MIGRAINE

Migraine headaches have been associated with food allergies/hypersensitivity. Studies on children with migraine showed that 93% of 88 children recovered on oligoantigenic diets. The causative foods were identified by sequential reintroduction, and the role of the foods provoking migraine was established by a double blind controlled trial in 40 children. Most patients responded to several foods. Many foods were involved suggesting an allergic rather than metabolic pathogenesis. Associated symptoms which improved in addition to headache included abdominal pain, behavior disorder, fits, asthma and eczema. In most of the patients in whom migraine was provoked by nonspecific factors like blows to the head, exercise and flashing lights, this provocation did not occur while they were on oligoantigenic diet.[14]

TREATMENT/MANAGEMENT

Management of food allergies are best done by 'avoidance'. Dietary elimination of the offending food(s) is the simplest methods to manage allergies/ intolerances. Other modalities include medical management and in case of emergencies, injectable epinephrine and oral antihistamine should always be readily available at hand. Prompt administration of epinephrine at the first signs of a severe reaction must be stressed since delayed attention has been associated with fatal and nonfatal food allergic reactions.[13]

Identification of the offending food(s) is very crucial since successful management involves life long avoidance of foods in any form, directly or indirectly. Following points need to be considered in the dietary management of any food allergy/ intolerance.

1. Elimination of the offending food.
2. Read all the labels on food products carefully and the ingredients mentioned there in. Any word indicating any close resemblance to the offending food should be checked for, e.g. in a milk free diet, not only milk in any visible form should be avoided but any indication of words like 'casein', 'whey', lactose, or 'flavoring colors', etc. should also be kept in the mind since these are also indirect signs of milk protein being present in some form. It may be a part of ingredient in recipes like in bakery products; chocolates, etc. egg protein may be present in a number of commercial products available over the counters, all of which may not necessarily indicate its inclusion.
   In case of protein allergy, where, peanut based products like butter is used along side with any non-peanut product, but the spatula used or the bowls used may not be separate for these products, chances of allergic reactions can be possible.
   Some of the hidden allergens which can go unnoticed are:
   - Eggs—baked foods, noodles, puddings
   - Milk—pies, cheese, bakery products
   - Soy—baked foods, candy
   - Wheat—soups, snacks, savories
   - Fish—seafood flavors.
3. It is safer to avoid use of all artificial foods or dining out.
4. In case of infants and toddlers, avoiding of any such food in the maternal diet is advisable, e.g. eggs, cow's milk, peanut, etc. Continuation of exclusively breastfeeding at least till 6 months is encouraged. Solid foods should be introduced only after 6 months.
5. Introduction of known hyperallergic foods can be delayed, e.g. cow's milk can be delayed till about 10–12 months, eggs till about 2 years and peanuts/nuts/fish can be delayed even up to 3 years.
6. Smoking should be refrained by elders in and around the periphery of the child's environment,

since smoking increases the risk of recurrent wheeze and asthma. This is also known to lead to life threatening food allergy.

7. If traveling take specially packed foods.
8. When dining out ask for information on ingredients.
9. In case if a child does react to any allergenic food, give medication immediately, seek medical help and keep injectables epinephrine at hand.
10. In case of peanut allergy, if any peanut containing food is handled by the mother or care giver or cutlery, etc. used, they should be washed thoroughly.
11. Roasting of peanut has been known to increase allergic properties.

Probiotics have been also considered to have beneficial effects on the host by improving its intestinal microbial balance, e.g. yogurt which contains Lactobacillus and bifidobacterium species.[15]

RECOGNIZING ALLERGIES IN CHILDREN

Generally most allergies can be detected by visible signs or symptoms in children. They may give indirect 'feelers' which should not be ignored since these may well be warning signals of some allergy commonly described signs by children could be

- Putting hands to mouth, pull or scratch tongue or voice may change
- Food is too spicy
- My tongue is hot or something is pricking it
- My mouth is tingly, itches or feels funny
- My tongue feels full or my throat feels thick.

REFERENCES

1. Bruijinzeel-Koomen C, Irtolani C, Aas K, et al. Adverse reactions to food. Allergy. 1995;50:623-35.
2. Geha RS. Regulation of IgE synthesis in humans. J Allergy Clin Immunol. 1992;90:143-50.
3. Bock SA, Atkins FM. Patterns of food hypersensitivity during sixteen years of double blind, placebo-controlled challenges. J Pediatr. 1990;117:561-7.
4. Wesley Burks. J Peanut Allergy: a growing phenomenon. Clin Invest. 2003;11(7):950-52.
5. Katrina J Allen, David J Hill, Heina RG. Food allergy in childhood. MJA. 2006;185(7):394-400.
6. Scott H, Schierer MD. Clinical aspects of gastrointestinal food allergy in childhood. Pediatrics. 2003;111(6): 1617-24.
7. Wesley Burks. Respiratory manifestations of food allergy. Pediatrics. 2003;111(6):1625-30.
8. Sampson HA, Albergo R. Comparison of results of skin test, RAST and double blind placebo controlled food challenges in children with atopic dermatitis . J Allergy Clin Immunol. 1984;74:26-33.
9. Block SA, Lee WT, RemingioL, et al. Appraisal of skin tests with food extracts for diagnosis of food hypersensitivity. Clin Allergy. 1978;8:559-64.
10. Scott H, Stcherer MD. Manifestations of food allergy. Evaluation and Management, Mount Sinai School of Medicine, New York. American family physician, Pub. By the American academy of family physician. Jan 15, 1999.
11. Irtolanic C, Ispano M, Pastorello E, et al. The oral allergy síndrome. Ann Allergy. 1988;(6112):47-52.
12. Beck SA, Burks AW, Woody RC. Auriculotemporal syndrome seen clinically as food allergy. Pediatrics. 1989;83:601-3.
13. Sampson HA, Mendelson LM, Rosen JP. Fatal and near fatal anaphylactic reactions to food in children and adolescents. N Engl J Med. 1992;327:380-4.
14. Eqqer J, Carter CM, Wilson J, et al. Is migraine food allergy? A double blind controlled trial of oligoantigentic diet treatment. Lancet. 1983 Oct 15;2 (8355):865-9.
15. Majamaa H, Isolauri E. Probiotics: a novel approach in the management of food allergy. J Allergy Clin Immunol. 1997;99:179-85.

13 Vitamin A Deficiency in Children

Vitamin A deficiency affects more than 127 million preschool children.[1,2] It is estimated that 20%–50% of infant mortality can be reduced by improving the status of vitamin A levels in this group of population.[3] Deficiency of vitamin A can extend through school age and adolescent years into adulthood. In India the prevalence is more than the WHO critical limits in most states. However, as per the National Nutrition Monitoring Bureau (NNMB) estimates it is higher in the states of Andhra Pradesh and West Bengal.[3]

Surveys carried out by NNMB in India, and Integrated child development services (ICDS) indicate that the prevalence of bitot's spot (the common indication of vitamin A deficiency) in preschool children (1–5 years) ranges between 1%–5% in different parts of the country. Incidence of corneal lesions is uncommon. Corneal xerophthalmia is reported to be about 0.05–0.1 per 100 preschool children in South India.[3] As per their estimates about 50,000 children become blind every year in India due to vitamin A deficiency.

The main causes of vitamin A deficiency in children are known to be:

Mother deficient in vitamin A: Maternal vitamin A deficiency exists in a good magnitude with serious and long-term implications. Infant and maternal morality is a common outcome of this deficiency. Deficient mothers obviously will produce breast milk low in vitamin A, thus adversely affecting the health of the offspring. The main cause of maternal deficiency in women is consumption of diets poor in this vitamin besides prolonged breastfeeding due to high fertility rates. In addition to consuming diets low in vitamin A, women in developing countries spend a substantial proportion of their lives breastfeeding, when vitamin A requirements are very high. In industrialized countries, women have on an average 1.6 babies and breastfeed them for 5 months. These women spend 8 months or 2.2% of their 30 reproductive years (ages 15–45) breastfeeding. But, in the lesser developed countries, women have on an average 5 children and breastfeed each for 2 years. Therefore, rural Bangladesh women spend one third of their reproductive years breastfeeding, when their dietary intake of vitamin A provides less than one third of their RDA.[4,5]

Maternal vitamin A deficiency although has little impact on the fetus, during lactation, healthy mothers transfer about 250 μmol of vitamin A (130 lt. of breast milk consumed, containing1.92 μmol of vitamin A per lt.), where as women in underdeveloped countries transfer only about half that amount, since the average milk vitamin A concentrations are about 1.05 μmol/l.[6,7] Therefore all babies are physiologically depleted of vitamin A at birth.

But, during lactation, breastfed babies of well nourished women accrue adequate stress, whereas babies of poorly nourished mothers remain depleted. In addition, if weaning foods are poor in vitamin A than the breast milk, the child's risk of deficiency increases further when breastfeeding stops.

Poor dietary source of vitamin A in children: A major factor of vitamin A deficiency in children is their poor dietary sources. In general, children in the developed countries receive a major percentage of their vitamin content from animal sources, where as poor children from the developing countries, consume mostly less expensive and poor plant sources. Studies from Egypt, Mexico and Kenya[8] and India[9] have shown that median intakes of animal sources of vitamin A were 174, 119, 50 and 33 µg/d, respectively providing only 11%–58% of the RDA and leaving these children largely dependent on the plant sources. In a study from Bangladesh where the only source of vitamin A (preformed) was breast milk, weaned children consumed only negligible amounts of vitamin A from animal sources.[10]

Childhood illness and infections: It is well known that illness worsens vitamin A status primarily by reducing intake due to anorexia and malabsorption and increasing utilization through greater catabolism and urinary loss. Anorexia is a major determinant of reduced dietary intake during episodes of diarrhea. Studies have shown that malabsorption of vitamin A can occur during diarrheal illness and lower respiratory infection.[11]

The two most common childhood diseases, chicken pox and measles, can severely compromise vitamin A status. Measles results in markedly depresses circulating vitamin A concentrations and can precipitate xerophthalmia.[12]

Vitamin A supplementation during acute measles episode consistently and dramatically reduces their fatality rates. Therefore high dose vitamin A is recommended for treatment of all cases of severe measles in places where measles case fatality rate exceeds 1%.

Ignorance and poverty: Lack of awareness among the rural illiterate regarding the importance of supplementing essential vitamins and minerals along with a healthy diet is another factor for deficiency in the rural masses especially in the under privileged classes.

Poverty and poor purchasing power in most communities prevents them from processing adequate food especially the healthy foods like dairy products and other animal foods which are rich in preformed vitamin A. They are mainly dependent on preformed vitamin A in the form of plant sources.

FUNCTIONS OF VITAMIN A

Vitamin A is a group of compounds that play an important role in vision, bone growth, reproduction, cell division and cell differentiation. It also helps regulate the immune system which helps prevent or fight off infections. It also helps lymphocytes fight infections more efficiently.

Growth

Lack of vitamin A prevents normal growth, as the bony structure will suffer a growth failure before the soft tissues manifest the stunting effect. The cessation of bone growth can lead to overcrowding of the brain and the central nervous system. At times there can be pinching of the optic nerve, leading to blindness.

Role in Monitoring Healthy Epithelial Tissues

Vitamin A has a crucial role in maintaining the healthy epithelial lining. It helps the skin and mucus membrane function as a barrier to bacteria and virus. In the absence of vitamin A, the specialized functions of the tissue are suppressed and is transformed to a keratinized (dry horny) type of epithelium. Excessive dryness of the skin may fail to secrete normally and becomes less resistant to bacterial invasion.

Red Cell Production

The red blood like all other cells are derived from precursor cells called the stem cells. These are dependent on retinoids for normal differentiation into red blood cells.

Antioxidant or Immune Functions

Vitamin A is also commonly referred to as an antioxidant for normal immune functions. As mentioned earlier in this chapter, retinol and its metabolites are required to maintain the integrity and function of the cells that line the airways, digestive tract and the urinary tract, and thus function as a barrier against any infections. Vitamin A and retinoic acid (RSA) is known to play an important role in the development and differentiation of white cells like lymphocytes, which play a critical role in the immune response. Activation of T-lymphocytes, the major regulatory cells of the immune system appears to require all trans RA binding of RAR.

Pathogenesis

The pathology involves dryness of the cornea, since the tear glands fail to secrete, causing severe ulcer like lesions and if untreated this can lead to blindness. The retina is the light sensitive inside layer at the back of the eye. There are two kinds of receptor cells in the retina—the 'rods' which function in dim light and the 'cones' that function in bright light and color vision in rods and rhodopsin in cones. In bright light rhodopsin changes to retenine plus protein with a possible loss of some vitamin A to resynthesise rhodopsin. Vitamin A is reoxidized to retinine and combined with a special protein opsin. In the absence of adequate vitamin A, night blindness may occur. This is a condition characterized by inability to see in dim light and the necessity of a prolonged time to adjust to dim light after exposure to bright light (Fig. 13.1).[13] 'Night blindness' is a stage prior to complete blindness where inadequate retinol available to the retina results in impaired dark adaptation. This is then followed by total blindness, where inadequate retinol available to the retina results in impaired dark adaptation. This is then followed by total blindness, if left undiagnosed.

In ancient egypt, it was known that night blindness could be cured by eating liver, which was later found to be a rich source of the vitamin.[14] Majority of the cases occur in children of 2–6 years of age. Initially, the condition may be left undiagnosed, when the child begins to stagger and find difficulty in seeing after dusk. This is characterized by mothers typically describing that the child has to grope his way towards evening or in dim light and needs help to find his way. Initially parents may over look these signs and by the time the child begins to literally lose vision, do they realize the gravity of the disease. Therefore early intervention helps in not only reversing this condition, but also prevents from total loss of vision.

Ninety percent of vitamin A is stored in the liver with small amounts in the lungs, body fat and kidneys. The stores being nil at birth, increase gradually with age. These stores are dependent on the amount absorbed from the diet and that absorbed. It has been estimated that a normal liver may contain as much as 600,000 IU of vitamin A enough to supply vitamin needs of one year.[15]

DEFICIENCY SIGNS OF VITAMIN A

Nutritional deficiency of vitamin A leading to blindness has been regarded as a major national health problem. WHO has recommended the

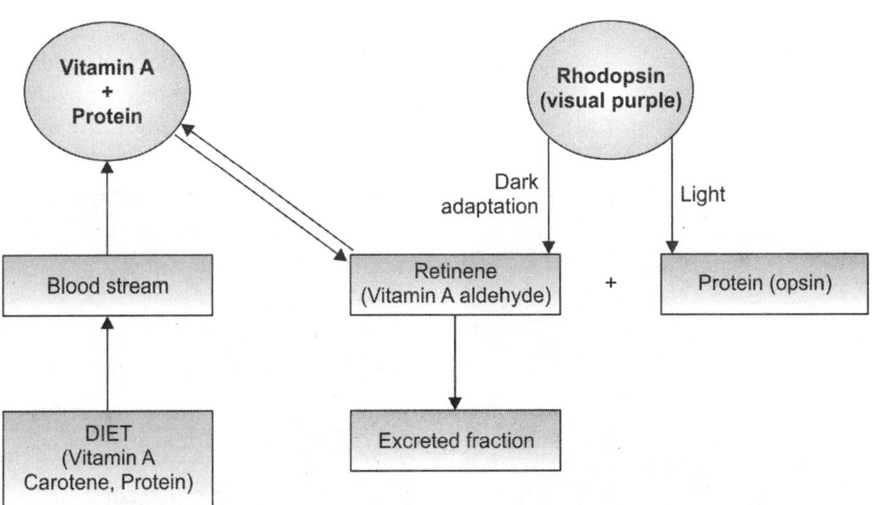

FIGURE 13.1: Diagram of formation of rhodops in xerophthalmia
(Adapted from Eddy and Dalldorf (1944), The Avitaminosis, The Willims & Wilkin Co, Baltimore p 66)

following classification of xerophthalmia, a term covering all ocular manifestations of vitamin A deficiency.[16] These include structural changes affecting conjunctiva, cornea and at times the retina including the biophysical disorders of retinal rod and cone function.

- Night blindness (XN)
- Conjunctival xerosis (XIA)
- Bitot's spots (XIB)
- Corneal xerosis (XZ)
- Corneal ulceration / Keratomalacia (<1/3 corneal surface × 3A)
- Corneal ulceration / Keratomalacia (>1/3 corneal surface × 3 A)
- Corneal scar (XF)
- Xerophthalmia fundus (XN).

Night Blindness (XN)

This is the first sign of vitamin A deficiency observed in children and history can be elicited by detailed questioning of the parent giving history of the child groping in dim light or they are unable to see the food in their plate in front of them.

Conjunctival Xerosis (XIA)

This is seen as dry patches on the conjunctiva. The tears in the child appear to emerge like sand at receding tide. There may be varying degrees of thickening, wrinkling and pigmentation of the conjunctiva.

Bitot's Spots (XIB)

This is an extension of the xerotic process. The spots are raised, muddy, and dry with triangular patches (Fig. 13.2). These spots are very early diagnosed, and may tend to remain as sequale of earlier corrected vitamin A deficiency even after therapy.

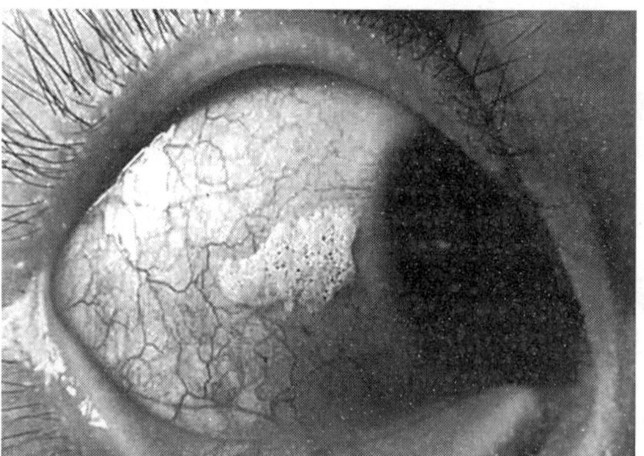

FIGURE 13.2: Eye with bitot's spot

Corneal Xerosis (X2)

This is diagnosed by the presence of haziness or dryness of cornea on clinical examination. The cornea gives the appearance of ground glass followed by corneal ulcers. Treatment reverses these symptoms except in cases where the stoma is deep rooted which can lead to blindness.

Keratomalacia (X3B)

This is the last stage, if left undiagnosed leading to irreversible blindness. It is marked by progressive necrosis and death of tissue affecting the full thickness of the cornea (Fig. 13.3).

Vitamin a Deficiency in Specific Conditions

There is increased interest in the early forms of vitamin A deficiency described as storage levels of Vitamin A that do not cause obvious deficiency symptom. This mild degree of vitamin A deficiency may increase children's decrease likelihood of survival from serious illness.[17] In the United states children are considered to be at increase risk for subclinical vitamin A deficiency in the following conditions.

- Toddlers and preschool age children
- Children living at or below poverty level
- Children with inadequate health care or immunization

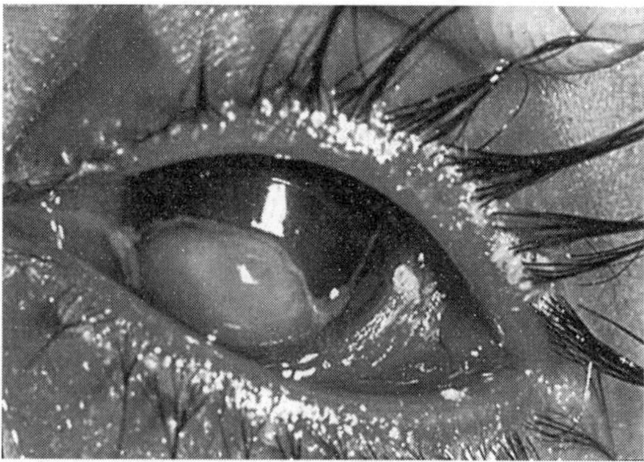

FIGURE 13.3: Eye with Keratomalacia

- Children living in areas with known nutritional deficiency
- Recent immigrants or refugees from developing countries with high incidence of Vitamin A deficiency or measles
- Children with diseases of the pancreas, liver or intestines of the pancreas, liver or intestines or with inadequate fat digestion on absorption.

Vitamin A deficiency can occur when there are losses through chronic diarrhea or when the total dietary intake is inadequate as in PEM. It has been suggested that vitamin A deficiency can also occur due to inadequate intake of vitamin itself or also due retinol binding protein (RBP). Iron deficiency too can affect vitamin A metabolism. It as seen that iron supplements provided to iron deficiency individuals may improve body stores of vitamin A and iron.[18]

HYPERVITAMINOSIS A

Excessive consumption of vitamin A may lead to toxicity called hypervitaminosis. Acute toxicity although rare, is marked by symptoms like nausea, headache, fatigue, anorexia, dizziness, dry skin and cerebral edema. Bone and joint pain may also be present. In infants symptoms of toxicity include bulging fontanels. Severe cases of hypervitaminosis may result in liver damage, hemorrhage and coma. However, such signs are associated only with long term consumption of the vitamin and in excess losses. On the other hand the toxicity can also occur by consuming large doses of preformed vitamin A over a short period. Such incidents generally tend to occur when taken as supplements. Dietary sources alone do not run the risk of toxicity.

Target Group for Vitamin A Supplementation

The WHO and the United Nations children funds (UNICEF) recommend vitamin A administration for all children where vitamin A deficiency is a serious problem and where death from measles is greater than 1 percent. In 1994 the American Academy of Pediatrics recommended vitamin A supplements for two subgroups of children likely to be at high risk for subclinical vitamin A deficiency; children aged 6 months to 24 months who are hospitalized with measles, and hospitalized children older than 6 months.[19]

Fat malabsorption can result in diarrhea and prevent normal absorption of vitamin A gradually leading to vitamin A deficiency. Some of the conditions involved would be:

- *Celiac disease*: genetic disorder where patients are allergic to the gliadin fraction of wheat protein.
- *Chron's disease*: this is an inflammatory bowel disease characterized by fat malabsorption and malnutrition.
- *Pancreatic disorders*: these include conditions like cystic fibrosis where due to the deficiency in enzyme secretion, fat malabsorption occurs causing huge losses of vitamin A. Supplementation of vitamin A helps prevent deficiency.
- *Vegetarians:* strict vegetarians not consuming eggs or even dairy products run the risk of developing of this vitamin A.

Requirements

The RDAS for vitamin A for infants and children are calculated on the basis of vitamin A intake through breastfed infants and extrapolated for children.[20] The daily intake of vitamin A by Indian infants through breast milk is about 140 μg during the first 6 months of life.[21] Since it was observed that children of such communities often develop deficiency signs during early childhood, intakes of 140 μg/d seem to be inadequate. Therefore based on the observations of breast milk intake by well nourished mothers, the expert group[22] has recommended a daily intake of 350 μg retinol up to 6 months of age. The same level is recommended for the next 6 months also, i.e. the later half of infancy, since no specific data is yet available on the needs of this group.

In view of the high incidence of vitamin A deficiency signs and low serum levels among Indian children with dietary intake less than 100 μg, the daily intake for preschoolers has been fixed at 400 μg and 600 μg for school children and adolescents. Table 13.1 gives the requirements suggested for different age groups of children and pregnant and lactating mothers, including the conversion factor of β carotene

TABLE 13.1: Recommended intake of vitamin A (μg/dl)

Group	Vitamin A	β Carotene
Adult women (NPNL)*	600	4800
Pregnant women	800	6400
Lactating women	950	7600
Infants 0–6 months 6–12 months	350	–
Children 1–6 years 7–9 years	400 600	3200 4800
Adolescents 10–17 years	600	4800

*non pregnant non lactating
A conversion ratio of 1:8 is used (for β carotene)
ICMR 2010[20]

to vitamin A. Studies have shown that when vitamin A was supplemented with a total of 300 μg/d over a period of 6 months, serum vitamin levels were found to be around 30 μg/dl and clinical deficiency signs were absent.[23]

Prevention of Vitamin A Deficiency

'Prevention is better than cure', so it is said and rightly so.

Deficiency of vitamin A is one disease which can easily be prevented. Education and awareness of the gravity of the problem, if explained to the parents can definitely help avoid this preventive disease with grave consequences. Nature has a bounty of food sources to provide vitamin A, both as preformed vitamin and β carotene, the precursor of the vitamin. Mostly all colorful fruits and vegetables, especially the yellow and the green ones provide the provitamin A, i.e. the carotenoids. These can be converted into the retinol form for absorption in the body. Common provitamin A carotenoids found in foods that come from plants are beta carotene, alpha carotene and beta cryptoxanthin. Among this β carotene is the most easily converted into retinol. Some of the provitamin A carotenoids have been shown to function as antioxidants also. Dark green leafy vegetables like spinach, etc. are affordable good sources. Retinol is found in foods that come from animal sources like, whole eggs, milk and liver. Most fortified foods like butter, margarine and breakfast cereals and fats and oils are converted to retinol.

TABLE 13.2A: Animal sources of vitamin A (μg %)

Foods	Retinol	β carotene
Animal sources		
Milk (cows)	53	
Curd (cows)	31	
Cottage cheese (cow milk)	110	
Cheese	82	
Butter	960	
Ghee (cow)	600	
Ghee (buffalo)	270	
Refined oil (fortified)	750	
Egg (hen)	420	
Liver (sheep)	6690	

TABLE 13.2B: Vegetarian sources of vitamin A

Foods	Retinol	Carotene	
		Total	β
Vegetable sources		15,700	
Colocasia leaves		15,000	5,920
Coriander leaves		42,000	4,800
Drumstick leaves		11,800	19,690
Fenugreek leaves		7,000	9,100
Lettuce		18,950	1,100
Mint		13,000	5,480
Radish leaves		9,400	2,200
Spinach		8,840	2,740
Carrot		2,100	6,460
Pumpkin		2,430	1,160
Chillies green		690	1,007
Chillies giant (capsicum)		400	140
Guava country		2,210	0
Mango (ripe)		2,240	1,990
Orange		2,740	190
Papaya (ripe)		3,010	880
Tomato (ripe)			590

(ICMR 1990)

Vitamin A sources from animal origin are absorbed more efficiently by the body. A list of vitamin A and provitamin sources are given in Tables 13.2A and 13.2B.[24]

Other strategies which can help prevent vitamin A deficiency are periodic supplements to the vulnerable groups and fortification of food products which are widely consumed. Nutrition counseling is simultaneously required to create awareness among the masses especially the lower socioeconomic sections. Education regarding making use of low cost, seasonally available fruits and vegetables can go a long way in prevention of the serious consequences of deficiency of this vitamin.

Another point to be stressed during education is the right cooking methods to be used while preparation of foods rich in vitamin A. Being fat soluble vitamins, it is important that for these foods deep frying for prolonged duration be avoided, since maximum losses can occur during this process.

TREATMENT

Treatment involves administration of large doses of vitamin A for all stages of active xerophthalmia including corneal lesions.

For children aged 1–6 years, an oral dose of 200,000 IU or oil miscible vitamin A is administered. This is followed by another dose of 200,000 IU, one to four weeks later. For infants below 12 months of age weighing less than 8 kg the same schedule is followed using half the dose of the vitamin. Children suffering from associated problems like diarrhea, acute respiratory infections and measles should be monitored closely and treated as medical emergency.[25]

Some Controversies About Vitamin A

Vitamin A, Beta Carotene and Cancer

Studies exist to suggest role of vitamin A rich diets in lowering risk of many types of cancer.[26]

However, there are other studies which contradict these observations. In fact, in one of the studies, where researchers provided supplements to subjects with lung cancer, they found a 46% higher risk of deaths occurring among them, therefore this study had to be abandoned.[27]

It was hence felt that beta carotene supplements are not advisable for general population, except in those with inadequate vitamin A.[17]

Vitamin A and Osteoporosis

There is no evidence of an association between beta carotene intake, especially from fruits and vegetables, and increased risk of osteoporosis. Current evidence suggests a possible association with vitamin A as retinol only. Similarly no association was found between blood levels of beta carotene and risk of hip fracture. However, it was also observed by some researchers that retinol intakes greater than 2,000 μg/d were associated with an increased risk of hip fracture as compared to intakes less than 500 mg.[28]

REFERENCES

1. West KF. Extent of vitamin A deficiency among pre school children and women of reproductive age. J Nutr. 2002;132:28575-665.
2. Humphrey JH, West KP Jr, Sommer A. Vitamin A deficiency and attributable morality among under 5 year olds. Bull WHO. 1992;70:225-32.
3. Vijayaraghavan K. Vitamin A deficiency, In: Textbook of Human Nutrition, Eds. Mahtab S Bamji, Prahlad Rao N and Redddy V. Oxford and IBM Publishing Co. Pvt Ltd. New Delhi. 1996;287-97.
4. UNICEF (200). State of the world children 2000. www. unicef org/sowc002000 UNICEF New York.
5. WHO Complementary feeding of young children in developing countries: a review of current scientific knowledge. 1998 WHO Geneva, Switzerland .Publ No WS 13098 Co. 1998.
6. Walling Ford JC, Underwood BA. Vitamin A deficiency in pregnancy, lactation and the nursing child. Eds. Bauerufeind J, Vitamin A Deficiency and its control. Academic Press New York. 1986:101-52.
7. Chappel JE, Francis T, Clandinin MT. Vitamin A and E content of human milk at early stages of lactation. Early human Dev. 11:157-67.
8. Calloway DH, Murphy SP, Beaton GH, et al. Estimated vitamin A intakes of toddlers: predicted prevalence of inadequacy in village population in Egypt, Kenya and Mexico. Am J Clin Nutr. 1993;58:376-84.

9. Ramakrishanan U, Martorell R, Latham MC, et al. Dietary vitamin A intakes of pre school age children in south India. J Nutr. 1999;2021-27.
10. Zeitlin MF, Megawangi R, Mara Kramer, et al. Mother's and children's intakes of vitamin A in rural Bangladesh. Am J Clin Nutr. 1992.
11. Sivakumar B, Reddy V. Absorption of labeled vitamin A by children with diarrhea during treatment with oral rehydration solution. Bull WHO. 64:721-4.
12. Reddy V, Bhaskaram P, Raghuramula N, et al. Relationship between measles, malnutrition and blindness: a prospective study in Indian children. Am J Clin Nutr. 1986;44:924-30.
13. Eddy walter Hollis, gilbert Dalldorf. The Avitaminosis, the chemical, clinical and pathophysiological Aspects of the vitamin deficiency disease 3rd ed. Baltimere. The Williams and Wilkins co.
14. Gerster H. Vitamin A functions, dietary requirements and safety in humans. Int J Vitam Nutr. Res 1997;67: 71-90.
15. Wilson ED, Fisher KE, Fuqua HE. Introduction to the vitamins and the fat soluble vitamins. In: Principles of Nutrition. Wiley Eastern Pvt Ltd. 1968.
16. Tielsch JM, Sommer A. The epidemiology of vitamin A deficiency and xerophthalmia, In: Annual Review of Nutr. 1984;4:183-205.
17. Stephens D, Jackson PL, Gutierrey Y. Subclinical vitamin A deficiency: A potentially unrecognized problem in the United States. Pediatr Nutr. 1996;22: 377-89.
18. Institute of Medicine. Food and Nutrition Board. Dietary reference intakes for vitamin A vitamin K, arsenic, boron, chromium, copper, iodine, iron, manganese, molybdenum, nickel, silicon, vanadium and zinc. National Academy Press, Washington DC. 2001.
19. Committee on Infectious Diseases. Vitamin A treatment of measles. Pediatrics. 1993;91:1014-15.
20. ICMR, Nutrient requirement and recommended dietary allowances for Indians, A report of the expert group of the ICMR. NIN, Hyderabad. 2010.
21. Belavady B and Gopalan C. Chemical composition of human milk in poor Indian women. Ind J Med Res. 1959;47:234.
22. WHO, Requirements of vitamin A, thiamine, riboflavin and niacin; WHO Tech Rep Sr no 362. 1967.
23. Reddy V. Vitamin A deficiency and blindness in Indian children, Ind J Med Res. 1978;68(suppl):26.
24. Gopalan C, Rama Sastri BV, Balasubraminiam SC. Nutritive Value of Indian Foods, National Institute of Nutrition, ICMR, Hyderabad, 1990.
25. Vijayraghavan K. Vitamin A deficiency. In: Textbook of human Nutrition, Ed. Bamji, MS, Rao NP, Reddy V, Oxford and IBH Publishing Co. Pvt Ltd. 1996.
26. Fontham ETH. Protective dietary factors and lung cancer. Int J Epidemiol. 1990;19:532-4.
27. Pryor WH, Stahl W, Rock CL. Beta carotene: From biochemistry to clinical trials. Nutr Rev. 2000;58:38-53.
27. Feskanich D, Singh F, Willet WC, et al. Vitamin A intake and hip fractures among post menopausal women. J Am Med Assoc. 2002;287:47-54.

14 Nutritional Anemia in Children

"Health is not valued till sickness comes"

Dr Thomas Fuller (1732)

IRON DEFICIENCY ANEMIA (IDA)

Iron deficiency anemia has been considered as one of the major national nutritional problems in our country. In view of the various consequences of inadequate iron stores in children, it poses a major health problem for all pediatricians and dieticians. The incidence is found to occur in significant proportions among both urban and rural populations. Because of the fact that mild to moderate forms of anemia are not recognized by parents, it goes untreated for a considerable length of time, till the child is brought to a clinician for any other illness or just for inadequate weight gain. Most often, among the rural groups or the lower socio-economic population, children are not taken for a regular routine check up and therefore the problem, even if existing in milder forms may go unnoticed. Even if they are taken for the routine immunization schedule, clinical examination is often missed out.

A number of studies at various times have demonstrated that IDA is one micronutrient deficiency, the prevalence of which is up to 53% of children surveyed.[1] Prevalence rates are generally found to be more among girls compared to boys among older age groups but among the below 6 year age group, it has been found to be as high as 64.8% in most of the cities in India.[2]

It has been well documented that breastfeeding exerts a protective effect in preventing or reducing the incidence of iron deficiency. The fact that exclusive breastfed babies maintained higher Hb levels than infants on formula feeds, has been well established. This is because the maternal stores of iron are adequate to suffice for their needs till 6 months through the breast milk. But beyond 6 months these stores are inadequate and serial supplements are required to meet the increased demands of the infant.

Moreover, the bioavailability of iron in human milk is also superior compared to other milk sources which can take care of the growth needs of the child. But a premature infant is unable to assimilate adequate iron from breast milk and hence have to be given iron supplements by 6–8 weeks of age. This is adequately absorbed when given along with breast milk.

There are studies to show that infants when fed whole cow's milk, the risk of gastrointestinal bleeding can cause loss of iron, therefore unmodified cow's milk is best avoided in early infancy.

Functions of Iron in the Body

Iron is widely distributed in the body. About 55%–60% of iron is in the blood; about 3% exists in the muscle tissue while a variable amount is stored in the liver, spleen, kidney and bone marrow, ranging from 1–2 grams.

In the Blood

Iron is located in the form of erythrocytes in the red blood cells. Hemoglobin is the compound formed by the union of an iron containing pigment, heme, and the protein globin. Iron is incorporated into hemoglobin after its absorption. Hemoglobin is involved in the function of carrying oxygen from the lungs to the tissues.

About 0.2% of iron exists in the blood plasma, which is in transport form. Plasma iron comes from

a. that absorbed from the gastro- intestinal tract
b. that salvaged from the breakdown of hemoglobin
c. that released from the stores in the body.

It is estimated that about 27–28 mg of iron per day is derived from hemolysis (destruction of red blood cells), whereas only 1 mg comes from dietary source. Under normal conditions, the plasma iron level may vary from 50–180 mg per 100 ml of plasma. In iron deficiency anemia, this level is reduced.

In Muscle Tissue

Iron is present in the muscle tissue in the form of

a. myoglobin
b. as a constituent of a combination of an iron pigment and a protein and is a carrier of oxygen. The iron containing enzymes in muscle tissue makes possible the oxidation of carbohydrates, fat and protein within the intact cell. Iron serves in a double capacity in cellular oxidation, it carries oxygen to the cells and makes possible oxidation in the cells through the iron containing enzymes.

Definition

Iron deficiency anemia (IDA) has been defined when the Hb concentration of the blood is lower than the given standard for the specific age and sex group. As per WHO,[3] IDA is categorized into 3 groups based on the level of Hb present in the blood for all age groups and both sexes as seen in Table 14.1.

Iron deficiency is actually the end result of a well defined sequence of changes that account for iron depletion. These are:

TABLE 14.1: WHO criteria for diagnosis of anemia

Age/sex group	Hb (g/dl)
Children (6 months–6 years)	< 11
Children (6 years–14 years)	< 12
Adult males	< 13
Adult females (nonpregnant)	< 12
Adult females (pregnant)	< 11

Source: WHO, 1968

1. Disappearance of storage forms from bone marrow (iron ferritin) and the reticuloendothelial tissues.
2. A decrease in serum iron level and simultaneous increase in the serum iron binding protein transferrin.
3. A decrease in the mean red cell volume and increase in free erythrocyte porphyrin levels.
4. A decrease in concentration of hemoglobin.

Clinical Features of Iron Deficiency Anemia

As mentioned earlier in this chapter, mild to moderate forms of anemia may go unnoticed by parents or other care givers. This is because the fall in the Hb level is usually gradual and by the time it actually falls very drastically, it generally comes to severe type.

Some of the common features encountered are:

- Pallor, irritability, anorexia
- Palpitation, fatigue, shortness of breath
- Decreased exercise intolerance, congestive heart failure
- Koilonychia (spoon shaped nails)
- Vitamin B deficiency signs in severe chronic conditions
- Pica (craving to eat clay, laundry starch, etc.)
- Alterations in small bowel mucosal functions
- Lowered IQ and decreased attentiveness are also frequently observed in children with anemia.

Implications of Iron Deficiency Anemia

Iron being an integral component of several enzymes which have an important role in metabolic processes and cell proliferation, a number of variable changes are observed in various organs and systems. Some significant adverse affects observed on various systems are:

Failure to Thrive/Growth Retardation

This is a common finding in most iron deficient children and could be due to the existing anorexia and altered intestinal functions. It is observed that very often children who are anemic are predominantly milk fed on prolonged breast feeding without adequate cereal supplementation. Milk being a poor source of iron, the child's reserves gradually gets depleted resulting in loss of appetite. This becomes a vicious cycle that of faulty feeding leading to anemia and this condition further resulting in loss of appetite. Iron supplementation is the only way to break this cycle which further helps in return of appetite.

Activity

Another very obvious outcome of iron deficiency anemia is decrease in work capacity and this is directly proportionate to the severity of iron deficiency. Studies from Hyderabad have shown that school children, who were anemic, did poorly in physical activity.[4]

Ever among housewives early signs of anemia can be foreseen by symptoms like easy fatigue ability during the course of routine household chores or weakness or loss of energy at the calves of their legs.

Temperature Regulation

Children with anemia are known to experience hypothermia and feel uncomfortably cold at normal temperatures too.

Mental and Psychomotor Response

It is well established that children who are inclined to be anemic, also show poor mental performance, are not able to concentrate or even comprehend in academics and suffer from loss of memory. Studies have shown that children with anemia are unable to meet the desired standards of scholastic tests besides having impaired motor development.

Immune Response

Iron deficiency leads to defect in cell mediated immunity which could result in recurrent infections. The leukocytes are adversely affected and unable to kill ingested microorganisms. They are also known to have depressed skin test response to common antigens.

Maternal Iron Deficiency

Maternal iron deficiency adversely affects fetal outcome. WHO studies have demonstrated that 20%–40% of all maternal deaths ascribed to childbirth every year, are due to anemia among the pregnant mothers.[5]

Infants born to anemic mothers have less than half the reserves compared to those born to non-anemic mothers. They are likely to remain deficient in iron during their early years and suffer from long term consequences.

Gastrointestinal Affects

Children with anemia are also likely to suffer from increased acid production leading to atrophic gastritis encouraging further infections.

Etiology of Iron Deficiency

Iron deficiency can occur due to three main mechanisms which may be either solely responsible or in combination. These are:

Inadequate Intake or Absorption

Adequate supply of iron to the body stores is essential to meet the demand of the body from time to time, under variable conditions. It is well known that for an infant breast milk can provide adequate stores of iron till 6 months of age. But beyond that it fails to meet the increasing demands of growth of the baby. Firstly because after 6 months, the iron stores in the breast milk diminish and secondly because the demand increases. Therefore cereal pulse supplements are strongly advocated after 6 months, so that the iron requirements can be met with (Refer Chapter 2, Table 2.1). However, we also know that absorption of iron from cereals and pulses is not very good. Addition of green leafy vegetables can improve the iron content of the diet. Therefore, if in a vegetarian diet the quantity of cereals, pulses and green leafy vegetables is increased and used in combination, the absorption is likely to increase by about one third. Intake of non-vegetarian foods like fish, meat or egg yolk, not only help increase the available iron in the diet but also increases the absorption. The bioavailability of iron from these sources is about 20%–30% and they also help in better absorption from other food sources.

Very often it is observed that children are continued to be exclusively breastfed well up to even one year. Even if they do supplement their diet, it is very insignificant, in the form of biscuits, rusks or very small quantities of cereals, pulses or vegetables which hardly contribute any iron. Milk being a very poor source of iron, the child if fed pre-dominantly on it, either breast or formula or even dairy source, can gradually be left with very poor of iron stores leading to nutritional anemia.

Besides poor intake, there are other factors which may inhibit the absorption of dietary sources like the presence of phytates which when bound with iron may make it unavailable. Similarly the presence of tannin in tea can also inhibit its absorption from food. Therefore, it is very important that children should be strongly discouraged to have tea especially with meals. A common practice observed in the northern part of the country, is that mothers generally tend to feed the infant with tea right from 6–12 months of age. Tea is considered as beneficial in providing relief from colds and coughs and even digestion, therefore widely encouraged. On the contrary, the prolonged consumption of tea can make the children addicted to it, to the extent of causing gastritis and loss of appetite.

On the other hand, cooking of infant feeds in iron pans can help in better absorption from the dietary sources.

The food intake of children can also be compromised with the existence of infections. Any infection, whether respiratory or gastrointestinal decreases the appetite leading to inadequate intake. Again mothers tend to feed them with milk or tea. 'Starving a fever' is a very common belief which contributes to poor food consumption, thus indirectly being a causative factor for anemia.

Increased Losses

Even if the intake or supply of iron from the diet is adequate or if there are simultaneous losses, IDA can occur. The losses can be in the form of parasitic infestations which can result in gastrointestinal bleeding, e.g. hookworm infestations in which case blood losses can vary from 2–100 ml/day depending upon the severity of infection.[6]

Another common cause of iron losses in children is malabsorption which can be due to defective absorption of iron, folic acid, B_{12} or pyridoxine.

Other sources of blood loss can be due to bleeding from any other source like gums, piles and fissures, polyps, peptic ulcers which could be drug induced or otherwise or in any other conditions like esophageal varices, ulcerative colitis, dysentery, etc.

Increased Demands

There can be certain physiological conditions when despite adequate intake and no losses or adequate absorption, the body demands increase like in pregnancy and in children during the growth period, i.e. during infancy and childhood. All the conditions mentioned in the earlier two causative factors can indirectly exert increased demands on the body reserves of iron.

TREATMENT OF IDA

In children, reversal of the iron deficiency state is generally achieved by iron supplementation orally. However, diet counseling regarding adequate cereal and pulse, green vegetables, etc. is also reinforced for long term management. Infants and children being fed on excessive milk are advised to restrict the milk intake, not exceeding 500 ml per day which is even otherwise the recommended allowance. Iron rich dietary sources like ragi, wheat, whole pulses especially black gram, green leafy vegetables are advised. Jaggery and dates are good sources which can be complemented in the routine meals of children. A list of iron rich sources are given in Table14.2.[7] Nonvegetarian foods like meat, fish and egg yolk are better sources of iron, besides having higher bioavailability in the body.

There are certain foods which act as iron enhancers, i.e. they promote better absorption in the body. These are ascorbic acid and nonvegetarian foods.

Ascorbic acid when ingested with a highly available iron salt can increase the bioavailability by almost 33%. Moreover, added in the food, it also lessens the inhibitory effect of other compounds present in the food. This is due to its reducing effect and preventing the formation of insoluble ferric hydroxide. Iron absorption, as we know, is always in the ferrous form. It also helps in formation of soluble complexes with both ferrous and ferric forms at low pH, which then preserves iron solubility at the more alkaline duodenal pH.

Meat, Fish and Amino Acids

The enhancing effect of meat and fish is well known. Unlike other enhancers, meat and fish increase the absorption of both heme and nonheme iron though the mechanism may differ in both. For nonheme iron, it is unlikely to be due to protein presence, as egg

TABLE 14.2: Iron content of common foods

Foods	Iron Content (mg %)		
	Poor < 2.0	Average > 2–4	Rich > 4.0
Bajra			8.0
Ragi		3.9	
Wheat flour whole		4.9	
Bengal gram dal			5.3
Bengal gram washed			9.5
Black gram dal		3.8	
Soybean			10.4
Rajma		5.1	
Other dals		2–4 mg	
Amaranth			18.4
Beet greens			16.2
Celery leaves			40.0
Colocasia leaves			10.0
Mustard leaves			16.3
Root vegetables	0.5–2.0		
Other vegetables	0.5–2.0		
Onion stalks			7.43
Plantain green			6.27
Almonds			5.09
Walnut		2.6	
Peaches		2.4	
Pineapple		2.4	
Raisins			7.7
Custard apple (seethaphal)		4.31	
Watermelon			7.9
Dates (dried)			7.3
Apricot (dry)			4.6
Other fruits	0.6–1.5		
Fish (hilsa)		2.1	
Pomfret (black)		2.3	
Sardine		2.5	
Surmai (dried)		2.0	
Egg (hen)		2.1	
Liver (sheep)			6.3
Milk	0.2–0.3		
Jaggery (cane)		2.64	

Source: NIN, ICMR, Hyderabad, Nutritive value of Indian Foods. Revised and updated by Narsingha Rao BS, Deosrhal IG and Pant KC. (2002).Gopalan C, Rama Sastri BV and Balasubramanian SC.

albumin has been shown to have no promoting effect. It is thought that it could be linked to amino acids composition. Amino acids like cysteine, histidine and lysine have also been known to enhance iron absorption. The action of cysteine is thought to be due to its chelating and reducing powers.

Prevention of Iron Deficiency

In the light of the issues discussed above, it seems obvious that the problem of IDA, which is widely prevalent among the preschool and older children, needs to be tackled right from the beginning with a right guidance and counseling to the parents related to good diets. Prevention is better than cure, so if certain preventive steps are taken into account the prevalence of anemia can be avoided to a large extent.

These may be summarized as follows:

Enhancing/inhibitory factors: As discussed earlier due to high iron requirements in infancy and a rather monotony of the infant diet, i.e. predominately milk, which is a poor source of iron, this deficiency is widely prevalent in the developing world.

We know, that bioavailability of iron from different foods varies widely. Iron enters into two common pools that differ in their mechanism of absorption—the heme and the nonheme iron pools. Heme iron present in the hemoglobin and myoglobin is well absorbed and even helps absorption from nonheme sources. The nonheme iron which is present in vegetables, cereals and pulses, etc. is poorly absorbed and is greatly affected by enhancing or inhibiting factors in the diet (Table 14.3). Since most food iron is nonheme, the presence or absence of these substances play a vital role in the availability of dietary iron.

Breastfeeding: Infants can be prevented from falling into the pit of iron deficiency anemia right

TABLE 14.3: Factors affecting bioavailability of non-heme iron

Enhancing	Inhibiting
Meat, fish, chicken	Carbonates, oxalates, phosphates,
Ascorbic acid	phytates
Certain amino acids	Bran, vegetable fiber
	Tea
	Egg yolk

from birth itself thanks to nature's greatest gift to them that of breastfeeds. It is well established. Now that breastmilk though low in iron has a superior bioavailability compared to cows, milk. But this is only up to 6 months of their life. Beyond this breast milk is inadequate to meet the increasing demands and it is here that introduction of iron rich foods need to be introduced. So till 6 months an exclusively breastfed child can be prevented from developing anemia. Infants on cow's milk or other dairy milk run high risk of iron depletion thus leading to anemia. Again when solid food is introduced, care should be taken to take into consideration the enhancers or inhibitors of iron bioavailability. In most of the northern rural areas and even in a large section of the urban population, offering tea is a common practice. It is infact given as a medicinal drink to children suffering from respiratory problems, fevers, indigestion, etc. Thus practice of feeding tea to children should be avoided.

In our own country cooking food in iron pans is very common. This is a good practice as it is known to enhance the iron content of the food cooked in them children can be fed food cooked in these pans.

Another common practice among Indian households is use of lemon or tomatoes in their cooking. This also can help enhance the iron bioavailability of the food cooked this way. Consumption of citrus fruits or fruit juice is another simple way of enhancing iron bioavailability. Nonvegetarian families can take the advantage of using fish or meat preparations in the diets of their children to enhance the bioavailability even from nonheme iron sources.

Avoiding excess iron losses: In infants and children the commonest source of iron losses is through parasitic infections. Infants with acute or chronic diarrhea may also lose significant amounts of blood. The cumulative loss of iron occurring from repeated episodes of gastrointestinal infections can be very significant. Therefore, prevention of such infections through better sanitary conditions can significantly help in preventing iron deficiency anemia. Another contributory factor for iron losses is use of cow's milk in early infancy which in some can cause gastrointestinal bleeding. Therefore avoiding use of cow's milk or any other dairy milk in early infancy can help prevent bleeds and hence iron losses.

Food fortification: Food fortification serves as the most preferred and simple method of preventing iron deficiency anemia. Today, we can see a range of products especially the baby foods fortified with iron. Some of the infant formulae available in the market are fortified with iron which can take care of a good percentage of infants or children and help prevent anemia.

A suitable vehicle is required to do the fortification and ensure palatability and acceptance. Foods commonly preferred for fortification are either salt or cereal flour. Though not yet practiced routinely, in common household foods, extensive studies need to be undertaken to successfully ensure their availability. It is important to ensure good bioavailability, of our fortified products without compromising on the color, taste or shelf life of the food product.

Folate and B_{12} Deficiency—Megaloblastic Anemia

Besides iron deficiency anemia, another common type of anemia observed among infants and children is the folic acid deficiency. Also known as megaloblastic anemia and

B_{12} deficiency which manifests as pernicious anemia (a genetic disorder) due to the absence of the intrinsic factor in the gastric secretion. Intrinsic factor is a protein that facilitates Vitamin B_{12} absorption. The name 'megaloblastic' is due to the fact that the peripheral smear exhibits large oval red cells and hyper segmented nuclei in polymorphs.

Folate Deficiency

This is a very common cause of megaloblastic anemia in children. Initially, the needs of the infant are adequately met by human or cows milk but babies fed on goats milk generally tend to get deficient, due to negligible content of folic acid in it. This type of anemia is also termed as 'goat's milk anemia'.

Causes of Deficiency

Food folate is susceptible to heat and cooing processes, therefore, pasteurized milk reheated served times for sterilization can get deficiency in folic acid. Fresh uncooked fruits and vegetables and juices, etc. when added to the diet of children fed on pasteurized milk helps in preventing this deficiency. All unprocessed and raw foods are good sources of folic acid.

Inadequate absorption: Absorption of folic acid occurs from the upper third of the small intestine. Therefore any destruction (structural or functional) of their area can result in Megaloblastic anemia.

Certain food compounds like those found in beans which when activated by heat inhibits absorption of folic acid.

Some drugs are also known to block folate absorption like the anticonvulsants dilantin. Most children on such drugs tend to be deficient in Folate. But treating them with B_{12} can antagonize the effect of the anticonvulsant action and thereby increase the tendency for recurrent seizures.

Increased requirements: Requirements are known to increase during infancy which is the period of rapid growth and particularly so in the mature infants. Conditions causing an increase in metabolic rates, e.g. hyperthyroidism can also exert an increased requirement of folate. Children with sickle cell anemia, in which in there is increased hematopoiesis, also tend to have increased requirements. In conditions like tropical sprue also the requirement increase since the plasma levels of both vitamin B_{12} and folic acid are low, deficiency is commonly found.

Increased excretion: In conditions like renal dialysis or recurrent episodes of vomiting, folate deficiency is usually found due to the reduced ability to incorporate folate into the cells due to lack of Vitamin $B_{12.}$ It is both heat labile and water soluble.

Increased destruction: Oxidative destruction can diminish the levels of folate but they can be preserved by use of reducing substances. In scurvy, folate deficiency can be observed since low vitamin C foods are also low in folates.

CLINICAL MANIFESTATION

Classical manifestations of folate deficiency existing along with leucopenia are thrombocytopenia since folic acid deficiency affects all proliferating cells in the body rather than red cells alone. There may be presence of smooth and sore tongue. About 10% of them might have hyperpigmentation splenomegaly and or low grade fever. Features of mental changes and other neurologic signs like irritability, forgetfulness and sleeplessness may exist but there can be found in vitamin B_{12} deficiency.

Vitamin B_{12} Deficiency/Cobalamin (Pernicious Anemia)

Vitamin B_{12} is also termed as cyanocobalamin due to the fact that it is composed of cyanide group and cobalt. It is slightly water soluble, therefore likely to be leached out during prolonged cooking processes. Deficiency of B_{12} is not routinely found in infants and children since maternal stores are adequate to take care of requirements during the first year of life. Moreover, human or cows milk also does provide small amounts. Beyond 6 month when cow's milk is increased, the requirements are usually met (Refer Chapter 2, Table 2.1 for requirements of B_{12} and folic acid).

However, in mothers from families who are strict vegetarian, i.e. not even consuming milk, this, deficiency may be encountered. In these, B_{12} producing micro-organisms and animal foods are the sole source of vitamin B_{12}. So a diet devoid of even milk can produce manifestation of megaloblastic anemia of B_{12} deficiency.

B_{12} the extrinsic factor (provided by diet) absorption takes place in the presence of another protein called the intrinsic factor, a glycoprotein which is present in the gastric secretion produced by the gastric parietal cells. In pernicious anemia, vitamin B_{12} is not absorbed due to the atrophic changes in the stomach wall and scanty secretion of the intrinsic factor. The absorption of B_{12} takes place in the ileum in pH 6–8 in the presence of a divalent ion like calcium. Therefore in conditions like ileal inflammation due to tuberculosis or resection of the ileal malabsorption or absorption can be impaired. However, diffuse absorption does occur throughout the length of the small intestine.

Clinical Manifestations

Deficiency of vitamin B_{12} generally occurs due to the absence of the intrinsic factor of the stomach leading to malabsorption of orally consumed vitamin $B_{12.}$ Specific manifestations of B_{12} deficiency occurs in the form of hematological and neurological changes.

The hematological changes are evidently by macrocytic anemia where in the blood smear shows variation in size and shape of the red cells. Neurological changes generally manifest in the form of spinal cord degeneration. These are however not very common among children. Mental changes like, depression psychosis and loss of mental energy may be seen in some cases which respond to B_{12} therapy.

Treatment involves intramuscular injection of B_{12} in therapeutic doses.

REFERENCES

1. Indian Council of Medical Research Studies on Pre-School Children. Technical Report Series No.26, New Delhi, ICMR. 1977.
2. Report of the Working Group on Fortification of Salt with Iron. Use of common salt Fortified with Iron in the Control and Prevention of Anemia. A collaborative study. Am J Clin Nutr 1982;35:1442-5.
3. Nutritional Anemias': Report of a WHO Scientific Group. WHO Technical Report series No.405, Geneva, World Health Organization. 1968.
4. Satyanarayana K, Pradhan DR, Ramnath T, et al. Anemia and physical fitness of school children of rural Hyderabad: Ind Pediatr. 1990;27:715-21.
5. World Heath Organization. Causes of death. Anemias Wld Hlth Stat Q. 1962;15:594-604.
6. Layrisse M, Rocke M. The relationship between anemia and hookworm infestation. Amer J Trop Med Hyg. 1964;79:279-301.
7. Narsingha Rao BS, Deorshall IG, Pant KC. Nutritive Value of Indian Foods. National Institute of Nutrition, ICMR, Hyderabad. 2002.

15 Iodine Deficiency Disorders in Children

Iodine is an essential micronutrient that occurs in soil and seawater in the form of iodides. It is oxidized by sunlight to iodine, which is a volatile substance. The concentrate of iodine in seawater is only 0.05 mg/l. If there are excessive losses of this nutrient from the sea without any correction, it may ultimately lead to deficit in the soil which can persist indefinitely. Crops grown in soil or water produced from such areas then tend to be deficient in iodine. Consumption of food produced form such crops can lead to deficiency of iodine, which is responsible for an array of disorder commonly termed as iodine deficiency disorder (IDD). Goiter and cretinism are the two clinical manifestations of endemic iodine deficiency, prevalent in many parts of the developing world.

Hetzel first used the world iodine deficiency disorder (IDD) in 1982 to denote all the effects of iodine deficiency on a population growth and development, which could be totally prevented by correction of the deficiency.[1] Though these effects can be evident in all stages of life, the most affected stages of human life are the fetus, neonate, infancy and pregnancy also to some extent.

Estimates exist, that about 800 million people living in iodine deficient environment throughout the world are exposed to the risk of IDD. Out of them 190 million are known to suffer form goiter and another 3.15 million from cretinism.[2]

FUNCTIONS OF IODINE

Iodine is considered an essential micronutrient due to the fact that it is a constituent of the thyroid hormone, thyroxine T4 and triiodothyronine T3, essential for normal mental and physical development in humans and animals and also for development of the brain and maintenance of body temperature. Deficiency of the hormone can lead to severe retardation and growth maturation of almost all organ systems. The total iodine content in healthy adult man is about 15–20 µg, 70%–80% of which is present in the thyroid gland. Daily requirement of iodine is about 150 µg.[2]

IN ENERGY METABOLISM

The thyroid hormone has an important role in the rate of oxidation in the cells of the body. An increased secretion of thyroxine speeds up the rate of energy metabolism. On the contrary, lack of it can retard the rate. Besides basal metabolic rate as a method for assessing the state of thyroid function, there are two other parameters used to assess the thyroxine function which are:

a. Determining the protein bound iodine (PBI) in the blood serum.
b. Observation on the utilization of radioactive iodine.

The PBI is chiefly thyroxine. It is found to be low in hypothyroidism and elevated in hyperthyroidism.

GROWTH AND DEVELOPMENT

Thyroxine is essential for the normal growth and development of the young. Inadequate levels can lead to growth retardation, which if severe and prolonged results in failure to mature physically and mentally. In children, this form of growth retardation is known as

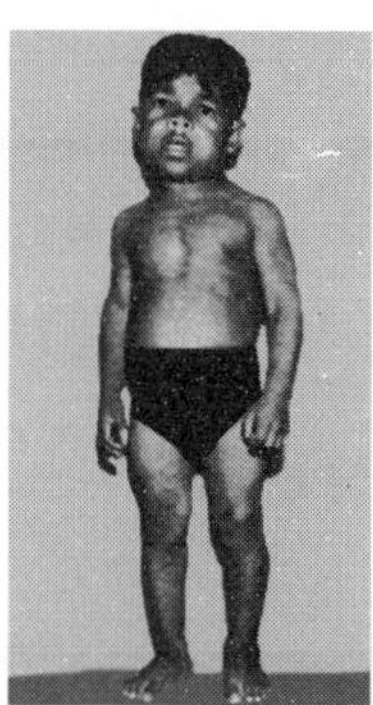

Figure 15.1: A child suffering from cretinism (Adapted from Scrimshaw NS. Endemic goiter, Nutr Rev. 1957;15:161)

'cretinism'. Besides as shown in Figure 15.1[3] arrested growth, their facial features appear coarse and swollen, the skin is thick, dry and pasty in appearance and deeply wrinkled. The tongue is enlarged and lips appear thickened and stay ajar usually.

In adults thyroxine deficiency is known as 'myxoedema'. The skin and subcutaneous tissue, particularly of the face and extremities are thickened and puffy. The face is characteristically expressionless and the person appears lethargic and inactive.

Iodine deficiency disorder (IDD) has been described as the world's single most significant cause of preventable brain damage and mental retardation. It affects about 14% of the world's population and 834 million persons are affected by goiter. There exist 43 millions cases of preventable brain damage caused by iodine deficiency.[4]

IN PREGNANCY AND LACTATION

Iodine has an important role in normal reproduction in both sexes. Goiter is generally known to occur in pregnancy, indicating a greater need for the thyroid hormone.

Metabolism of Iodine

Iodine is readily absorbed both in organic and inorganic form. Most of the iodine is absorbed form the small gut and excreted by the kidney. Iodine enters the circulation and is taken up by the thyroid gland and other tissue. The thyroid gland concentrates the element and serves as a storehouse for it. Iodine is oxidized by hydrogen peroxidase from the thyroid peroxidase system. This oxidized iodine combines with the amino acid 'thyroxine' present in the thyroglobulin to form monoiodotyrosine (MIT) and diiodotyrosine (DIT).

By the coupling of the MIT and DIT, T4 and T3 are formed. The iodized thyroglobulin is absorbed back into the thyroid cells, where it undergoes proteolysis, releasing T4 and T3 into the blood. This entire process of absorption, synthesis and release of thyroxine is regulated by thyroid stimulating hormone (TSH) secreted by the pituitary gland.

The body can auto regulate its iodine supply. When thyroxine levels are down, it is assumed that some of the iodine is saved for reuse. This salvaged iodine joins that absorbed form the gastrointestinal tract (GIT) in a common pool for use.

Spectrum of IDD

As mentioned earlier, some stages of life are affected adversely by the deficiency of iodine. There can be grouped as

Fetus	: Abortions Stillbirths Congenital anomalies Increased perinatal mortality Increased infant mortality Neurological cretinism Myxoedematous cretinism Psychomotor defects
Neonate	: Neonate goiter Neonate chemical hypothyroidism
Infancy	: Goiter, thyroid deficiency (loss of energy) Impaired school performance, Retarded Physical development
Adults	: Goiter with its complications Hypothyroidism Impaired mental functions.

Goiter

Goiter is a term applied for an enlargement of the thyroid gland, which, if is due to iodine deficiency is also termed endemic goiter. In this condition, the thyroxine level in the blood is lower than normal, which stimulates the thyroid gland to greater action,

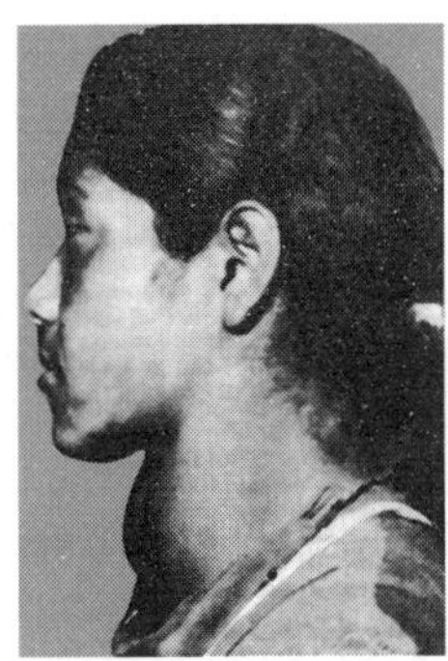

FIGURE 15.2: A young woman showing endemic goiter
(Adapted from Scrimshaw NS. Endemic goiter, Nutr Rev. 1957;15:161)

tending to cause it to enlarge as seen in Figure 15.2.[3] This condition is characteristically associated with children. The rate of incidence of goiter increases with age and reaches the maximum level by adolescence. The prevalence rate is more among girls as compared to boys. A large percentage of children in a population could be suffering from iodine deficiency leading to lethargy, which in the long run can cause irreparable losses due to fall in output in households and in the work place.

These can ultimately have its toll on high costs of medical and institutional care. Mental disability leads to poor school performance by children thus producing long term effects in their lives.[5]

Cretinism

Cretinism is a term used to denote severe iodine deficiency during intrauterine life. This includes a wide range of disorders like mental deficiency, deaf mutism and spastic paralysis of legs in varying degrees are associated with this condition. There are two types of cretinism which are known clinically:

a. Neurological cretinism: This involves mental retardation, deaf mutism, squint and spastic rigidity affecting the lower limbs.
b. Myxedematous cretinism: In this condition, sings of hypothyroidism are observed, e.g. coarse, dry skin, swollen tongue, deep horse voice, apathy and mental deficiency. Signs like, sluggish bowel sounds and weak abdominal muscles may also be observed.

Hypothyroidism

This condition is characterized by signs like course dry skin, husky voice and delayed tendon reflexes.

Psychomotor Defects

Low or inadequate iodine levels in school children have shown poor scholastic performance and lower IQ levels, besides poor motor coordination.

Imparied Mental Function

Reduced mental functions have been observed in populations with low iodine levels. They have low intelligence levels and high degree of apathy which is evident by lack of initiative and decision making capacity in people.

Assessment of IDD in a Community

The parameters helpful in assessing the extent of prevalence of IDD in a community can be gauged by a few simple signs and laboratory tests like:

- Prevalence of goiter
- Prevalence of cretinism
- Urinary iodine excretion
- Serum T4 levels
- Serum TSH levels
- Prevalence of neonatal chemical hypothyroidism
- Iodine levels in drinking water
- Iodine levels in the soil.

Classification of IDD

Based on the severity of the problem IDD has been graded into three categories as follows:

Mild IDD: When in an endemic area, urinary iodine level ranges from 5.0–9.99 µg/dl and goiter prevalence is 10%–30%, it is considered as mild. At this stage mental and physical growth are not affected and the thyroid hormone levels too may be normal.

Moderate IDD: In moderate IDD, the median urinary iodine excretion level is 2.0–4.99 µg/dl and prevalence rate of goiter is about 20%–50%. Thyroid hormone levels may be reduced with increased risk of hypothyroidism. Sings of cretinism however may be absent.

Severe IDD: Areas with median urinary iodine levels of 2.0 µg/dl or less and goiter prevalence of 30–100% are considered to be severe. Here presence of marked hypothyroidism, mental retardation and cretinism are obvious.

Causes of IDD (Antithyroid Factors)

Geoclimatic Factors

Iodine deficiency disorder (IDD) occurs mainly due to geoclimatic factors. It is mainly the low content of soil which is responsible for the environmental iodine deficiency. This is particularly seen in hilly areas, where iodine content is lost due to years of washing of the soil by glaciers and heavy rains and in plains by recurrent flooding. These conditions tend to leech out the iodine form the soil which further result in lower levels of all vegetation grown in that soil. Deforestation and soil erosion add to compound the problem further.

Drugs

In Kerala studies conducted by Kerala agricultural university revealed that frequent consumptions of tapioca could be one reason for prevalence of goiter in that area. It is due to the presence of hydro-organic acid which blocks the uptake of iodine by thyroid causing gland. (Tapioca and goiter incidence of Kerala, 1998).[6]

A second group of drugs which appear to block thyroxine synthesis even in the presence of adequate iodine are thiourea, thiouracil, phenol derivatives and cobaltous chlorides.

Antithyroid Compounds in Foods

There are certain dietary factors which can inhibit the uptake of iodine. These are termed as "goitrogenic" due to the fact that they increase susceptibility to goiter resulting from iodine deficiency.

Cabbage is known to have an antithyroid compounds as also the seeds of most of the mustard family. The substance is known as goitrin.[7]

A precursor of goitrin, progoitrin is also present in the seeds of some plants and has been identified in plants like white turnips. Progoitrin is active only when converted to goitrin. These compounds are not heat labile and hence raw and cooked form both can be potentially goitrogenic.

Continuous ingestion of small amounts of goitrin or other unidentified goitrogens that may exist could alter normal thyroid hormone synthesis.

Polluted water with presence of *E. coli* tends to produce goitrogenic substances.[8] Organic chlorine insecticides widely used in agriculture can cause goiter.

Endemic goiter is also found where sandstone type of soil which is rich in lime and calcium is present.[9]

Faulty cooking and dietary practices which reduce the bioavailability of iodine make Keralites prone to IDD.[6]

Prevalence of more than 4% goiter in a given place indicates iodine deficiency in the soil or in the food grain grown in that place.

Prevention of IDD

Dietary sources of iodine although exist, are too small in amounts to present deficiency in endemic areas.

The WHO study group on endemic goiter in the early fifties had recommended that all food salts should be iodized compulsorily in any country or area where goiter is endemic, local variations in incidence of disease being disregarded.[10]

The easiest way of prevention of goiter in an endemic area is found to be fortification of food items with iodine or iodine supplementation

IODINE FORTIFICATION

Fortification of salt has been the most successful way of preventing goiter. Other food items like wheat flour, methi, sugar or drinking water have also been practiced in different parts of the world.

The reason why salt has been widely used is due to the fact that it is universally consumed by all sections of the community irrespective of economic status and is consumed in the same level throughout the year. Production of salt is confined to a few production centers. By adding a dose of fixed iodine to salt at centralized locations, the majority of the population can have access to adequate amounts of iodine. The mixing of salt is simple with no adverse chemical reactions. Nor is there any change in color, taste or odor, besides being cost effective also.

Certain studies have shown that nonvegetarians have higher levels of iodine as compared to vegetarian though there are other reports which have not been consistent with these findings.[11]

Salt can be fortified either with potassium iodate or potassium iodide. Fortification with potassium iodide is more stable, hence commonly used. Daily consumption of 10 gm of iodate salt (25 ppm of potassium iodate), provides about 150 μg of iodine. This level of fortified salt if used on regular basis can help prevent mild to moderate degree of deficiency disorders.

Certain Points to be Considered While Using Iodized Salt

- According to nutrition advisory ministry of family welfare of the government of India, the date of manufacturing should be stamped on salt packets, which must be moisture proof. This is done, since iodized salt needs to be consumed within one year of iodization. According to NIN (Hyderabad), under standard conditions including transportation by rail or road, 25–30% of iodine is lost within 3 months and 40–60% within one year of iodization.[12]
- Salt should not be stored in open space or damp places and never beyond 6 months. It should be protected from moisture, sunlight and high temperature. Containers should be air tight and prevent from humidity in the air. The moisture content in the salt, humidity in the air, acidity of the salt and chemical form of iodine are important factors limiting the stability of iodine.[12]
- Salt should be added the food after cooking to reduce the loss of iodine. Addition of salt before cooking hastens the loss of other nutrients including iodine. Cooking losses and extent of absorption are some of the factors, which determine the availability of iodine to the body.

Non-iodized salt has been banned in most of the states in the country. Therefore only iodized salt alone should be used.

Iodized Oil Injecions

Oil injections of iodine can provide iodine for 4 years but is used only in selected populations. But this practice had been strongly opposed by Goplan since thousands of disposable syringes would be used and a whole array of 'injectors'.[13]

Iodine Tablets

Although iodine tablets of 100–500 μg of potassium iodate are available for daily use, it is difficult to implement their use regularly and ensure its proper utilization regularly. Oral administration needs direct target contact therefore, their method has not been very popular.

Iodized Water

Fortification of water by iodine was introduced by Dr Rosaiuwanik of Bangkok. Since water is a daily necessity like salt, potassium iodate is added to the water stored in vessels for drinking purpose. However, again it had many limitations, like water consumed varies from day to day and season to season, the water may also not be totally safe for drinking if not stored hygienically. More over the iodine mixed in water may not be acceptable in taste and odor.[14]

IDD the Indian Scenario

Iodine deficiency disorder (IDD) has been described as the world's single most significant causes of preventable brain damage and mental retardation. It affects about 14% of the world's population and 834 million people are affected by goiter.[15] The average goiter prevalence in Asia is about 7.3%.[16]

In India, estimate made in 1989 suggested that 150 million persons are at risk form IDD, 54 million people had goiter and 2.2 million people suffered from cretinism.[17] Table 15.1 gives an estimate of a total of 275 districts surveyed in the country in 1998, of which 235 have been found endemic for IDD.[18]

Nearly 90,000 still births or neonatal deaths occur in India due to IDD. The Himalayan goiter belt is the worlds' greatest IDD affected area, and spread to 2400 Km form Jammu in the North West and Kashmir to Manipur in the North East. As per estimate in 1997 no state in India was found to be IDD free.[19]

Biochemical hypothyroidism has been reported up to 10% among neonates in northern India.[20]

The National Goiter Control Program (NGCP) which was initiated in 1962 by the Government of India, to survey the magnitude of this problem was redesignated as National Iodine Deficiency Disorder Control Program (NIDDCP) in 1992. In 1996, the

WHO declared 90% iodization of edible salt in its member countries.

TABLE 15.1: Prevalence of iodine deficiency disorders in different states/UTs of India

State	Total number of districts	No. of districts surveyed	No. Districts endemic
Andhra Pradesh	23	7	6
Arunachal Pradesh	10	10	10
Assam	18	18	18
Bihar	38	22	21
Goa	02	02	02
Gujarat	19	16	08
Haryana	16	09	08
Himachal Pradesh	12	10	10
Jammu and Kashmir	15	14	11
Karnataka	20	17	06
Kerala	14	14	11
Madhya Pradesh	45	16	16
Maharashtra	31	29	21
Mizoram	04	04	04
Manipur	08	08	08
Meghalaya	05	02	–
Nagaland	07	07	07
Orissa	30	02	02
Punjab	12	03	03
Rajastan	27	03	03
Sikkim	04	04	04
Tamil Nadu	21	12	12
Tripura	03	03	03
Uttar Pradesh	67	34	29

Ministry of Family Welfare, Government of India (1998)[18]

The objective of this project was to reduce the prevalence of goiter in the age groups of 10–14 years to less than 5% and to bring down to zero, the number of cretin born by the year 2000. It was aimed to provide iodized salt to 100% population by strengthening the monitoring system from production to consumption level.[21]

The effects and benefits of iodine intervention indicated were:

Effects	Benefits
Reductions in:	
1. Mental deficiency	1. Higher work output in the household and in work place
2. Deaf mutism	2. Reduced cost of medical care and custodial care
3. Spastic diplegia	3. Reduced education cost from reduced absenteeism and grade repetition and higher academic achievement by students
4. Squint	
5. Dwarfism	
6. Motor deficiency	

DIETARY SOURCES OF IODINE

Iodine content from dietary sources depends to a large extent on the soil and fertilizer conditions from soil of one region to that of another. Marine or deep sea fish and shell fish are high in iodine content. Sea water contain about 0.05 mg/l (0.05 ppm) of iodine. People consuming sea weed which is grown along the coastal areas can get adequate quantities of iodine.

The leaves and flower of plants (spinach, turnip green and broccoli) appear to have higher iodine concentration than the root vegetables.

Drinking water provides about 10%, and about 90% comes from the food consumed depending upon the soil on which the crop is produced.

Although fish is rich in iodine, but since the thyroid gland which is rich in it, is located in the head, it is of little value if the head part of the fish is discarded. Sea salt is also considered rich in iodine, containing 0.28 ppm of iodine.[22]

REFERENCES

1. Hetzel BS. Iodine deficiency disorders (IDD) and their eradication. Lancet. 1983;11:1126.
2. GNV Brahmam. Iodine deficiency disorders. In: Textbook of Nutrition, Eds. Mahtab S Bamji, Prahlad Rao N, Reddy V. Oxford & IBH Publishing Co. Pvt. Ltd. New Delhi. 1996;278-86.
3. Scrimshaw NS. Endemic guitor, Nutr Rev. 1957;15:161.
4. World Health Organization 1998, Iodine deficiency Disorders, In: J Trop Pediatr. 1998;44(5):270-74.
5. Jayakrishna T, Jeeja MC. Iodine deficiency disorders in school children in Kannur Dist. (2002), Kerala Research Level Development Center for Development Studies, Thiruvananthapuram Iodine deficiency disorders in school children in Kannur Dist. (2002), Kerala Research Level Development Center for Development Studies, Thiruvananthapuram.
6. Kerala Sastra Sahihtya Parishat, Keralathile Samakaika Arogya Prasnangal. KSSP. 1998.
7. Greece MA. The significance of naturally occurring anti thyroid compounds in the production of goiter in man. Border's Rev Nutr Res. 1960;21:61.
8. Kulkarni AP, Bharath JP. Textbook of Community Medicine. 1998.
9. Mahajan BK, Gupta MC. Textbook of Preventive and Social Medicine, Jaypee Brothers, New Delhi. 1995.
10. WHO Study Group on Endemic Goiter. Bull Wrld Hlth Orgn. 1953;9:293.
11. Remer T, Neubert A, Manz F. Increased risk of iodine deficiency with vegetarian nutrition, Br J Nutr. 1999;81(1).
12. Narsingha Rao BS. Fortification of salt with iron and iodine to control anemia and goiter: Development of a new formula with good stability and bio availability of iron and iodine, National Institute of Nutrition, ICMR Bulletin, Hyderabad. 1996.
13. Gopalan C. Micronutrient malnutrition, SAARC. The need for food based approach. Nutrition Foundation of India (NFI) Bull, New Delhi. 1998.
14. John T Dunn. Iodine supplementation and the prevention of cretinism. Annals of the New York Academy of Sciences. 1993;678(1):158-68.
15. World Health Organization Report,1998,1999.
16. World Health Organisation. Iodine Deficiency Disorders in South East Asia, WHO/SEARO Regional Health papers, No. 10, WHO, New Delhi. 1985.
17. Kochupillai N. Organisation and Implementation of neonatal hypothyroid screening program in India. A primary health care approach, Ind J Ped. 1985;52:223.
18. Government of India, National Iodine Deficiency Control Program. Ministry of Family Welfare. 1998.
19. Park K. Textbook of Preventive and Social Medicine, Bonarside's Bhanot Publishers. 1997.
20. Kochupillai N, Pandav CS. Neonatal chemical hypothyroidism in iodine deficient environments. In: The Prevention and Control of Iodine Deficiency Disorders. Eds. B S Hetzel, JT Dunn and JB Stanbury, Amsterdam: Publ; Elsevier.
21. International Council for Control of iodine deficiency disorders (ICCIDD), Proposed guidelines for assessment of progress towards IDD elimination. IDD Newsletter. 1995;1192:19.
22. Pandav CS, David P, Hunton, Hema Viswanathan. Partnership to end hidden hunger, Collaboration of the stakeholders in sustaining elimination of iodine deficiency disorders. SOS a Billion. 1997.

16 Zinc in Infant Nutrition

Zinc is one of the numerous trace elements which are known to have a significant role in the growth and development of an infant. In fact its role has been attributed right from the antenatal period, as deficiency of this micronutrient can have a crucial bearing upon the health of the new born. Prasad defined the role of zinc in human nutrition in 1991. It was the observation between increased susceptibility to infectious diseases and nutritional zinc deficiency which led to the increased interest in the importance of this trace element.[1]

Zinc is required in over 200 enzymes and hence likely to affect a number of various systems in the human body. Severe to moderate zinc deficiency has been found to cause oxidative damage to the proteins, lipids and DNA in rat testes[2] which may be due to iron accumulation or a reduction in zinc dependent antioxidant processes.

Zinc is present in all organs, tissues and other body fluids. It is primarily an intercellular ion with intracellular zinc contributing to more than 95% of the total body zinc. Skeletal muscle and bone together contain 80% of the total body zinc. It is widely distributed within the cells bound to protein. It governs a wide range of body functions:

1. ***Cell division and growth***: Zinc has vital role in cell division and growth. It governs cellular growth and differentiation. Early zinc deficiency reduces cell division which in turn affects growth as an adaptive mechanism.
2. ***Membrane Function***: Zinc has an important role in the stabilization of biomembranes by binding sulfhydryl groups and forming mercaptides. Decrease in biomembrane zinc is suggested as one of the early biochemical lesions of zinc deficiency.
3. ***Protection against free radical change***: Zinc is believed to have a role as an antioxidant against free radical related diseases. Liver injury, chronic inflammatory conditions, essential fatty acid deficiency, cancer and radiation damage are all associated with decreased levels of zinc in the body.
4. ***Zinc and sex hormones:*** Deficiency of zinc is known to impair testosterone production in humans. In pregnant females difficult labor is believed to be a manifestation of zinc deficiency.
5. ***Zinc and immune functions***: Animal studies have confirmed the role of zinc in maintaining the immune levels in the body. This is considered to be due to its role in cell proliferation and other cellular functions. Zinc is essential for the function of many enzymes, which are vital for the growth, and regulation of immune cells.
6. ***Zinc and mental development***: In experimental animals it has been demonstrated that zinc deficiency has on impact on the fetal outcome. This affect is however dependant on the degree and duration of deficiency. The adverse affects on fetal outcome could be in the form of congenital malformation and fetal resorption. In humans however, such affects are not well established in case of mild or border line deficiency states.
7. ***Zinc and brain development***: Deficiency of zinc is known to have adverse affects on the cerebral

morphology and also on behavioral development of animals.

8. ***Zinc and vitamins***: Zinc is present in high concentration in the retina and other ocular tissues, therefore considered to be interrelated with vitamin A metabolism especially in relation to vision. Its deficiency can also affect night vision despite adequate amounts of retinol concentration.
9. ***Zinc and metals***: Zinc is considered to be adversely affected by interaction by certain metals like iron, calcium and copper if present in excess.

METABOLISM

Zinc is absorbed from the proximal bowel. 60% of the circulating plasma zinc is found loosely bound to albumin and amino acids, while the remaining 40% is tightly bound to alpha globulins and is not free to diffuse into the tissues. The total zinc content in the human body is about 2–3 grams. Almost 50% of the total body zinc is in bone and is not readily available for metabolic needs. Zinc is not stored as such in the body which implies that there has to be a continuous provision of this micronutrient through the diet for tissue growth and repair.

Excretion of zinc is mainly through the stool. In fact the total zinc content is around 54 mg, 60% of which is passed to the fetus in the last trimester at the rate of about 30 micrograms per kg. of body weight per day. Inadequate amounts of dietary zinc or increased losses may place the infant at increased risk of developing deficiency.

The zinc content of breast milk is quite high, the concentrations in Indian mothers being about 36.1 μmol/l during the first week of lactation and gradually decreases to 24.4, 22.6 and 20.2 μmols/lt by 3, 6 and 9 months respectively.[3]

This concentration can vary from one mother to another although not significantly. The average daily intake of zinc in an infant works up to about 1.75 mg at 4 weeks, 0.83 mg at 12 weeks and 0.40 mg at 24 weeks.[4]

Zinc Requirements

Zinc deficiency in humans is mainly due to a lack of bioavailable zinc in the diet, general malnutrition or malabsorption.[5]

Nutritional zinc requirements are influenced by many dietary factors that affect its bioavailability and physiological requirements which vary greatly between different age groups. On the basis of current evidence, the suggested recommended dietary intake of zinc during the first half of infancy is 3–4 mg/d, between 6–12 months is 6 mg/d and during later childhood it becomes 10 mg/d.[6] The requirements increase in the preterm low birth weight and children recovering from malnutrition. These requirements are considered for Indian children as well. For adults the zinc requirement has been set as 15.5 mg/d[7] which are in accordance with the values suggested by WHO.[8]

Implications of Zinc Deficiency

Zinc is perhaps one trace element, the deficiency of which has been implicated with a wide variety of problems like acrodermatitis enteropathica, sickle cell anemia, immunological disorders, and neurological disorders and even in the outcome of pregnancy. Its role has been well described in the treatment of diarrheas, infections and protein energy malnutrition.

In children moderate to severe zinc deficiency is known to depress skeletal growth and gonad development which were found to reverse on zinc therapy.[1,9]

Zinc Status in Pregnancy

Zinc deficiency in pregnancy not only affects the mother, but it also has immunological consequences for the fetus. Various immune defects have been reported in animal studies. One of the earliest and clinically most relevant signs of maternal zinc deficiency are low levels of natural immunoglobulins including a persistent defect in IgM and transiently diminished levels of IgA and IgG2 in neonates. The explanation proposed for this is diminished transport of immunoglobulins. Besides, the reduction in total amount of antigen, there is in addition, depressed repertoire of antigens recognized by these antibodies. This effect has been described even in mild transient deficiency.[10]

Prenatal zinc deficiency might also have an important effect on child immunity as observed in animal studies. Hypogammaglobulinemia together with altered antibody repertoire and decreased T cell proliferation in response to T cell dependent antigens may lead to impaired success of vaccination in the infant, which in turn can have important consequences for the health status of the population. In humans, immunological defects may possibly have a bearing on subsequent generations as suggested by animal studies which may be irreversible.[11]

Supplementation trials on pregnant women who can be at risk of zinc deficiency have not been conclusive. Controversy exists between different authors regarding the role of supplementation in this group, therefore no extra dose, is required except, when there might be some definite indication for deficiency.

Zinc and Childhood Infections

Zinc and diarrhea: Zinc deficiency has been associated with high rates of infectious diseases including skin infections, diarrhea and respiratory infections besides malaria and delayed wound healing. In the developing countries extensive studies have been done regarding diarrhea and respiratory infections. These trials were done in pre-school children who were representative of poor country population. The results from all the groups showed that zinc supplemented children have lower rates of diarrhea than those of normal children.[12] Trial studies of zinc supplementation during acute persistent diarrhea have shown consistent benefits of zinc supplementation. These benefits were in the form of shorter episode duration of diarrhea. More significantly, there were large reductions in the rate of 'treatment failure' or death in these trials.

Zinc supplementation is known to significantly reduce lactulose excretion in persistent diarrhea and this effect was seen to be more marked in malnourished children. Therefore, zinc has a significant effect on intestinal integrity and is likely to contribute to a better recovery. Besides, children with diarrhea who received supplementation 15 mg of zinc acetate per day had significantly greater gains in height and weight in the following 9 weeks than unsupplemented children.[13] It was therefore suggested that for preventive use of zinc, there is need to evaluate various ways to improve the zinc nutriture in children in developing countries. These include dietary sources and availability of zinc, fortifying foods with zinc and supplementation programs.

Zinc and respiratory infections: Several field studies have shown that zinc supplementation is beneficial in preventing pneumonia in children in developing countries. A pooled analysis (Zinc Investigators Collaborative Grouup, 1999) has shown that zinc supplemented children have a 41% reduced rate of pneumonia compared to the controlled group.[14]

Zinc in protein energy malnutrition: Rehabilitation from severe protein energy malnutrition requires the provision of adequate quantities of macro and micronutrients. Zinc deficiency has been implicated as a limiting factor in recovery[15] and WHO recommends that all severely malnourished children be treated with zinc along with other micronutrients.

A study from India[16] has shown that though there was no difference in weight gain between zinc supplemented and placebo group, the former showed an increase in plasma zinc which rose to normal levels. In the latter group, the plasma zinc decreased significantly during the period of rapid growth. This indicates that though dietary zinc may be sufficient for efficient weight gain, it is not able to compensate for the extra requirements demanded in the process of new tissue deposition.

Zinc and cognitive development: The role of zinc in the cognitive development and behavior of a child has been explained based on its critical role in the function of several structural regulatory and catalytic proteins. It is present in the brain bound to proteins and is important for its structure and function.[17,18] There is also some evidence to suggest that zinc deficiency results in lowered levels of ω-3 and ω-6 chains possibly causing impaired fatty acid metabolism in the neurons.[19]

Moreover, it seems to be important for neurogenesis, neuoral migration and synaptogenesis and its deficiency could interfere with neuro-transmission and subsequent neurophysiological development. Besides zinc is also understood to be involved in the metabolism of thyroid hormones, receptor functions and transport of other hormones that could influence the central nervous system.[20]

Findings from studies in monkeys suggest that the zinc deprived group showed progressive decline in day time activity and attention performance. The study also indicates that zinc deprived adolescents may be more susceptible to behavioral changes before the onset of growth retardation.[21] Studies from India have shown a positive association between zinc deprivation and activity in malnourished children. Reduced activity inhibits exploration which may contribute directly to diminished cognitive development. It was observed from this study that children randomized to receive 10 mg/d of zinc gluconate in addition to the vitamins A, B_1 B_2, B_6, D_3, E and niacinamide, spent 72% more time performing high movement activities like running. The effects were greater in boys and this could be due to extra zinc requirement in them. Among the zinc supplemented group, the activity rating was 12% and 8% higher by a previously validated children's activity rating and the energy expenditure score respectively.[22]

There is evidence to prove the association between zinc status and neurophysiological behavior also. Supplementation with zinc have resulted in alteration in fetal neurobehavior, better motor development in very low birth weight infants, more vigorous physical activity in malnourished infants and toddlers and improved neuropsychological functions in school age children.

Zinc deficiency affects cognitive development by alterations in attention, activity, other features of neuropsychological behavior and motor development. These effects vary by age and may be influenced by the care giving environment, particularly the behavior of the mother and the social context.[23]

Acrodermatitis enteropathica: The most extreme forms of zinc deficiency can be studied in zinc specific malabsorption syndrome 'acrodermatitis enteropathica'; a rare autosomal recessive inheritable disease[24] which appears to be more common in girls.

This disorder manifests insidiously from the age of weaning, characterized by severe skin lesions, alopecia, failure to thrive and diarrhea. The lesions appear typically on the cheeks, knees and elbows. The hair becomes reddish in color. Even ocular manifestations in the form of photophobia, conjunctivitis and corneal dystrophy can be observed. Associated characteristics like chronic diarrhea, stomatitis, glossitis, personality changes, intercurent bacterial infections are also commonly seen. Administration of oral zinc therapy in doses of 50–150 mg/d reverses the symptoms dramatically.

A possible role of zinc involving metabolic inters relationship with other micronutrients has also been postulated.[25] Some of these are:

- Zinc deficiency may lead to poor mobilization of hepatic stores of vitamin A and thus cause hypovitaminosis.
- Zinc absorption may be affected by inorganic iron.
- Zinc may also depress copper absorption which can lead to biochemical evidence of copper deficiency.

Zinc Toxicity

Although toxicity of zinc is not common, it is known to occur if ingested in large quantities in the form of inhaled fumes of zinc. Vomiting follows about 3 hours after ingestion of excess zinc. Dehydration, electrolyte imbalance abdominal pain, nausea dizziness and lethargy are some of the other symptoms known to occur if taken in large amounts. If taken over a prolonged period, it interferes with copper metabolism which results in severe anemia, neutropenia reduced serum levels of iron and even immunosuppression. If taken in excess during pregnancy, it can adversely affect the fetus too.[24]

Dietary Sources of Zinc

If a normal balanced diet is taken the requirements are generally met with. Good sources of zinc are whole pulses, nuts like almonds and cashew, oilseeds like gingelly, mustard, safflower and poppy seeds.

CONCLUSION

As per evidence available from Indian data, it was suggested that since isolated zinc deficiency rarely exists in pregnancy or in new borns' and older children, routine supplementation of zinc is not warranted. However, during treatment and rehabilitation phase of severe PEM or persistent diarrhea, zinc supplementation in the required doses is justified, where even other micronutrient supplement is also given in view of coexisting deficiencies.

REFERENCES

1. Prasad AS. Discovery of human zinc deficiency and studies in an experimental human model. Am J Clin Nutr. 1991;53:403-12.
2. Oteza PJ, Olin KL, Fraga CG, Keen CL. Zinc deficiency causes oxidative damage to proteins, lipids and DNA in rat testes, J Nutr. 1995;125:823-29.
3. Bhaskaram P, Hemalatha P. Zinc status in breast fed infants. Lancet. 1992;2:1416-17.
4. Zlotkin SH. Assessment of trace element requirements (zinc) in new borns and young infants, including the infant born prematurely. In: Trace Elements in Nutrition of Children-II Ed. Chandra RK, Nestle Nutrition Workshop New York, Raven Press. 1991;(23):49-77.
5. Prasad AS. Zinc: an overview, Nutrition 1995;11:93-99.
6. Hambidge KM. Zinc in the nutrition of children. In: Trace elements in Nutrition of children-II Ed. Chandra RK. Nestle Nutrition Workshop, New York, Raven press. 1991;(23):9965-77.
7. ICMR, Nutritional requirements and recommended dietary allowances for Indians. A Report of the Expert Group of the Indian Council of Medical Research. 2002;41-42.
8. World Health Organization. Trace Elements in Human Nutrition (WHO Tech Rep Sr No. 532).
9. Agget PJ, Severe zinc deficiency In: Zinc in Human Biology. Ed. Mills CF. Berlin, Springer Verlag. 1988;259-79.
10. Prasad AS. Discovery of human zinc deficiency and studies in an experimental human model. Am J Clin Nutr. 1991;53:403-12.
11. Shankar AH, Prasad AS. Zinc and immune function: the biological basis of altered resistance and infection. Am J Clin Nutr. 1998;68:447S-63S.
12. Beach RS, Gershwin ME, Hurley LS. Persistent immunological consequences of gestational zinc deprivation. Am J Clin Nutr. 1983;38:579-90.
13. Sazawal S, Black R, Bhan M, et al. Zinc supplementation in children with acute diarrhea in India. N Eng J Med. 1995;333:839-44.
14. Behrans RH, Tomkins AM, Roy SK. Zinc supplementation during diarrhea: A fortification against malnutrition. Lancet. 1990;2:442-3.
15. Zinc Investigators Collaborative Group. Prevention of diarrhea and pneumonia by zinc supplementation in children in developing countries: pooled analysis of randomized controlled trials. J Pediatr. 1999;135: 689-97.
16. Hemalatha P, Bhaskaran P, Khan MM. Role of zinc supplementation in the rehabilitation of severely malnourished children. Eur J Clin Nutr. 1993;47: 395-9.
17. Fierka C. Function and mechanism of zinc. J Nutr. 2000;130:1437S-46S.
18. Hambidge M. Humanzinc deficiency. J Nutr. 2000;130: 13445-95.
19. Wauben PM, Wainwright PE. The influence of neonatal nutrition on behavioral development: a critical appraisal. Nutr Rev. 1999;57:35-44.
20. Morley JE, Gordan J, Hershman JM. Zinc deficiency, chronic starvation and hypothalamic pituitary-thyroid function. Am J Clin Nutr. 1980;33:1767-70.
21. Golub MS, Takeruchi PT, Keen CL, Hendricks AG, Gershwin EM. Activity and attention in zinc deprived adolescent monkeys. Am J Clin Nutr. 1996;64: 905-15.
22. Sazawal S, Bentley M, Black RE, Dhingra P, George S, Bhan MK. Effect of zinc supplementation on observed activity in preschool children in an urban slum population. Pediatrics. 1996;98:1132-7.
23. Black MM. Zinc deficiency and child development. Am J Clin Nutr 1998;68(Suppl):464S-9S.
24. Bhaskaram P, Krishnaswamy K. Trace elements of clinical significance. Zinc and Selenium, In: Textbook of Human Nutrition Eds. Bamji MS, Rao NP, Reddy V; Oxford & IBH Publishing Co Pvt Ltd. New Delhi. 1996.
25. Gopaln C. Micronutrient deficiencies- Public Health Implications. NFI. 1994;15:1-6.

17 Role of Other Micronutrients in Children

POTASSIUM

Potassium in the human body constituts almost 98% within the cells, most of which is in the skeletal muscle. After calcium and phosphorous, it is the third most common mineral in the body.[1] It is involved in many body processes like fluid balance, protein synthesis, nerve conduction, energy production, muscle contraction, synthesis of nucleic acids and control of heart beat. In many of its roles, potassium is opposed by sodium and the two positive ions are jointly balanced by the negative ion chloride.

Functions

Potassium has an important role in various functions:

- It plays an important role in energy production in the cells in the body.
- It helps maintain blood pressure at normal levels.
- Essential for protein and nucleic acid synthesis.
- Maintains fluid balance.
- Involved in normal nerve function—nerve transmission, muscle contraction and hormone secretion from endocrine glands.
- Converts glucose into glycogen (muscle fuel).
- It is involved in kidney functions.
- It helps elimination of carbon dioxide from lungs.
- It helps in maintaining acid/alkali balance.
- It helps in rhythmic contractions of the heart muscle.

Potassium Deficiency

Deficiency of potassium can lead to fatigue and muscle weakness. Severe potassium deficiency can lead to electrolyte imbalance affecting all muscles, nerves and many other bod functions. The main risks of potassium deficiency are:

- Diarrhea/vomiting, e.g. in inflammatory bowel disease.
- Chronic renal failure sharply increases potassium excretion.
- Change in body pH (metabolic acidosis/alkalosis).
- Many diuretics may increase potassium losses in urine leading to depletion of the mineral.
- Deficiency of magnesium also can contribute to depletion of body stores of potassium.

Signs and Symptoms of Potassium Deficiency

Deficiency of potassium may manifest in the form of any of the following signs and symptoms:

- Fatigue, lethargy
- Delayed gastric emptying
- Decreased blood pressure
- Muscle weakness
- Constipation
- Cardiac arrhythmias

Certain factors can lead to increased potassium accretion like

- Sweating can account for loss of almost 3 g/d
- Vomiting
- Diarrhea.

Potassium is excreted mainly by the kidneys. In renal disorders, Potassium may be reduced in which can lead to toxicity.

TABLE 17.1: RDA for potassium in infants and children

Age group (years)	mg/d (potassium chloride, g)
0–0.5	350–925 (1.8)
0.5–1	475–1275 (2.5)
1–3	550–1650 (3.2)
4–6	775–2325 (4.5)

Refer. ICMR, 2010

Requirements

The recommended dietary allowance (RDA) as per ICMR, 2010, for infants and children which are considered as safe and adequate is as given in Table 17.1.[2]

Sources of Potassium

Plant foods are the major dietary sources of potassium. In fact they contain more potassium as compared to sodium. Good sources are cereals, pulses, fruits, green leafy vegetables nuts and oilseeds. A normal mixed diet can provide approximately 4–7.5 g of potassium per day. Processed foods are poor sources of potassium due to its being leached out during the processing.[2]

CALCIUM

The role of calcium in a growing child cannot be over stressed. Maintaining adequate levels of calcium during childhood is essential for the development of a maximum peak bone mass, which has future implications in adulthood by reducing the risk of osteoporosis.[3]

In children with chronic illnesses, fracture may occur during childhood secondary to mineral deficiency associated with the disease process or the effects of therapeutic interventions (e.g. corticosteroids) on calcium metabolism.[4]

Functions of Calcium

Bone and tooth structure: Calcium with phosphorous forms hydroxyapatite crystals which give strength and rigidity to the bones and tooth enamel: 99% of the calcium in the body is in the skeleton.[5]

Blood clotting: Calcium is an important component of the blood coagulation cascade.

Muscle Contraction: In skeletal and heart muscles cell, calcium is an intercellular messenger that triggers contraction of the muscle fibers.

Nerve transmission: Calcium plays a vital role in nerve cells through depolarization of membranes and nerve transmission.

TABLE 17.2: Signs and symptoms of calcium deficiency

- Osteoporosis
- Dental caries with poor quality enamel
- Muscle cramping and spasm
- Increased irritability of nerve cells
- Abnormal blood clotting and increased bleeding after trauma

Refer. 3

Risk Factors of Calcium Deficiency

Low levels of calcium in children over a prolonged period can lead to various long term problems like:

- Demineralization of the skeleton and increased risk of osteoporosis, resulting in poor mobilization from skeleton to maintain adequate circulating levels.
- Chronic use of certain drugs like antacids, laxatives, steroids, etc. produce a negative calcium balance by decreasing absorption and increasing excretion.
- Gastrointestinal disorders like malabsorption drastically decreases fat absorption which in turn decreases the bioavailability of calcium from dietary sources, making it unavailable for absorption from the diet. Vitamin D deficiency especially in dark winter months, reduces absorption of calcium from the diet.
- The common signs and symptoms of calcium deficiency are summarized in Table 17.2

Role in Infants

Premature infants have higher calcium requirements than full term infants. These may be met by using human milk fortifier (HMF) with additional minerals or with specially designed formula for premature infants,[6] while in the hospital. On discharge, also, it is advised to provide formula fed premature infant formula with higher concentration than those of routine cow's milk based formula.

The optimum primary nutritional source of calcium during the first year of life is human milk. It has been demonstrated that the bioavailability of calcium from human milk is relatively greater than that from infant formula or cow's milk. It is therefore considered justifiable to increase the concentration of calcium in all infant formulae like soya and casein hydrolysates, to account for the potential lower biovailability of the calcium from these formula relative to cow's milk based formula.

Role in Children

Calcium retention is relatively low in toddlers and gradually increases with approach of puberty. It is observed that calcium intake levels of 800 mgs/d are associated with adequate bone mineral accumulation in prepubertal children. It is important that children be encouraged to develop eating patterns that will be associated with adequate calcium intake later in life.

Role in Preadolescence and Adolescence

There is enough data to show that efficiency of calcium absorption is increased during puberty and the majority of bone formation occurs during this stage. An intake of 1200–1500 mg/d is shown to achieve maximal net calcium balance and intakes beyond this level is excreted and hence wasted. Studies have shown that supplementing calcium only for a short duration of say 1–2 years, may not exert long term benefits in establishing and maintaining a maximum peak bone mass.[7] This emphasizes the importance of diet in achieving adequate intake and in establishing dietary patterns consistent with a calcium intake near recommended levels throughout childhood and adolescence.

TABLE 17.3: Calcium requirements of infants and children

Category	Age (years)	Calcium (mg/d)*
Children	1–3	600
	4–6	600
	7–9	600
Boys/Girls	10–12	800
	13–15	800
Boys/ Girls	16–17	800

*A minimum of 200 ml/d of milk is essential to maintain this level on a cereal legume diet.

Refer. 6 (ICMR, 2010)

Calcium Requirements

The calcium requirements for children of various age groups and sexes are as shown in Table 17.3.[8]

Dietary Sources of Calcium

Milk is one of the richest sources of calcium which is bioavailable. In general calcium bioavailability from milk products and most calcium supplements is approximately 25%–35%. Calcium from plant sources tends to be less bioavailable due to the presence of fiber, phytic acid and oxalates. But milk also being a good source of protein, phosphorous and sodium, there is a tendency of increased losses from the body as these are known to increase losses. Other dietary sources are ragi among cereals, legumes (gram, soybean), green leafy vegetables, certain nuts and oilseeds, dry fruits and (See chapter 11, Table 11.2). Factors which could inhibit calcium absorption from dietary sources are:

- Protein intake > 20% total calories
- Phosphorous (milk products, meat, colas)
- Phytic acid (whole grains)
- Sodium
- Coffee and black tea.

For children who are lactose intolerant or allergic to milk, other alternatives need to be considered, like soya based milk, tofu and other products. In case of children who are mildly lactose intolerant, a combination of milk with cereal or yoghurt can be attempted as it is known that the lactose load or concentration in the diet can also influence the tolerance.

Children may not always be inclined to consume milk in which cased parents can try to incorporate more calcium in their diets by:

- Making custard, pudding, rice kheer, etc.
- Adding milk to cooked cereal, soups and gravies.
- Making a smoothie with milk and fruit.
- Altering the flavors by adding strawberry, chocolate or making eggnog, cocoa, milkshakes, etc.

MAGNESIUM

Magnesium is an essential mineral for human nutrition, and serves several important metabolic functions:

- It plays a role in the production and transport of energy. The breakdown and oxidation of glucose, fat and proteins all require magnesium dependent enzymes.[9]
- It regulates calcium triggered contraction of heart and muscle cells and is a physiologic calcium channel blocker.
- It has a preventive role in management of hypertension by causing vasodilation of the coronary and peripheral arteries.
- In combination with calcium and phosphorous, it is important for the structure of the bones and teeth.
- It is involved in the synthesis of nucleic acids and proteins (cell reproduction).
- It can help prevent kidney and gall stones by its effect on calcium levels.
- It is also known to have a role in prevention of diabetes mellitus.

Deficiency of Magnesium

- Magnesium deficiency can be caused by a lack of magnesium in the diet, by an excess of calcium or by other factors which may increase excretion or limit absorption.
- Athletes and children involved in sports activities and doing strenuous activities have increased requirements.[10]
- Intestinal malabsorptive conditions like chronic diarrheas, pancreatic diseases, etc. tend to reduce absorption of dietary magnesium.
- Certain drugs or medicines can inhibit magnesium absorption by way of increased retention like diuretics, laxatives and chemotherapy.

Signs and Symptoms of Magnesium Deficiency

Magnesium can manifest in the form of following signs and symptoms:

- Muscle cramps and spasms, trembling
- Increased potassium and calcium losses leading to hypocalcemia and hypokalemia
- Fatigue, tiredness.
- Anorexia, vomiting and nausea
- Sodium and water retention

TABLE 17.4: RDA for magnesium in children

Group	Age	mg/kg/d	mg/d
Infants	0–6 months 6–12 months	6.0 5.5	30 45
Children	1–3 years 4–6 years 7–9 years	4.0 4.0 4.0	50 70 100
Boys	10–12 years	3.5	120
Girls	10–12 years	4.5	160
Boys	13–15 years	3.5	165
Girls	13–15 years	4.5	210
Boys	16–17 years	3.5	195
Girls	16–17 years	4.5	235

Refer. ICMR 2010.

- Impaired action of vitamin D
- Anemia
- Hypoglycemia
- Childhood hyperactivity (attention deficit behavior).

The above deficiencies could be due to either low intake or as a result of increased absorption or decreased absorption.

Requirements

The recommended dietary allowances (RDA) as laid down by Indian Council of Medical Research (ICMR), 2010 for magnesium in children are as given in Table 17.4.[3]

Dietary Sources of Magnesium

The main dietary sources of magnesium are nuts and seeds like peanuts, almonds, raisins, seafoods like habitude, legumes and wheat cereals.

VITAMIN D

Vitamin D is the only vitamin whose biologically active form is a hormone. The term' vitamin D' refers to a family of related compounds. It is a fat soluble vitamin that is naturally present in very few foods. It is also produced endogenously when ultraviolet rays from sunlight strike the skin and trigger vitamin

D synthesis. Therefore exposure to sun for some time is recommended to meet the requirements. However, it is biologically inert and has to undergo two hydroxylations in the body for activation. The first occurs in the liver and converts vitamin D to 25 hydroxy vitamin D [25(OH)D] also termed as 'calcidol'. The second occurs in the kidney and forms the physiologically active 1, 25, dihydroxy vitamin D also termed as 'calcitriol'.[12]

Functions of Vitamin D

Calcium regulation: It promotes calcium absorption in the gut and maintains adequate serum calcium phosphate concentration, thereby enabling mineralization of bone and also prevent condition of hypocalcemic tetany. A fall in blood calcium will trigger production of active vitamin D which will then stimulate calcium absorption from the diet, increases release of calcium from the bone and slows renal excretion.

Skeletal health : It is essential for normal bone growth during childhood and for maintaining bone density and strength during adulthood. Adequate levels of vitamin D in children helps prevent deficiency states like rickets in children and osteomalacia in adults.[12]

Cell growth and development: Vitamin D has an important role in the body including modulation of cell growth, neuromuscular and immune functions and reducing inflammatory conditions.[12,13,14] Many genes encoding proteins that regulate cell proliferation, differentiation and apoptesis are modulated in part by vitamin D.[12]

Immune system: Vitamin D enhances the activity and immune response to white blood cells in the body and therefore also considered to play a role in prevention of cancers in the body.

Vitamin D Deficiency

Deficiency of vitamin D can occur consequent to dietary inadequacy, impaired absorption and use, increased requirement or increased excretion. Rickets and osteomalacia are classical vitamin D deficiency states. In children vitamin D deficiency causes rickets, characterized by failure of bone tissue to mineralize adequately resulting in soft bones and skeletal deformities.[15] Prolonged exclusive breastfeeding without any vitamin D supplements is a significant cause of deficiency in children, especially in dark skinned infants breast-fed by mothers with low levels of vitamin D.[15]

Some common signs and symptoms of deficiency of the vitamin in children are listed in Table 17.5.

Deficiency of vitamin D can be assessed using serum concentrations as given in Table 17.6.[15]

TABLE 17.5: Signs and symptoms of deficiency of vitamin D

Children	Adolescents
• Delayed growth and development (delayed crawling and walking) • Irritability and restlessness • Rickets: softening of bones, spinal deformities • Bowed legs and knock knees, enlargement of rib sternum joints • Delayed tooth eruption and poorly formed tooth enamel • Impaired immune response with increased risk of infection	• Impaired growth of bones and musculature • Swelling and pain at the end of long bones, especially the knees • Impaired immune response with increased risk of infection

Refer. 15

TABLE 17.6: Serum 25 hydroxyvitamin D concentrations as in health

ng/ml*	Health status
< 12	Associated with vitamin D deficiency leading to rickets in infants and children and osteomalacia in adults
12–20	Generally considered inadequate for bone and overall health in healthy individuals
≥ 20	Generally considered inadequate for bone and overall health in healthy individuals
> 50	Emerging evidence links potential adverse effects to such high level, especially >150

Refer. 15

*Serum concentrations of vitamin D are reported in nanograms/ml.

Requirements of Vitamin D

The recommendation of 400 IU (10 μg) as a daily supplement (only under situations of minimal exposure to sunlight) has been made by the Expert Group Committee.[16] In view of the increasing trend of limited outdoor physical activity by children leading to inadequate exposure to sunlight and obesity, it was felt that outdoor physical activity is the best means of achieving both adequate vitamin D status and controlling overweight and obesity in the population. Increasing the recommended daily intake was not a solution, neither food supply can be considered as a substitute for the vitamin D available from exposure to sunlight .

Sources of Vitamin D

Food: Dietary sources of vitamin D are limited. Fish liver oil and flesh of certain fish, like salmon, tuna and mackerel. Liver, cheese and egg yolk also contain small amounts of the vitamin D. Dairy milk as also certain oils are fortified with vitamin D.

Sunlight: Exposure to sunlight as is one of the commonest sources of vitamin D.[12] Ultraviolet (UV) B radiation with a wavelength of 290–320 nanometers penetrates the skin and converts cutanous 7 dehydrocholesterol to previtamin D3 which in turn becomes vitamin D3.[12] It is suggested that approximately 25–30 minutes of exposure between 10 am to 3 pm at least twice a week to the face, legs, arms and back without sunscreen usually can provide adequate synthesis of the vitamin.[13]

REFERENCES

Potassium

1. Luft K. Potassium and its regulation. In: Ziegler EE, Filer LJ eds. Present knowledge in Nutrition. 7th edn. Washington DC ILSI Press. 1996.
2. ICMR. Nutrient Requirements and Recommended Dietary Allowances for Indians. A Report of the Expert Group of the Indian Council of Medical Research. 2010.

Calcium in Children

3. Institute of Medicine, Food and Nutrition Board National Research council. Recommended dietary reference intakes for calcium, phosphorous, magnesium, vitamin D and fluoride. Washington DC, National Academy Press. 1977.
4. Abrams SA. Studies of calcium metabolism in children with chronic illnesses. In: Wastney Me, Siva Subramanian KN. Eds Kinetic models of trace element and mineral metabolism during development. Boca Raton FL: CRC Press. 1995:159-70.
5. Weaver CM, Heaney RP. Calcium In: Shills ME, Olson JA, Shike M, Ross AC eds. Modern nutrition in Health and Disease. Baltimore: Williams and Wilkins. 1999.
6. Schanler RJ, Abrams SA. Postnatal intrauterine macromineral accretion rates in low birth weight infants fed HMF. J Pediatr. 1995;126:441-47.
7. Lee WT, Leung SS, Leung DM, et al. A follow up study on the effects of calcium supplement withdrawl and puberty on bone acquisition of children. Am J Clin Nutr. 1996;64:71-77.
8. Indian Council of Medical Research. Nutrient Requirements and recommended Dietary Allowances for Indians. A report of the Expert Group of the Indian Council of Medical Research. 2010.

Magnesium in Children

9. Shils M. Magnesium. n: Ziegler EE, Filer LJ, et al. Present knowledge in nutrition. 7th ed. Washington DC ICSI Press. 1996.
10. Clarkson PM. Minerals: Exercise performance and supplements in atheletes. J Sports Sci. 1991;9:91.
11. Nutrient Requirements and Recommended Dietary Allo wances for Indians; A Report of the Expert Group of the Indian Council of Medical Research. ICMR. 2010.

Vitamin D

12. Institute of Medicine, Food and Nutrition Board. Refernce intakes for calcium and vitamin D, Washington DC. National Academy Press. 2010.
13. Holik MF. Vitamin D In: Shils ME, Shike M, Ross A. C, Callabero B eds. Modern Nutrition in Health and Disease, 10th edn, Philadelphia: Lippincott; Williams and Wilkins. 2006.
14. Norman AW, Henry HH, Vitamin D. In: Bowman BA, Russel RM eds. Present knowledge in nutrition. 9th edn. Washington DC, ISLI Press. 2006.
15. Wharton B, Bishop N. Rickets. Lancet. 2003;47:107-13 (PubMed abstract).
16. Nutrient Requirements and Recommended Dietary allowances for Indians; A Report of the Expert Group of the Indian Council of Medical Research. ICMR. 2010.

18 Nutrition Counseling—Role in Children

INTRODUCTION

Nutrition counseling is an ongoing process in which the counselor, in this context, the dietician works with an individual to assess his/her routine dietary intake and identify areas where any modifications may be required. The nutrition counselor provides information, educates and provides material to guide the recipient (parents or care givers in this context), and maintains a follow up to help the child and parent maintain the required dietary changes.

GOAL

The goal or purpose of nutrition counseling is to help parents plan age appropriate diet for the children or to modify the existing dietary pattern as per the condition of the child, e.g. if suffering from any disease state. Nutrition counseling is an integral part of treatment with eating disorders, gastro-intestinal problems, cardiac ailments, neurological disorders, growth and development abnormalities or a case of any surgical interventions which may be required.

The counselor works with the parents and the child to assess the existing eating patterns and family life style, and identifies areas where modifications are required. Adults are usually are able to identify their concerns and express them to the counselor, where as children are more likely to express their concerns and feelings either indirectly, through 'play or directly through behavior'.

Nutrition Counseling Characteristics

The main characteristics of nutrition counseling are:

- Assessing and analyzing various health needs with regard to diet and activity.
- Helping or counseling people to set achievable health goals and teach various ways of maintaining these goals over a prolonged period.
- Assisting or guiding parents of children or adolescents with eating disorders, e.g. anorexia nervosa or bulimia.
- Providing education material in the form of charts or pamphlets, brochures, etc. and help maintain the required changes.
- Educating and assessing regarding qualities of nutrition in a diet.
- Educating regarding modifying eating habits, dietary patterns, allergies and weight management.
- Helping modify lifestyle pattern not only of the target child or adolescent but the entire family.

Learning Process in Children

The children usually learn through information which is processed through attention, perception, memory, thinking and problem solving.[1] A child is known to process information using 5 stages:[2]

Attention

For an infant recognition of anything begins with recognizing the parent by way of responding to their facial expressions by smiling or looking up for security and comfort. Recognizing something brings the child to focus his/her attention first.

Perception

After the child has recognized something, the next step is trying to perceive or comprehend, like the first perception a child will have is for food as he or she grows. The sight of a bottle or breast for the infant or the bright colors of the cereal bowl for the toddler will attract attention and elicit response based on the meaning associate with that item. Therefore, counseling strategies should focus on attracting attention, for instance, bright colored pictures or food models can gain the attention of the child and impress upon his mind the concept of food.

Memory

One of the goals of nutrition counseling is retention of information over a period of time. In children this is done by[3]

1. Familiarizing the objects in the form of food model or pictures.
2. Involving the child actively by encouraging him/her to hold and play with the objects of food models or pictures.
3. Repeated exposures of the same concept of food items.
4. Making the information playful so that the attention of the child is retained, e.g. involving them to make belief by cutting, cooking or distributing food models.

Thinking

An older child after the initial stages gets into a decision making phase, where in he/she will choose to either select or reject the information given. This stage can be made use of by encouraging the child to be involved in group activity, e.g. including food from each food group and getting him/her involved in planning a meal.

Problem Solving

This stage is more applicable to older children, whereby they can learn and comprehend the consequences of their actions and decisions. They can learn to modify their actions based on their experience and consequences they have encountered through them.

Counseling Techniques

The counselor needs to follow a given set of techniques or steps to interview the parent or and child. The commonly accepted technique is the five stage model which comprises the 5 A's[4] as listed below. These steps organize the tasks of the provider (counselor) and act as a reminder where emphasis needs to be placed during a particular session.

Step 1: Assess

The counselor first selects and analyses information to make decisions, which can be provided by the receiver, e.g. in case of life style problems, it is important to assess the chronicity of the recipient's relevant behavior. Creating rapport between the two is crucial, which can be done by a simple way of using facial expressions (in the form of a smile, laugh), play activities or drawing.

Step 2: Advise

For counseling to be more effective, it is important to identify a specific target behavior on which to focus. The first target should be concrete, avoiding abstract talk, identifying positive aspects. The counselor should help with the decision making process with his/her knowledge of the situation or condition.

Step 3: Agree

The child should be allowed to explore the ideal world, but the target should be short-term and a way out needs to be tracked which can most easily divert him/her from the current situation.

Step 4: Assist

The various possible course of action should be discussed together with the recipient to achieve the desired goal. The onus of the responsibility rests with the recipient (parent or child), who tries to follow the suggestions agreed upon as per plan and bring back experiences for discussion and evaluation together. Behavioral tactics like model support, skill, training, environmental change, relapse prevention and training, environmental change and maintenance techniques are generally used by counselors to achieve the target goal.

Step 5: Arrange

This step comprises monitoring for evidence for change and assessing the extent or degree of compliance or adherence the recipient has achieved through the previous sessions.

Principles of Counseling

There are 5 essential principles involved in counseling:

1. *Express sympathy*: Counselors should reflect a level of understanding regarding the challenges faced by the recipient, but not sympathize with him/her.
2. *Avoid argumentation*: Arguing can pose a barrier to counseling and can put off the recipient permanently.
3. *Roll with resistance*: There is bound to be resistance posed by the recipient in which condition the counselor should pause and respond to queries or resistance posed by them.
4. *Support self efficacy*: Inculcating self confidence in his/her ability to cope with modifications or changes the recipient is an important job of the counselor.
5. *Develop discrepancy*: Behaviors and beliefs are usually at odds and so it is important to guide them to recognize their responsibility which will facilitate change smoothly.

The Counseling Process

The counseling process involves the following steps:

Assessing Dietary Habits

The counselor first interviews the parent or the care giver and the child regarding his/her typical food intake. This is done by using different methods like estimate of all the foods and beverages consumed over the day. For this the counselor records all the detailed intake of the previous day, which is generally done by 24 hour recall method, which is repeated for 3 consecutive days to elicit an average of the 3 days to give a more accurate picture. A food frequency questionnaire is also maintained which can complement the average of the 3 days 24 hours recall estimate, thereby representing a more accurate food intake and eating pattern (See Chapter 3). This involves asking the responder the frequency of any given food consumed over a daily, weekly or monthly basis, thereby eliciting the detailed diet record. Another method involved is maintaining a daily food diary over a period of time and then assessing and analyzing the actual energy and nutrient intake.

In case of toddlers it is the parent who provides the dietary history of the child which could include either breastfeeding or complementary foods or both. As the child grows, the intake can be totally from home based diet. Parents respond best when information is focused on their specific needs.[5]

Identifying Changes Required

Verbal suggestions are required to convey brief, concrete nutritional concepts but clearly written or printed information also should be provided to reinforce the message and for detailed information. Modeling or role playing by parent is an important technique for parents to convey the desired message regarding eating pattern and lifestyle. Inactivity is associated with poor eating habits during childhood and can lead to a lifetime or health problems. Therefore, benefits of an active lifestyle for children can be brought out by families exercising together and finding activities that can be accomplished by varying skill levels and enjoyed on regular basis. Parents should be counseled to discourage children from watching television, by restricting the number of hours spent before it to less than 2 hours per day.

Setting Goals

The counselor can help guide the child through an age and developmentally appropriate play experience to learn basic health concepts and can assist parents to discover the correct balance of independence for the child. Any limitations required by family structure and therapeutic dietary modifications may also need to be communicated.[6] The nutrition counselor and the parent or child set behavior oriented goals together, which focus on the need to achieve the desired dietary changes, rather than on an absolute value, e.g. if achieving a set target body weight. For a child to prevent weight gain associated with certain modifications, for instance, his/her goal must be to increase the amounts of fruits, vegetables and whole grains daily. Such changes can help prevent weight gain while emphasizing on needed behavior rather than on actual weight.

Making Dietary Changes

While briefing about dietary changes it is worth considering the child's background and other factors affecting decisions. The process may need to be a gradual one, beginning with one or two dietary changes initially and slowly making additional more difficult ones over a period of time.

Identifying Barriers to Change

There may be certain potential problems in bringing about the identified changes which need to be kept in mind. Changing eating behavior could mean modifying the lifestyle or routine life, e.g. purchasing different foods, planning ahead, foreseeing any social events, food preferences, lack of knowledge or time and cost, etc.

Finding Support

Parents or care givers are encouraged to attend nutrition counseling session along with the children or adolescents so that they can share responsibility for food selection and preparation. Family support and understanding can help achieve the goals more easily and successfully.

Maintaining Changes

Maintaining the dietary changes over a long term period is an actual challenge. Parents and family members need to be encouraged to ensure the modified changes in the dietary habits be continued without too many breaks, although occasional slips may be acceptable. The counselor can help them to identify situations that may lead to relapse and plan ways to handle the situations ahead of time. The parent should be advised to maintain regular meal timings for the child so that he/she is tuned to the routine, rather than allowing the child to eat as and when he/she feels like. This helps the child to avoid developing an erratic eating behavior. It is for the parent to decide what and when the child should eat, but the amount to be eaten should be left to the child to eat, e.g. the amount planned for one particular meal should be served at the designated time of the meal and the child should be asked to complete the meal within a span of about 15–20 minutes. If he is not inclined to eat or complete the amount served to him, the plate should be withdrawn from him, rather than forcing or coaxing him to complete it over a prolonged period of half to one hour. But then it should be also ensured that he would not be served any food before the next designated timing of meal if, he demands food in between. That would train the child to get more disciplined with regard to eating pattern.

Secondly, distractions while eating also act a barrier to eating behavior, e.g. watching television or video games while eating. The parents should discourage the children to watch television while eating and also follow the same principles for themselves to. One cannot expect the child to refrain from watching television, if they themselves do not follow the same behavior.

Counseling the Child

The initial goal of nutritional counseling would be to increase the receiver's awareness of risks associated with their existing eating habits. In situations where there is an adolescent with diabetes, they may be aware of the need to change dietary habits but may be reluctant initially. In such cases, the goal should be small and achievable along with concrete strategies to facilitate the required dietary changes. This is the initial stage of nutritional counseling. Adolescents learn best when they are actually involved in the counseling in any of the following ways:

- A larger group of teens can be counseled in topics like making healthy food choices at fast food outlets, class room presentations or group education sessions are some effective measures of counseling.
- Smaller groups can be used to provide counseling those who are at risk and would benefit from modifying eating behavior, e.g. weight management or sports nutrition.
- Individual approach like one to one counseling is required for those at a higher level of nutritional guidance, e.g. initial education related to diabetes, hyperlipidemia, hypertension or any other specific problems like cystic fibrosis, nephritic syndrome, celiac disease, etc.

The initial component of nutrition counseling should involve developing a positive rapport and getting to understand the psyche of the adolescent. Adolescent should be made to get involved in decision making process during the counseling sessions, by allowing them to provide inputs as to what aspects of their eating habits they think need to be changed and what changes they are more likely to occur when they have identified specific behaviors that they feel need to be changed, thus expressing willingness to change.[7] Follow-up sessions should be scheduled to change in order to provide feedback and monitor progress towards individual goals.

Role of the Parent

Besides assessing the developmental level of the child, it is important to assess that of the parent too. Initially the counselor should consider having all material provided to parents in simple language which is clearly legible, since they may not be able to grasp any complex information which could only cause more stress on the family environment. This is likely to decrease the compliance or adherence to the advice. With the passage of time more complex information may be provided.

Cultural Influence

The counselor should be sensitive to the ethnic and religious facets of the child's environment which is critical for long term compliance to the nutritional advice. The meal plan suggested should incorporate foods which are used in their particular culture or environment. Knowledge of cultural and ethnic religious traditions becomes essential for the counselor, so that these can be integrated into the day to day meals.

Feeding Relationships

For children with feeding difficulties enrolled in rehabilitation programs, observation of a feeding session with a speech therapist can provide valuable information on the parent child relationship. Maintaining food diary with food record of 2–3 days with meal timings can provide useful information on the structure of the family lifestyle. In-depth probing on the parent's feelings towards food and the child's feeding issues can help in developing a successful nutritional care plan.

Psychosocial Relationship with the Child

Food can become the center of power struggle between the child and the parent for which intervention by a counselor can help. One parent sabotaging the efforts of the other in feeding in a particular way or a particular food, is picked up by the child which he tries to exploit in his favor, thus creating a barrier to effective counseling.

Model Behavior

Parents can act as role models who mould for their child, especially when it comes to eating behavior. Modifying the dietary pattern of the entire family can make it easier for the child to follow and accept the changes advised, e.g. in case of an overweight child, who is advised to follow a low fat high fiber diet, would do better if the modifications are made for the whole family. At times the nutrition counselor herself can act as a role model for the child if it may not be possible for the family situation.

Counseling the Child with Special Needs

Children with any physical disabilities may require specialized counseling which must be attuned to the developmental stages. The counselor should be aware of the specific disability and the level of parental environment. Play therapy allows many children with special needs to discover what strengths they have in relation to their disabilities. The involvement of parents/caregivers becomes very important in this population and may require coordination of efforts with other health care professionals.

REFERENCES

1. Yusson SR, Santrock JW. Child Development: An Introduction. Dubuque IA: WC. Brown Co. 1982.
2. Gullo DF. Developmentally appropriate teaching in early childhood. Washington DC: National Education Assoc. 1992.
3. Jackson NE, Robinson HB, Dale PS. Cognitive development in young children. Washington DC. National Institute of Educ. 1976.
4. Ivey AE, Ivey MB, Simek-Morgan L. Counseling and psychotherapy: A multicultural perceptive. 3rd Boston, MA: Allyn and Bacon, 1993.
5. Glascoe FP, Oberklaid F, Dworkin PH, et al. Brief approaches to educating patients and parents.
6. Bridget M, Klewitter. Nutrition Counseling, In: Handbook of Pediatric Nutrition. Eds. Samour PQ, Helm KK, Lang CE. 2nd ed, Jones and Bartlett Publishing Co. Massachusetts. 2004; 121-132.
7. Croll J, Neumark-Sztaina D, Story M. Healthy Eating: What does it mean to adolescents? J Nutr Educ. 2001;33:193-8.

19 Probiotics—Role in Child Health

INTRODUCTION

The role of probiotics is generally considered as a functional food capable of altering or modifying the gut flora for beneficial effects in the human gut. The origin of use of probiotics, dates back to the 20th century, when it was first introduced by a Russian scientist and Nobel laureate Elj Metcnikoff, who suggested its possible role in modifying the gut flora by replacing harmful microbes with useful ones.[1] He suggested that the aging process results from the activity of putrefactive microbes, producing toxic substances in the large bowel. He attributed this effect to 'intestinal autointoxication' which caused the physical changes associated with old age.

The practice of fermenting milk with lactic acid bacteria (to inhibit the growth of proteolytic bacteria due to the low pH produced by fermentation of lactose) was prevalent in that era too in certain rural populations of Europe, e.g. Bulgaria and Russia. People who lived largely on milk fermented by this process also had an exceptionally long life. Based on this theory it was proposed that consumption of 'fermented milk' would 'seed' the intestine with harmless lactic acid bacteria and decrease the intestinal pH, which would further suppress the growth of proteolytic bacteria. This 'sour' milk was consumed by Methnikoff himself which called 'Bulgarian bacillus' and fond that his health benefited.

The term probiotic was first introduced in 1953, by Kollath, which was described as microbially derived factors that stimulate growth of other microorganisms.[2] The definition used widely used now was suggested by Roy Fuller in 1989, which is 'a live microbial food supplement which beneficially affects the host animal by improving its intestinal microbial balance'.[3] On the other hand, another term 'prebiotic' is also used which is described as nonabsorbable food components that beneficially stimulate one or more of the gut beneficial microbial groups and thus have a beneficial effect on human health.[4]

The most commonly used prebiotics are carbohydrate substrates, e.g. dietary fiber, which has the ability to promote the components of the normal intestinal microflora which may evince a health benefit to the host.

When probiotics and prebiotics are administered in combination, it is termed as 'synbiotics'. The combined effect has a definitive benefit by synergestic action (Table 19.1).

TABLE 19.1: Definitions

Probiotics	A live microbial food ingredient which is beneficial to health
Prebiotics	A nondigestible food ingredient which beneficially affects the host by selectively stimulating the number of bacteria in the colon having the potential to improve host health
Synbiotic	A mixture of pre and probiotics which beneficially affects the host by improving the survival and implantation of live microbial dietary supplements in the gastrointestinal tract (GIT), thereby improving host health and well being

Refer. 2, 3, 4

Source of Probiotics

The microbiota of a new born develops rapidly after birth. It is initially dependent on the mother's microbiota, mode of delivery, birth environment and rarely genetic factors.[5,6] The maternal vaginal and intestinal flora constitutes the source of bacteria, which colonizes the intestine of the new born, the dominative strains being facultative anaerobes like the enterobacteria, coliforms and lactobacilli. By the time the child is weaned, the microflora alters gradually and begins to resemble that of an adult. Although there are almost 500 different microbial species in the GIT, the ones with beneficial properties include mainly bifidobacteria and lactobacilli. Others include bacteroides, clostridium, bifidobacterium, escherichia and veillonella. The initial compositional development of the gut microflora is considered a key determinant in the development of normal gut barrier functions.[7]

Intestinal mucosal defence mechanisms acting in the lumen and mucosa restrict colonization by pathogenic bacteria by interfering with the adherence of micro-organisms to the mucosal surface. The normal gut microbiota can prevent the overgrowth of potential pathogenes in the GIT.

Probiotics—Criteria

For organisms to be considered as probiotic the criteria needed to be fulfilled are:[8]

- Should be isolated from the same species as its intended host.
- Should have a demonstrable beneficial effect on the host.
- Should be nonpathogenic.
- Should be able to survive transit through the GIT.
- On storage, large number of viable bacteria must be able to survive prolonged periods.

Mechanism of Action

The mechanism of the beneficial effects of pro-biotics is broadly based on:

1. Those arising from colonization and inhibition of pathogenic bacteria.
2. Those effects which arise from enhancement of the host immune response and intestinal barrier function.
3. Those which suppress growth or epithelial binding/invasion by pathogenic bacteria and production of antimicrobial substances.
4. Those which control transfer of dietary antigen
5. Those which stimulate mucosal and systemic host immunity.

There are known to be more than 400 bacterial species, both resident microbiota as well as a variable number of transient species existing in any given specific region of the intestine. The intestinal bacteria are controlled by the epithelial cells which form a physical barrier and are also capable of discriminating between resident flora and enteric pathogens. Specific glycoconjugates are released by the epithelium in response to the presence of bacteria which act as receptors for the attachment of bacteria. The intestinal epithelium completely inihibits the adherence of pathogens by increased production of bacteriocins, hydrogen peroxide, biosurfactants, mucin and defensin-β 2, an antimicrobial peptide. This antagonism of the pathogenic bacteria are most effective when the probiotic themselves adhere to the intestinal epithelium. The number of viable bacteria colonizing the intestine depends on factors like:

- Probiotic formulation.
- Coadministration with food or milk.
- Gastric pH.
- Intestinal motility.
- Composition of intestinal microbiota.

Probiotics are also known to modulate cytokine release from cells of the GIT, thereby providing immunity. By its interaction with epithelial cells, T cells and dendritic cells of the gut, produce anti-inflammatory and immune regulatory effects.

The action of one probiotic is also affected by the presence of another strain of probiotic and they also exhibit host specific and strain specific difference in action, ability to colonise the gut and clinical efficacy.[9]

The prebiotic acts as an alternative for probiotics or their cofactors. Complex carbohydrates pass through the lower gastrointestine where that become available for some colonic bacteria, but are not utilized by the majority of bacteria present in the colon. The commonly used prebiotics in human nutrition are galacto-oligosaccharides, fructo-oligosaccharides,

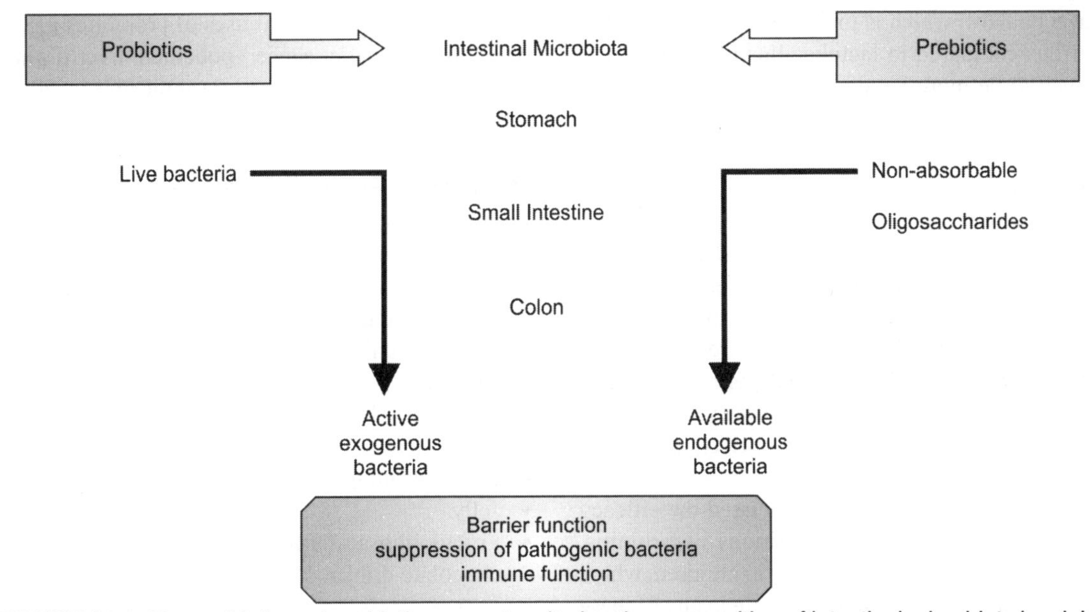

FIGURE 19.1: The probiotic and prebiotic concepts: altering the composition of intestinal microbiota by viable bacterial supplements versus nonabsorbable bacterial substrates
Refer. 8

inulin and its hydrolysates, malto-oligosaccharides and resistant starch.[8] Figrue 19.1 presents the concept of synergistic mechanism of pre and probiotics.

The probiotics have the ability to dampen inflammation of the gut which may require anti-inflammatory mediators. Chronic diseases like allergies and other autoimmune and inflammatory diseases are known to benefit from probiotics. The rationale of probiotic therapy involves normalization of the properties of unbalanced indigenous microflora by specific strains of the healthy gut microflora.[8]

Clinical Uses

In Infants

It is well known that breast feeding has a protective role in preventing infectious diseases which is done by multiple mechanisms. It is believed that there are certain components in breast milk which can modulate the composition of intestinal flora amongst which bifidobacteria comprise a significant number in the normal intestinal flora in breastfed infants.[10]

It is postulated that a combination of increased bifidobactreial counts and decreased concentration of other enterobacteria and luminal host factors may play a role in protecting premature babies and new borns from diarrheal diseases.[8]

Necrotising enterocolitis is one of the common devastating intestinal diarrhea occurring in 10%–25% of the premature infants and very low birth babies with a mortality of 20%–30%. Babies given supplements of lactobacillus GG daily is known to show reduction of this entity in some trials, which suggest a co-relation between the reduction of lactobacilli and the increased risk of necrotizing entero colitis.[11,12]

Diarrheal Diseases

Infective diarrhea: Acute infantile diarrhea due to rotavirus is the most common type of diarrhea encountered in infants worldwide for which oral rehydration solution (ORS) is the primary treatment. A systematic review of the results of various trials has revealed an overall reduction in the duration of diarrhea by 17–30 hours.[13,14,15]

Traveler's diarrhea: Travelers visiting high risk areas are prone to have acute episode of diarrhea, though most of them are self limiting. Several studies using probiotics (saccharomyces boulardii) for treating such diarrhea confirmed a significant beneficial effect on the duration of the diarrhea.[16,17] It is observed that S boulardi which is more effective on bacterial diarrhea compared to lactobacillus GG (LGG) has proven to be more beneficial in viral or idiopathic bacteria.

Allergy

Atopic disease, a manifestation of food hypersensitivities is generally due to the intestinal microflora which contributes to the processing of food antigens in the gut. It is believed that probiotics have a role in modifying the structure of potential antigens, reducing the intestinal permeability and the generation of proinflammatory cytokines that are elevated in patients with a variety of allergic disorders.[8]

A number of studies have evaluated the efficacy of probiotics in allergenic conditions like rhinitis, atopic dermatitis and food allergy in children, which are promising but their definitive role in any of these conditions is still not clear.[18,19]

Lactose Intolerance

Probiotics have been shown to have a positive role in the management of lactose intolerance, a condition widely prevalent in various sections of the population. The effect is observed by its action on lactose digestion by reducing the symptoms of intolerance and also slowly orocecal transit.[20]

The mechanism involved is that during fermentation the pathogenic bacteria, e.g. *Lactobacillus* (e.g. *L. bulgaricus*) and *Streptococcus thermophilus* produce lactase, which hydrolyses the lactose in dairy products to glucose or galactose. Their effect exerted on the lactase activity *in vivo* in the gut lumen facilitates digestion and decreases intolerance; this phenomenon has been demonstrated in children and adults.[21,22]

There are other clinical uses of probiotics e.g. in prevention of colon cancer, pouchitis, liver disease and sepsis, all of which are more applicable in adults, rather than in children.

Probiotic Food Supplements

Probiotics in the form of food are widely available, some of which are:

- Live yoghurts containing lactobacillus, streptococcus, etc.
- Ferments dairy products.
- Cheese.
- Freeze dried supplements.
- Fruit juices.
- Infant weaning foods.
- Jelly.
- Fructooligosaccharides as biscuits and powdered chocolate drinks.

Disadvantages of Probiotics

Despite their benefits, probiotics have not proven beneficial in some conditions in various trials. In case of childhood allergies, a trial designed to show the effectiveness of probiotics, in fact showed that the group given the good bacteria were more likely to develop sensitivity to allergens. There are reports indicating that yoghurt could be a possible cause for obesity, but this theory was contested on the ground that the obesity could be linked to the dairy products which may be high fat rather than the yoghurt per se. There is a possible risk of antibiotic resistance transfer by the use of probiotics to more pathogenic bacteria. Some strains of lactobacillus were found to be resistant to vancomycin, which can be of serious concern. Almost 68.4% of the isolates have been found to be resistant against multiple antibiotics.[9]

REFERENCES

1. Metchnik off E. Essais optimists. Paris The prolongation of life. Optimistic Studies. Translated and edited by P. Chalmers Mitchell. London. Heineman. 1907.
2. Hamilton—Miller JM. The role of probiotics in the treatment and prevention of H. pylori infection. Int J Antimicrobial Agents. 2003;22(4):360-6.
3. Fuller R. Probiotics in man and animals. J Appl Bactriology. 1989;66(5):365-78. PMID 2666378.
4. Gibson GR, Roberfroid MB. Dietary modulation of the human colonic microflora: introducing the concept of prebiotics. J Nutr. 1995;125:1401-12.
5. Fravier CF, Vaughan EE, De Vos WM, et al. Molecular monitoring of succession of bacterial communities inhuman neonates.
6. Bennot Y, Mitsuoka T. Development of intestinal microflora in human and animals. Bifidobacteria Microflora. 1986;5:13-25.

7. Hooper LV, Wong MH, Thelin A, et al. Molecular analysis of commensal host microbial relationships in the intestine. Science. 2001;291:881-4.
8. Harish K, Verghase T. Probiotics in humans – evidence based review. Calicut Med J. 2006;(4):e 3.
9. Kumar K. Probiotics In: Basics of Clinical Nutrition. Ed Joshi YK. Paypee publishers 2nd ed, New Delhi. 2008;397-403.
10. Yoshita M, Fujita K, Sakata H. Development of the normal intestinal flora and its clinical significance in infants and children. Bifido Microflora. 1991;10:11-27.
11. Sticker T, Braegger CP. Oral probiotics prevent necrotizing entero colitis. J Pediatr Gastroenetol Nutr. 2006;42:446-7.
12. Hoyos AB. Reduced incidence of necrotizing entero colitis associated with enteral administration of lactobacillus acidophilus and bifidobacterium in infants to neonates in an intensive care unit. Int J Infect Dis. 1999;3:197-202.
13. Allen SJ, Okoko B, Martinez E, et al. Probiotis for treating infectious diarrhea. Cochrane Database Syst Rev. 2004;2:CD003048.
14. Szajewska H, Mrukowiez JZ. Probiotics in the treatment and prevention of acute infectious diarrhea in infants and children: a systematic review of published randomized, double blind placebo controlled trials. J Pediatr Gastroenetrol Nutr. 2001;33(2):S17.
15. Van Neil CW, Feudtners C, Garrison MM, et al. Lactobacillus therapy for acute infectious diarrhea in children: a meta analysis. Pediatrics. 2002;109:678.
16. Katelaris PH, Salam I, Farthing MJ. Lactobacilli to prevent traveler's diarrhea: N Engl J Med. 1995;333: 1360-1.
17. Bleichener G, Blehaut H, Mentec H, et al. Sacchromyces boulardii prevents diarrhea in critically ill tube fed patients. A multi centre, randomized, double blind placebo controlled trial. Intens Care Med. 1997;23:517-23.
18. Miralgia del Giudice M, De Luca MG. The role of probiotics in the clinical management of food allergy and atopic dermatitis. J Clin Gastroenetrol 2004;38:S84-5.
19. Isolauri E, Arvola T, Sutas Y, et al. Probiotics in the management of atopic eczema. Clin Exp Allergy. 2002;30:1604-10.
20. Sandres ME. Summary of the conclusions from a consensus panel of experts on health attributes on lactic cultures: significance to fluid milk products containing cultures. J Dairy Sci. 1993;76:1819-28.
21. Saltzman JR, Russel RM, Golner B, et al. A randomized trial of lactobacillus acidophilus BG2F04 to treat lactose intolerance. Am J Clin Nutr. 1999;69:104-6.
22. Shermack MA, Saavedra JM, Jackson TL, et al. Effect of yoghurt on symptoms in hydrogen production in lactose malabsorbing children. Am J Clin Nutr. 1995;62:1003-6.

20 Nutrition for Dental Health in Children

Dental health in children in terms of nutrition is still not widely recognized by parents, nor has it been emphasized upon by the community. In fact, diet plays an important role in dental health especially after the eruption of teeth. It is only after the age of 3–4 years when teeth have erupted completely, or till ages 6–7 years when a child is brought to a pedodontist for any dental problems.[1] Now with increasing awareness of parents regarding the dental health of their children, they tend to bring them for examination as soon as any kind of abnormality or problem is detected. But before that period, the fact is generally ignored that a good diet and healthy eating practices can actually defer their visit to the pedodontist for any dental problem. It is here that the role of the pediatrician along with the dietician comes that of educating the parents regarding good dental health and the influence of the child's feeding behavior (right from infancy onwards) upon dental health of the child. Nutrition affects the teeth during development and malnutrition may exacerbate periodontal and oral infectious diseases.[2,3]

TOOTH DEVELOPMENT AND STRUCTURE

There are two sets of teeth which appear in one's life time. First is the primary set or the 'milk teeth' as they are known, which appear from age of 6 months onwards and the second one—the permanent set which gradually replaces the primary set between the ages of 6–12 years. The primary set comprises 20 teeth, while the permanent set comprises 32 teeth. The tooth consists of 3 types tissues (Fig. 20.1):

Enamel: This is a hard substance which forms the outer surface of the tooth and is composed of calcium and phosphate. This is the only part exposed to the oral environment.

***Dentin*:** It is the major component of the tooth which is supplied with nerves and blood vessels.

Cementum: The dentine is covered by a thin layer of bone like material which forms the cementum. This holds the teeth in the jaw.

The mineralization of the teeth begins before birth, with the process of enamel formation being completed during the first year of life. It is at this stage of infancy when the feeding pattern of the child can be influenced (e.g. fluoride in the water, bottle feeding or bottle caries), although diet can continue to influence the teeth after eruption through local effects.

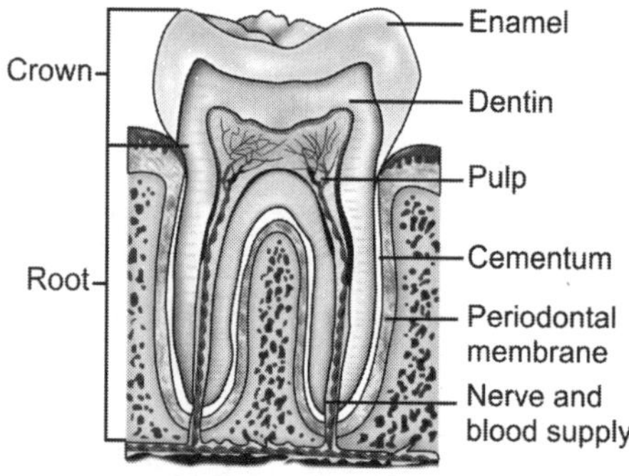

FIGURE 20.1: Structure of a tooth

NUTRITIONAL INFLUENCE ON THE PRE-ERUPTED TEETH

The teeth begin to develop at 6–8 weeks *in vitro* and continue to be influenced by systemic nutrition till they erupt. They go through 3 main stages of development before erupting into the oral cavity:

The proliferative stage: This is the initial stage when there is hyperplastic growth of the teeth, and requires adequate proteins for the process. Vitamins A and C are essential for the enamel forming cells (ameloblasts) and dentin forming cells (odontoblasts).

The matrix formation stage: The matrix is mainly collagen and for this vitamin C and adequate amounts of protein is required from infancy itself. Deficiency of these nutrients can lead to susceptibility to caries and altered or malformed teeth.

The pre-eruptive stage: This is a process of teeth maturation and hardening to increase the resistance of enamel to dental caries. Excessive sugar intake during the pre-eruptive stage can adversely affect the maturation process.

ROLE OF SPECIFIC NUTRIENTS ON TOOTH MATURATION

During the process of matrix formation liberal calcification of the ameloblasts and the odontoblasts occurs, forming a calcified mass of tricalcium phosphate. This calls for a good source of calcium, phosphate and vitamin D for adequate mineralization. If during the first 6–8 years of life any portion of these ameloblasts are injured or killed due to deficiency of vitamin D, high fever or administration of antibiotics like tetracyclines, enamel discoloration and disfigurement can result. It has been suggested that the most critical age is 10 months and between 2 and a half to 5 years, when the enamel cells are most sensitive to any stress.[4]

Demineralization and Remineralization—Role of Fluoride

When there is inadequate brushing or cleaning of the teeth, a sticky substance called plaque develops. This plaque bacterium produces acids by fermentation of sugars, decreasing the pH at the tooth surface. The sugars may be already present in the foods or produced by starch breakdown in the mouth. These acids dissolve the minerals in the enamel (calcium and phosphorous), a process which is known as demineralization. Enamel demineralisation takes place below a pH of about 5.5, which is called the 'critical pH'.

The acids produced in the mouth are gradually neutralized by saliva. This causes the pH of the tooth surface to rise above the critical pH. The increase in pH causes a return of the dissolved calcium and phosphate back to the enamel. This is called 'remineralisation'.

In the event of constant eating during the daytime, chance of remineralisation is greatly reduced. A gap of 2–3 hours between 2 meals can spare the damage done by demineralization and gives time for the teeth to repair themselves.[5]

Fluoride is an important nutrient required for mineralization of the tooth, and an adequate amount of it in the diet or water during the pre eruptive stage can ensure good teeth which can be caries resistant. The tooth enamel is known to become fully mineralized during the pre-eruptive maturation period and it is during this phase that a significant amount of fluoride is acquired. Out of the 1 mm (1,000 μm) thickness of the tooth enamel, only the outer 30–50 μm of the enamel surface acquires significant amount of fluoride.[6] Fluoride deposition continues in the external enamel surface during the late pre-eruptive period, well after calcification is complete. The higher the concentration of fluoride in the outer layers of the surface enamel, the more caries resistant is the tooth.

Fluoride is known to protect the teeth against dental caries. It can be incorporated into the teeth during formation. It can also act locally once the tooth has erupted making the enamel surface of the tooth more resistant to acid and it also reduces the production of acids by bacteria in the mouth, thereby increasing the remineralisation process.

Dental Caries

Dental caries is the progressive destruction of the teeth by acid produced by the bacteria on the tooth surface. This happens over a period of time when the process of demineralization exceeds that of remineralization. Dental caries is widely prevalent and is increasing in some developing countries undergoing nutritional transition.[7]

Epidemiological studies have demonstrated evidence between the amount and frequency of free sugars intake and dental caries. Other carbohydrates especially cooked starch, e.g. in crisps, which can be broken down by enzymes in saliva to component sugars, may also damage the teeth although to a lesser degree.

Sucrose is most commonly associated with caries, although glucose, fructose and maltose seem equally cariogenic. The amount of sugar consumed at one time is less important than how often sugar containing foods are consumed. The longer the teeth are exposed to sugary foods, greater is the time during which the tooth are exposed to low pH levels inducing demineralisation. The sugars present in complex forms or in combination with other foods, can reduce the impact of damage on the teeth, thus reducing the risk of caries, since other foods hinder the drop in pH.

Fruit juice compared to fruits can be more cariogenic. The explanation lies in the fact that sugars in fruits are held in cells of the fruit and are not released until chewing breaks down the cells. On the contrary, in fruit juice, sugars are no longer held in the cells of the fruit, thus causing development of caries. This can be aggravated more in children in whom the teeth are exposed for a longer time, e.g. in a feeding bottle.

The sticky nature of carbohydrates also tends to promote risk of caries, since foods like dry fruits or chocolates or certain sweets can stick to the mouth, thus reducing the pH in the mouth for a long time, leading to demineralization.

A common example of the effect of protracted exposure of teeth to sugar is the so called 'nursing bottle syndrome' leading to 'bottle caries'.[8,9] This is characterized by extensive and rapid loss of tooth surface in all the upper teeth including the lower molars. This is commonly prevalent in the 2–4 year old children who continue to nurse the bottle as a pacifier at bed time. The bottle is not only used for milk, but also for other beverages like tea, juices or sweetened water. The beverage tends to accumulate around the upper teeth. The interaction between the sugars and the teeth lowers the pH, encouraging demineralization, which decalcifies and destroys the teeth. While the child is asleep, lack of adequate salivary flow leads to stagnation of fermenting beverage and neutralizes its acids. This results in painful and broken down carious teeth.[7] It is therefore recommended that mothers be educated regarding measures to keep in mind while feeding their children which are:

Try to avoid use of feeding bottles, especially as pacifiers at bedtime

- In situations where a child has become emotionally dependent upon the bottle, plain water should be used which can gradually dissuade him away from the bottle.
- The plaque must be removed before offering the next feed by brushing or wiping it away with a gauze pad.

Dental Erosion

Dental erosion differs from dental caries, since the former is not caused by bacteria but by action of acid, which could be either gastric or foods and drinks. Erosion can also occur in children with gastroesophageal reflux where there is a recurrent problem of vomiting or regurgitation. The erosion of the enamel and the dentine from the tooth can cause exposure of the pulp leading to pain and sensitivity to hot or cold foods.[10]

Some of the common foods and drinks consumed by children like soft drinks, fruit juices or carbonated fizz drinks and vinegar based foods all are acidic to some degree and can contribute to dental erosion. Children between 5–14 years are most prone to dental erosion due to their increased tendency to rely on such foods.[11]

Prevention of Dental Caries

Avoidance of acidic foods and drinks is the only prevention for dental erosion. Moreover, the duration of contact the teeth are exposed to the acidic food or beverage also determines the degree of erosion the teeth undergo. Using a straw for beverages can help minimize the risk and duration of exposure the teeth are subjected to. Swishing drinks or fruit juice in the mouth as most children playfully do should be avoided. Secondly, after consuming such foods and beverages, the teeth should not be brushed for at least one hour, since immediate brushing (e.g. at bed time just after dinner), will prevent the remineralization of the enamel to take place.

REFERENCES

1. Nizel A E. Nutritional support for optimizing children's dental health. In: Textbook of Pediatric Nutrition ed. Suskind RM. Raven Press. 1981;583-95.
2. Infente PF, Gillespie GM. Enamel hypoplasia in relation to caries in Guatemalan children. J Dent Res. 1977;56:493-98.
3. Infente PF, Owen GM, Russel AL. Dental caries in preschool Apache Indian children. J Dent Res. 1977;54:915.
4. Massler M, Schour I. Am J Orthod Oral Surg. 1946;32:495-517.
5. British Nutrition Foundation. Dental Health. 2004.
6. Melberg JR. Fluoride in preventive dentistry. J Prev Dent. 1977;4:8-20.
7. Moynihan P, Peterson PE. Diet, Nutrition and the prevention of dental diseases. Public Health Nutr. Feb 2004;7(1A):201-26.
8. Bernick S. What the pediatrician should know about children's teeth IV. Baby-Bottle Syndrome. Clin Pediatr. 1971;10:243-44.
9. Castano F. Penn Dent J. 1972;39:8-11.
10. Gandara BK, Truelove EL. Diagnosis and management of dental erosion. The J of Contemporary Dental Practice. 1999;Vol. 1, No. 1 Nov. 15.
11. Dugmoro CR, Rock WP. A multifactorial analysis of factors associated with dental erosion. Brit Dent J. 2004;196(5):283-6.

SECTION 2

Nutrition in Disease

21 Diet in Fever and Infections

Fever has been described as an elevation of body temperature above the normal, resulting from an imbalance between the heat produced in the body and that eliminated from the body. Fever, by itself is not a disease, but should be considered as a sign of any underlying infection or inflammation.

Fevers may vary in the form of manifestation like:

1. May be of short duration or acute, e.g. in colds, coughs or any upper respiratory tract infections or any other viral infections. Most of the infections whether of viral or bacterial etiology have one common feature that being fever.
2. May be chronic, or lasting for months and even may be of variable pattern, e.g. in tuberculosis, enteric, viral hepatitis, diphtheria, etc.

PATHOGENESIS

Fever, be it as a result of any cause, involves certain metabolic affects, which are proportional to the elevation of the body temperature and the length of time the temperature persists. Some of the metabolic affects are:

1. An increase in the basal metabolic rate which is almost 7% for every degree rise in temperature.
2. Decreased glycogen stores from the adipose tissue.
3. Increased catabolism of proteins, e.g. in enteric fever, viral hepatitis which exert an increased renal load by increase in nitrogenous wastes.
4. Accelerated loss of body fluids owing to increased perspiration and excretion of wastes.
5. Increased excretion of sodium and potassium
6. The gastrointestinal metabolism too is altered due to altered motility of the gastrointestinal tract. Vomiting, if accompanied by fever can cause further imbalance of electrolytes and fluids.

Dietary Management

During the course of any fever, appetite is generally compromised, resulting in decreased intake. This leads to the child getting lethargic and weak. It is essential that adequate nutrients are provided during this period, as this will prevent him/her from slipping into a catabolic state. The older concept of starving a fever no longer holds good; on the contrary this will only accelerate the catabolic state of the child and delay convalescence.

Energy

Due to the increase in the basal metabolic rate, the energy requirements are proportionally increased—almost 50%, if the temperature is very high and prolonged. Conditions like tuberculosis, viral hepatitis, enteric fever, pyogenic meningitis, liver abscess or empyemas all require energy dense feeding to prevent further catabolism. Easy to digest cereals and pulses prepared with moderate amounts of fat and/or sugar, honey, etc. can help to enhance the energy content of the preparations offered.

Proteins

Normal to high protein diets are adequate to meet the requirements in conditions like the ones described above. Milk and milk products, whey proteins, egg, chicken and fish are some high class protein sources which can take care of the increased requirements.

Carbohydrates

Due to depletion of glycogen stores during fever, liberal intake of carbohydrates may be offered which will build up the required calories. Sweetened beverages, but not aerated ones can help build up the glycogen stores. Fruits and fruit juices help provide adequate reserves of glycogen.

Fats

The intake of fats may be modified such that the calorie requirements are adequately taken care of. Emulsified fats in the form of butter or cream may be better tolerated as compared to heavy fried foods which may cause nausea. Too much of fried foods like snacks, etc. are best avoided. Contrary to the common myth in conditions like viral hepatitis, slight increase in fat sources will actually enhance the energy intake and help in maintain the body reserves.

Minerals

Adequate amounts of minerals like calcium and iron also can be provided through the foods offered. Milk and milk products are good sources of calcium while green vegetables cooked along with the preparations can take care of the iron levels. Jaggery may be substituted for sugar, as it is a very good source of iron. Non vegetarians may be offered half boiled egg or poached egg with bread which can provide both calcium and iron. Fruits and fruit juices can help compensate for the sodium and potassium losses which are very commonly seen in prolonged fevers.

Vitamins

Requirements of vitamins, especially the water soluble ones like thiamine and riboflavin generally increase due to the long-term course of antibiotics used to treat the infective fevers. This group of vitamins is generally not absorbed during the course of antibiotics, therefore it would be worthwhile supplementing them if oral intake is inadequate. Deficiency of these could lead to signs like angular stomatitis, cheilosis, etc. Good servings of fruit juices can help prevent such deficiency states.

Fluids

Due to losses of fluid from the skin via perspiration, it is essential to provide liberal fluid intake in the form of milk, juices, soups, buttermilk and water. Tea is best avoided in the case of infants and children as it is likely to cause gastric acidity on an empty stomach, besides suppressing appetite. Adequate fluid intake also can help maintain adequate urine output which facilitates waste excretion.

Factors Involved in Feeding

The type of food offered would be determined by the age of the child, the type of illness, and of course the child's individual preference also should be taken into consideration. Small frequent feeding can be tried in case the child seems disinclined to eat anything. Taboos like 'hot' or 'cold ' foods or 'light' or 'heavy' foods should be broken and anything the child desires may be offered; e.g. rice is considered cold and avoided during fever or gram flour is considered hot or heavy and so not given. In fact, 'besan sheera' is a good option for a child with fever, being a good protein and energy source. Similarly banana is considered to be causing phlegm and so avoided, whereas on the contrary it is one of the most safe and nutritious fruits which can be given in almost any condition. Citrus fruits which are a good source of ascorbic acid and good anti-oxidants are generally avoided due to the fear of causing throat infection or is considered cold. Such myths only further deteriorate the already cachectic state of the child and result in delayed convalescence.

The consistency of the food offered may be modified as per the child's individual acceptance and suitability. Very high fiber foods may be avoided to facilitate easy digestion.

Diets in Specific Conditions

Fever may be prolonged in certain specific conditions as the ones mentioned below.

Tuberculosis

In this condition, fever may persist for quite some time despite initiation of antitubercular drugs. There may be associated anorexia too due to the fever, but attempt should be made to offer foods high in proteins and energy to compensate for the enhanced basal metabolic rate which increases the demand upon the body. Inadequate feeding is likely to lead the child to not only inadequate weight gain but also to weight loss. Consequently the child becomes quite emaciated with decreased muscle mass leading to a state of lethargy, decreased immunity and loss of stamina to perform the routine chores.

A high energy, high protein diet is recommended for tissue building besides the normal growth and development. First class proteins like milk and eggs should be encouraged. Other protein rich sources like pulses, especially soybean can also be incorporated in the meal planning. If required protein supplements may be considered. Fruits and juices also should be a part of the meal to provide the much needed antioxidants.

Enteric Fever

In the earlier times severe dietary restrictions were imposed in children with enteric fever (typhoid fever), with the view to give 'rest' to the intestines. But it was realized that such restrictions further deteriorated the condition causing prolonged delay in the healing process. All essential nutrients were deprived of resulting in completely emaciating the patient. Only foods like barley water, rice kanjee, weak tea, diluted milk, buttermilk or flavored water, etc. were fed for the entire period of illness. In case of children whose physiological demands are at the peak, such restrictions only lead to delayed or stunted development and growth failure.

It is therefore recommended that a complete normal diet as per requirements for the age of the child needs to be encouraged. A full balanced diet with all the food groups incorporated in different preparations can be offered to bring variety to the diet. Most important, the food preferences of the child should be the basis of meal planning in this condition. Any kind of food taboos or myths should be done away with.

Viral Hepatitis

Jaundice is commonly encountered among school going children which is mostly of viral etiology. Fever persists for a prolonged length of time and typically there is severe anorexia in most patients. Again due to certain food taboos many foods are avoided in this condition, especially fats. They are mostly made to thrive on boiled food and that too most of the yellow colored foods are avoided. Thus the food presented is a very bland looking and tasting equally bland, which only helps in creating more aversion to an already anorexic child. Here too the requirements are increased for the healing of the liver cells and restoring the liver to its normal function. Therefore a calorie dense diet with normal to high proteins and equally high fat diet should be planned to be able to meet the increased demands. Foods like milk based (casein) sweets (khoya), cheese, paneer, chocolates and such other tempting stuff can be given liberally to meet the requirements with minimum quantity (See Chapter 15). As mentioned for earlier conditions, anything that the child demands as per his/her taste can be offered. No food restrictions should be imposed. The only caution to be taken is that the food procured should be from a hygienic source, especially fruit juices or other snacks. Fried foods also may be offered if the child so demands, but fats like butter or cream are better options as these can be incorporated in different foods planned.

Finally the concept of 'starving a fever' would only translate in 'starving the child'.

22 Enteral Nutrition in Hospitalized Patient

Enteral nutrition (EN) is an alternative method of providing nutrition support to a patient who is otherwise unable or not in a condition to receive oral nutrition. In a child it becomes all the more essential that nutritional support is provided where there is inadequate oral intake or the child is very malnourished and unable to ingest the required amount of feeds orally. This nutrition support can be provided through the enteral route where the gut is intact. EN goes a long way in restoring the nutritional status of the child and plays an adjunctive role in the disease and immune process. It improves physical and mental functions, decreases the effect of catabolism and prevents further weight loss.

Feeding by the enteral route may reduce sepsis, blunt the hypermetabolic response to trauma and maintain gut integrity.[1] It is recommended that a child with malnutrition or likely to receive inadequate nutrient intake for a minimum of 7 days or more, should be offered EN.

Enteral nutrition (EN) has been successfully used within 24–48 hours after surgery or trauma to provide fluids, electrolytes and nutritional support. In case there is gastric ileus, nasogastric feeding can be replaced by nasojejunal or nasointestinal feeding. This allows successful post pyloric passage of the feeds.[2]

Enteral nutrition (EN) formulae can vary in composition and nutrient density. By and large these include standard whole protein formulae, elemental or peptide based or any disease specific formulations. These may also include certain specific nutrients like glutamine, arginine and omega 3 fatty acids. Apart from these indigenous formulates, feeds can also be administered by modifying the locally available commercial protein or MCT based formulae to the indigenous formulation (kitchen based feeds). These have also been successful in the developing countries. This can help in reducing the cost in an otherwise resource limited setting.

According to the British Medical Association (BMA), it is important to identify the need for enteral feeding, before deciding whether a child should be artificially fed.[3]

INDICATIONS FOR ENTERAL NUTRITION SUPPORT IN CHILDREN

- Enteral nutrition (EN) support may be used for children in any of the following conditions:
- Unable to suck/swallow, e.g. in ventilated patients.
- Swallowing may be unsafe, e.g. in cerebral palsy, seizures.
- Poor sucking, e.g. in premature infants.
- Increased requirements, e.g. in conditions of cystic fibrosis, burns, trauma or any congenital heart disease.
- Poor appetite secondary to illness like in disorders of the liver, kidney or cancer.
- Congenital abnormalities, e.g. in tracheo-esophageal fistula, orofacial malformation
- Unpalatability of specialized feeds, e.g. Crohn's disease.
- Continuous supply of nutrients required to prevent hypoglycemia or in glycogen storage disease Type 1.

Once the decision to provide nutrition entrerally is made, the patient needs to be explained regarding the objective of doing so. This can be done by explaining the proposed benefits of the treatment, i.e. weight gain, speedy recovery and prevention of starvation, explaining the possible risks and complications involved, e.g. infection, granulation, gastroesophageal reflux, tube displacement, leakage, vomiting, retching, diarrhea or constipation or blocked tube, explaining the impact of the treatment on the family, e.g. restricted freedom of mobility, monitoring of feeds and checking for aspirates.

Nutritional Requirements in Enteral Nutrition

Calories: The nutritional requirements can be calculated based on the RDA for age, as is done when planning an oral feeding. However, for bedside calculation, a minimum requirement may be determined which may be adequate for an average child. The formula used is 100 calories/kg up to 1 year, 1000 calories at 1 year and thereafter, 1000 +10 calories/each year up to puberty. At puberty, the requirement is equated to 1 unit of energy (2, 400 calories).[4]

Proteins: The protein requirement can be calculated as 10%–15% of the calories, which amounts to 1.5–2 g/kg/d. In case the child is very malnourished, protein may be increased gradually to 3–4 g/kg/d. In conditions of renal failure, the protein may be decreased to around 0.5 g/kg/d. The protein requirement may be met by utilizing either whole proteins, protein hydrolysates or as individual amino acids or a combination of these based on their absorptive capacity, requirement and tolerance. Whole proteins being less expensive can be given in patients with no suspected major absorptive defect or protein allergy. These also allow greater nutrient density. In patients who are able to tackle whole proteins or have any specific absorptive defect or deficiency, can be offered protein hydrolysate. However, hydrolyzed proteins have high osmolar load as compared to the whole proteins

Fats: The high caloric density of fats (especially triglycerides) makes it a highly desirable nutrient in the nutritional support of the hospitalized child. Three major considerations are involved in the use of dietary fats—the use and absorption of LCT, MCT and the requirement for EFA.

It has been recommended that if there are no defects in the absorption of fats, the choice should be LCT. Excessive use of MCT in patients with intact mechanisms can lead to osmotic diarrhea due to the rapid hydrolysis of MCT to free fatty acids and glycerol. A combination of LCT and MCT fats may be justified in order to gain maximal absorption in patients in whom increased calories are vital.[4] A total of 25–30% of calories can be provided by fats out of which up to 10–15% of the fats can be provided as visible fat. In case where there is suspected fat malabsorption, MCT can be provided as a safe source of fat e.g. in conditions of hepatobiliary diseases.

Carbohydrates: Ideally 50%–60% of the energy can be provided by carbohydrates. In diseases involving the mucosa of the small intestine, all of the disaccharides may be depressed. Lactase is one of the most sensitive to injury and the last to recover too. This may result in transient lactase deficiency. Starvation by itself is known to depress the disaccharide activity, therefore it is important to avoid or minimize dietary sources of lactose in treating the malnourished child.

Micronutrients: Since children who are malnourished with their intake compromised, there is an increased demand for all micronutrients, especially during the acute phase of illness. Supplementing these with the enteral feeds should be done as per the recommended doses.

Properties of an Enteral Feed

Enteral feeds although are formulated to provide more or less complete nutritional requirements, certain factors need to be kept in mind regarding their effects on the patient (Table 22.1).[5]

Physiologic effects: The effects of various types of food or acid secretion are proportionate primarily to the protein content. There is evidence to suggest that the carbohydrate fraction of the meal stimulates gastrin secretion. When amino acids are administered as mixtures, as in the defined formula diets, pancreatic stimulation occurs. This can be averted, if the feeds are given intrajejunally and at a neutral pH. This kind

TABLE 22.1: Special considerations in administering feeds through enteral route

Risk of aspiration
Comatose patient
Restrained patient
Small Infant
Depressed gag reflex
Palatability
Distorted N: calorie ratio
Inappropriate formulations
Osmolality—formulae with increased nutrient intensity

Reference: Leiko NS, Murray C and Munro HN. Enteral Suport of the hospitalized child. In: Textbook of Pediatric Nutrition. Ed. Robert M Suskind. Raven Press, New York. 1981.pp.352-74.

of therapy is particularly suitable in case of patients with fistulae or pancreatitis.

Nitrogen : Calorie Ratio

Generally the protein content of enteral feeds is 15%–17% of the energy content. In such a case the N: calorie ratio is approximately 1:150, which is considered adequate for recovery and growth in infants suffering from varying degrees of malnutrition. However, in cases requiring unusually high protein content due to excessive losses, higher protein ratio also can be provided for maintenance.

UNIFORMITY

Defined enteral diets are designed to be uniform in composition and this is the reason it can be used as a supplement to total parenteral nutrition. These formulae are devoid of fiber as a result of which there is a decrease in stool frequency, weight and bulk and the stools are usually dark green in color, watery and nonformed.

Osmolality

An important factor to be considered when choosing or formulating an enteral formula is the osmolality of the feed. An osmolality above 600 mOsm/l can lead to an increased incidence of gastro intestinal symptoms and intolerance to feeds. It has been shown that an osmolality of 560 mosm/l can cause a significant delay in gastric emptying.[5]

Carbohydrates electrolytes and amino acids are the major factors determining the gastrointestinal osmotic load of a formula. Smaller particles like glucose and free amino acids contribute to a higher osmolality than do larger particles such as polysaccharides or intact protein molecules. That is why hydrolysed proteins and monosacharides will tend to have a higher osmolality than will formula with intact protein and glucose polymers.[6]

An osmolality of less than 460 mOsm/kg has been recommended for infant formula, therefore for children younger than 4 years, the enteral formula should be < 400 mOsm/kg and for older ones, < 600 mOsm/kg.[7,8]

Contraindications of Enteral Nutrition

Contraindications to enteral feeding in most cases are relative rather than absolute. It is also dependent upon the appropriate feeding site administration technique, formula and equipment.[9]

Terminal illness: Potential problems include aspiration, diarrhea, overhydration, discomfort and cost.

Short bowel: Patients with a short bowel often require TPN for 1–3 months post surgery, while the remaining bowel adapts to allow adequate nutrient absorption. Adaptation of the gut is accelerated by early institution of some enteral feeding.

Obstruction: Complete mechanical obstruction of the GI below the duodenum or pseudo-obstruction like in GI motility disorders can be contraindication for EN.

GI bleeding: Chronic, slow upper GI bleed may not be an absolute contraindication for EN but frequent vomiting or nausea may require withholding of EN temporarily. In such cases, small bowel feedings rather than gastric feeding are a better option.

Vomiting and diarrhea: Vomiting may make it difficult to maintain the nasogastric feeding tube in place, in which case small bowel feeding can be done. Diarrhea may not be due to EN but could be associated with the type of feeding formula, e.g. lactose based or medications received as in case of antibiotics.

GI ischemia: GI ischemia may result due to the disease state itself or medical treatment which may reduce the blood flow to the gut, e.g. critically ill patients with a low cardiac output, patients with sepsis and those with multiorgan failure.

Ileus: In surgical conditions like perforation, anastomatic leaks, intraperitoneal hemorrhage, peritonitis and other intra-abdominal infections, ileus can occur. This is more frequently known to affect the stomach and large bowel. Therefore to overcome this hurdle postpyloric feeding tube placement can be done.

GI inflammation: In conditions like IBD (Inflammatory Bowel Disease), radiation or chemotherapy, inflammation or enteritis is commonly seen. In such cases, bowel rest is advised and parenteral nutrition may be resorted to. Bowel rest is advised in pancreatitis, although successful enteral nutrition support has been demonstrated to yield good results.

Routes of EN

After deciding upon the type of enteral nutrition to be administered, the next step is to evaluate the way to do it. Ideally 'where the gut works, it should be used.' Oral feeding whenever possible even though in small proportions must be preferred to maintain the gut integrity. Breastfeeding if possible should be continued. But in cases where oral intake is not possible due to various reasons like swallowing difficulty, esophageal atresia, gastrectomy, seizures or other neurological conditions, alternative route of feeding have to be made use of. This will depend upon the best available route and feasibility of administration at the available site. Some common routes used are:

- Nasogastric
- Nasojejunal
- Gastrostomy/Jejunostomy.

An illustration of protocol for decision making for selecting the route of feeding is illustrated in Figure 22.1.[10]

Nasogastric Feeding (NG Feeding)

This is the most preferred route used in most children with intact GIT or who are unable to swallow orally. The nasogastric feedings are used mainly for short term use (6–8 weeks). Formula or kitchen based feeds are generally given through this route either as bolus feeds at periodic intervals or as continuous drip method. The latter is a better option and acceptable since there is better tolerance as compared to bolus feeding. The rule is to begin with small feeds at periodic intervals and gradually increase the volume and density of the feeds as the tolerance improves. A common observation is that in case of malnourished children, who are unable to eat orally as per the required dose, if NG feeding is initiated and continued for a few days, the appetite of the child begins to improve and gradually they can be weaned off the NG feed completely. However NG feeding is contraindicated in patients with seven esophagitis or who have no obstruction between the nose and stomach.

Nasojejunal Feeding (NJ Feeding)

This method of feeding involved placement of the tube well beyond the stomach, into the jejunum, so that the feed is deposited beyond the pylorus, thus preventing regurgitation. This route is used typically for children who are at risk of aspiration which include diminished gag reflex, delayed gastric emptying, frequent vomiting or severe gastroesophageal reflux (GER). The intestinal wall having a larger surface area allows for rapid absorption of iso and hypoosmolar solutions. Some problems of pain, nausea, distension or hypermotility and diarrhea may result if the formula is hyperosmolar, has whole protein sources, complex carbohydrates and LCTs. Necrotising enterocolitis is one complication which could be related to use of hyperosmolar solutions in premature infants.[6]

Gastrostomy Feeding

Gastrostomy feeding is used in children expected to be on long term NG feeding, e.g. in severe neurological impairment, esophageal pathology or severe cardiorespiratory disease, who have an intact GIT. The rate and volume of feeding is done as is done in NG feeding. In conditions where the stomach or duodenum integrity is affected, Jejunostomy feeding tube is used. The considerations for using this route are same as for NJ feeding.

Methods of Administration of EN

The mode of feed delivery is based on the condition of the patient and the anatomic location of the tube (gastric or transpyloric). The feeds may be delivered either through intermittent bolus or continuous drip method. Intermittent bolus feeds are given 2–4 hourly

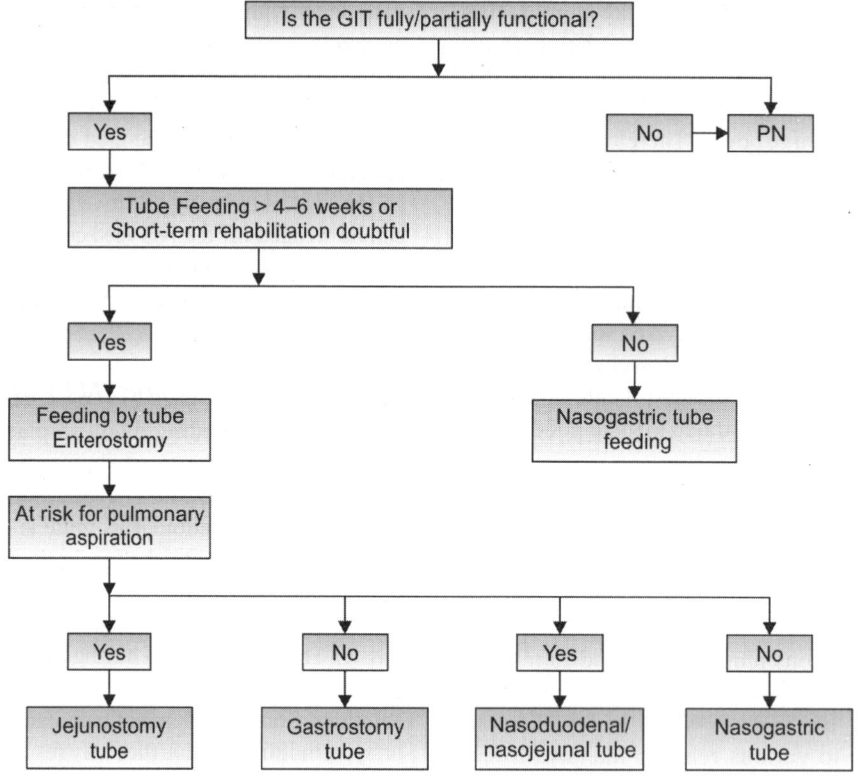

FIGURE 22.1: Decision making for selecting feeding

Reference: Rombeau JL and Caldwell MD, eds. Enteral and Tube Feeding. In: Clinical Nutrition,Vo; 1, 1984, WB Saunders Company.

over a period of 15–20 minutes by gravity, while continuous drip method involves infusion of nutrients at a constant rate over several hours. The choice of the type of delivery mode depends on a number of factors like:[11]

- Enteral access route
- Volume of feed required
- Stability of the patient
- Gastrointestinal tolerance of the feed
- Age of the patient
- Type of formula
- Nutrient requirement
- Patient cooperation and mobility.

Initiation of Advancement of Feeding

The rate of advancement of enteral feeding is contingent on the structure and function of the patients GIT. Children being weaned from PN to enteral nutrition or who are malnourished may require a more conservative feeding progression than what is typically administered to children with normal GI.

General Considerations

There are a certain general guidelines to be considered when advancing enteral nutrition in children, which have been laid down based on institutional practices and modifications of adult regimens as under.[6]

- Plan for a 2–5 day period to meet the nutritional goals.
- Use isotonic feedings initially.
- Avoid making a simultaneous change in volume and concentration.
- Use of dilute feedings in patients with altered GI functions or when weaning from PN to EN.
- Advance continuously and gradually in very critical or malnourished children.

- Increase volume before increasing concentration when administering transplyloric feeds.
- Advance concentration before volume when administering gastric feeds.

If not tolerated, revert back to the last tolerated concentration and volume and progress slowly again.

Continuous Drip Feeding

Begin at a rate of 1–2 ml/kg/h.

Advance in increment of 0.5–1 ml/kg/h every 8–24 hours.

Rate of feeding for various age groups as recommended in Table 22.2.[10]

Intermittent Feeding

Determine the total volume of formula needed to provide nutritional goal.

Begin delivery at 25% of the volume goal on the first day.

Space the formula volume equally between 6–8 feedings.

Increase formula volume by 25% per day as tolerated, with total volume equally divided between numbers of feedings.

Administer by gravity over 15–30 minutes.

A comparative picture of the advantages and disadvantages of the above modes of delivery of enteral nutrition are highlighted in Table 22.3.[6]

Complications of EN

Although administration of EN through tube feeding takes care of all the nutrient requirements of the patient and feeding can be ensured even when the child is sick or unable to take orally, there are certain factors to be borne in mind while administering EN, which if not considered may lead to complications. Some of the common complications known to occur while giving feeds are:

TABLE 22.2: Recommended rate of continuous drip feeding for children

Age	Weight (kg)	Initial rate (ml/h)	Max. rate (ml/h)
Infants	3–10	3–10	25–50
Toddler/Preschool	10–20	10–20	60–70
School age	20–40	20–40	80–100
Adolescent	> 40	40–50	100–150

Reference: Rombeau JL and Caldwell MD, eds. Enteral and Tube Feeding. In: Clinical Nutrition, Vol. 1, 1984, WB Saunders

TABLE 22.3: Advantages and disadvantages of different modes of enteral feeding

Continous Drip Feeding	
Advantages	**Disadvantages**
Ability to increase volume of formula more rapidly	More expensive feeding method since pump is required
Improved absorption of nutrients in infants with intestinal disease	Restricts patient ambulation
Reduced stool output in hypermetabolic patients	Less physiologic
Reduced incidence of vomiting in infants with gastro-esophageal reflux	
Greater energy intake when volume tolerance is a problem	
Intermittent Feeding	
Advantages	**Disadvantages**
More physiologic since resembles a normal feeding schedule	Associated with longer time of reach nutritional goals
Less expensive since pump not required	Reduced weight gain and nutrient absorption in infants with malabsorption
Greater flexibility in feeding schedule	Larger bore tube may be required for gravity administration
Freedom from infusion equipment	More time required for administration than for pump delivered feedings
Improved N retention with less fat and fluid accumulation	
Allows the gastric acidity to increase	

Reference: Nancy Nevin Folino and Murna Miller. Enteral Nutrition. In: Handbookok Pediatric Nutrition, 2nd edn. Patricia Queen Samour, Kathy King Helm and Carol E. Lang. Jones and Bartlett Publishers, Massachusetts, 2004. pp.513-49.

Mechanical Complications

Tube displacement: These may involve placement of the feeding tube which could be displaced or faulty placement resulting in lacerations along the esophagus, upper airway injury, GI injuries, bleeding ulcers, extrusion or migration of feeding tubes. Many of these problems occur with larger or stiffer tubes and can be minimized by using small bore feeding tubes and meticulous nursing care.

Tube clogging: This can occur with feeds which are protein based and viscous in nature. Mostly kitchen based feed may tend to have some residue settling down which is likely to clog while passing through the tube. Flushing of the tube with water after every feed or checking of aspirate can minimise the problem.

Aspiration: This is a serious complication of any enteral feeding. Aspiration pneumonia can occur in 5% of gastric fed patients, resulting in cough, bronchospasm, pulmonary edema, pneumonia, empyema and respiratory failure.[10,11]

GI Complications

GER: Reflux of contents from the stomach can occur in some patients when the gastric pressure exceeds that of the pressure of the lower esophageal stricture (LES) which prevents the gastric contents from pushing up towards the esophagus. In patients with large volume or ascites (due to the increased abdominal pressure), reflux can be encountered.[12,13]

Diarrhea: Diarrhea can be frequently seen in patients receiving enteral feeds. This could be either if feed is lactose based (e.g. in high volume milk based feeds) or could also be due to bacterial growth or presence of toxins, or medications, e.g. certain antibiotics, SBS, high fat based feeds or due to the nature of the disease itself.[5] Withdrawal of feeding is not recommended in such cases, but a change of formula or tackling the infective source could help minimize the complication. In extreme cases if no specific cause can be elicited for the problem, enteral feeds may be considered to be replaced by parenteral nutrition.

Constipation: This can result from inactivity, decreased small bowel motility, decreased fluid intake, impaction or lack of dietary fiber. Adequate hydration and use of fiber based formulae can help minimise the problem. Laxatives and enemas may also help relieve the problem.

Metabolic Complications

Hyperglycemia: This is not a very common problem because of enteral feeding, but could be encountered in patients who may be diabetic. At times high carbohydrate feeds may also cause increased blood sugar levels. Patient on IV fluids over a considerable period when fed enterally also may develop hyperglycemia. Increased blood glucose levels should be tackled immediately by use of insulin. The aim should be to maintain the blood glucose concentrations below 150–180 mg/d.[5]

Electrolyte and mineral deficiencies: Losses of electrolytes (sodium, potassium) through stools, ostomies, fistulae, urine and skin can result in considerable electrolyte and animal losses too. Mineral deficiencies like magnesium, calcium, phosphorous might also be encountered along with the above problems, coupled with lack of these minerals in the eneteral feeds. Adequate supplementation of these needs to be considered in such cases.[5]

Refeeding syndrome: This is a condition known to occur in malnourished children, where there are acute intracellular shifts of electrolytes or cell anabolism is stimulated.[14]

Vitamin deficiencies: Both water soluble and fat soluble vitamin deficiencies can be encountered in patients on EN. Children with pancreatic enzyme deficiency, e.g. in cystic fibrosis are prone to be deficient in vitamin A, D and E as these require bile and pancreatic enzymes for absorption.[5] Other conditions where such deficiencies can occur are in malabsorption. These vitamins need to be monitored and replaced along with the EN. Similarly among the water soluble vitamins are folate and ascorbic acid and thiamine, which could be deficient in the enteral feeds and may need adequate replacement.

Dehydration: Dehydration is commonly encountered among patients on enteral feeds. An average requirement of water is 1 ml/calorie consumed. The use of concentrated formulae or high protein feeds may result in decrease in fluids, e.g. loss of body fluids when there is urea dieresis with high protein feeds. Restoration of intravascular volume and water balance can reverse this condition.[5]

REFERENCES

1. A.S.P.E.N. Board of Directors. Guidelines for use of Parenteral and Enteral Nutrition in adult and pediatric patients. JPEN. 1993;17(4):1-52.
2. Kudsk KA, Croce MA, Fabian TC, et al. Enteral versus parenteral feeding on septic morbidity alter blunt and penetrating abdominal trauma. Ann Surg. 1992;215:503-13.
3. Dartford, Gravesham NHS Trust, Dartford Gravesham, Swanley Primary Care Trust. Pediatric Enteral Feeding Guidelines Operational Policy (Infants and Children). Jan 2007.
4. KE Elizabeth. Enteral and Parenteral Nutrition. In: Nutrition and Child Development, 3rd edn. Paras Medical Publishers. 2004.pp.188-217.
5. Leiko NS, Murray C, Munro HN. Enteral Suport of the hospitalized child. In: Textbook of Pediatric Nutrition. Ed. Robert M Suskind. Raven Press, New York. 1981. pp.352-74.
6. Nancy Nevin Folino, Murna Miller. Enteral Nutrition. In: Handbookok Pediatric Nutrition, 2nd edn. Patricia Queen Samour, Kathy King Helm and Carol E. Lang. Jones and Bartlett Publishers, Massachusetts, 2004.pp.513-49.
7. Kalawitter BM. Pediatric Nutrition Support. In: Williams CP, ed. Pediatric Manual of Clinical Dietetics. Chicago IL: The Am Dietet Assoc. 1998.
8. Cox JH, ed Nutrition Manual for At-Risk Infants and toddlers. Chicago IL: Precept Press. 1997.
9. Lingard CD. Enteral Nutrition. In: Handbook of Pediatric Nutrition, Queen PM and Lang CE. Eds. Gaithesburg MD. Aspen Publishers. Inc. 1993.pp.249-78.
10. Rombeau JL and Caldwell MD, eds. Enteral and Tube Feeding, In: Clinical Nutrition, WB Saunders Company. 1984.Vol.1
11. Lysen LK, Samour PQ, Enteral Equipment, Principles of Nutrition Support. WB Saunders Company. 1998.p.202
12. Hamaai E. Gastroesophageal reflex during gastostomy feeding. JPEN. 1995;19:172-73.
13. Gustke RF, Varma RR, Soegel KH. Gastric reflux during perfusion of the proximal small bowel. Gastroenterology 1970;59:890-95.
14. Solomon SM, Kirby DF. The Refeeding syndrome: A review. JPEN. 14:90-7.

23 Protein Energy Malnutrition

"Health is not simply the absence of sickness"
Hannah Green

The health and well being of any individual is based on a combination of various factors. Besides diet and good nutrition, a host of contributory factors go a long way in preventing disease and malnutrition. These may be environmental, socio-demographic, immunization programs, provision of clean water supply and even psychosocial.

Environmental factors include parental education, socioeconomic status, living standards and child rearing practices.

Sociodemographic factors include breastfeeding practices, diet during illness for mother and child, maternal malnutrition, low birth weight babies, recurrent infections, etc.

According to WHO definition, malnutrition involves a cellular imbalance between supply of nutrients and energy and the body's demand for them to ensure normal growth, maintenance and specific tissue functions.[1] Malnutrition accounts for more than 50% of all infant mortality in developing countries, especially in the below 5 year age group.

The most common form of malnutrition in children is protein energy malnutrition (PEM), which earlier was also called protein calorie malnutrition (PCM). It has also been defined as a pathological state characterized by inadequate intake of proteins and calories in varying degrees commonly associated with infections.[1] Children between 6–36 months old are generally at high risk of falling prey to this condition, since they are more vulnerable to infections, especially gastrointestinal and measles. Death rates are high among children with untreated PEM, and the risk of dying increases with severity of the condition. Electrolyte imbalance, hypothermia and complicating infections are some of the causes of mortality in these children.

Etiology of PEM: PEM occurs primarily due to food deprivation, but other factors play a major role also. These can be discussed as:

- ***Low birth weight and infections:*** Recurrent diarrhea, acute respiratory infections, other preventable infections like measles, tuberculosis, whooping cough and helminthes, can aggravate and complicate a pre-existing condition of low birth weight. Again maternal malnutrition is an important cause of low birth weight.
- ***Food deprivation:*** Poverty is one important cause of food deprivation in small children. Large families contribute to this problem and the priority of food distribution generally is for the male child followed by other male members in the family.
- ***Food taboos and myths:*** Even where resources are not a limiting factor, very often self imposed restrictions regarding intake of food, can affect provision of adequate nutrients to the child. Food fads and myths related to consumption of specific type of foods at different phases of pregnancy or lactation and subsequently weaning practices can be a sole cause of food deprivation. Very often these fads and myths are interlinked with various cultural beliefs and/or religious beliefs. A common observation made is pertaining to infant feeding

practices, where, in most rural classes colostrum is discarded as it is considered poisonous for the baby. The maternal diet is also restricted keeping in mind 'hot' or 'cold' foods which may be 'unsuitable for the infant. All such practices can go a long way to adversely affect the availability of essential macro- and micronutrients required for adequate growth and development of the child.

- ***Ignorance:*** Many rural and urban mothers are quite ignorant of their infant's need for adequate nutrition. It's a common belief that milk is the 'best and only' food for a child, even after he has crossed the first 6 months of his life. They continue to breastfeed exclusively, well upto 12–24 months, making little effort to offer cereal supplements. Alternatively, if breast milk is inadequate, they will continue to feed diluted milk without introducing cereals. Even during illness of the child, solid food is withheld and the baby is kept on undiluted milk or tea with an occasional biscuit or so. Cereal, pulse base foods are considered 'heavy' for the child's liver. These factors further contribute to inadequate nutrient intake and subsequently growth failure.

Pathogenesis of PEM

Gopalan in 1968 introduced a new hypothesis, that of 'adaptation'.[2] This was termed as 'dysadaptation', stating that kwashiorkor in fact was a failure of adaptation. This was explained on biochemical and hormonal factors. The malnourished child adapts himself to the unfavorable circumstances and to the calorie and protein gap. They reduce their activity, curtail their growth thereby bringing down the basal metabolic rate (BMR) and thus save energy for survival. This reduction in BMR and lack of insulating fat leads to hypothermia which may prove fatal.

The basic adaptation to explain the mechanism was that the gradual wasting of muscle and subcutaneous fat would also protect certain other metabolic processes. Like, the essential amino acids are made available, which it was assumed, would enable the liver to maintain the synthesis of components essential for homeostasis, like serum albumin and β lipoprotein. This could explain the absence of edema or fatty liver in marasmus.[3]

The high level of catabolic hormones including cortisol causes muscle and fat breakdown. The anabolic hormones like insulin and insulin like growth factors maintain near normal anabolism to prevent edema and fatty liver by enabling the synthesis of albumin and β lipoproteins from the available pool of amino acids.

Another theory postulated in the pathogenesis of PEM is that of free radicals which are assumed to play a role in edema, skin changes and fatty liver. The free oxygen radicals which are toxic to cell membranes are produced during infections.[2] In the malnourished child, deficiency of nutrients like vitamins A, C and E and selenium which are anti-oxidants can result in the accumulation of toxic free oxygen radicals. These further damage the liver cells resulting in kwashiorkor.

Classification of PEM

Various parameters are used to classify PEM like, weight for age, height for age or weight for height. The most widely used accepted criterion is the weight for age. This has been done by various workers of different times. Besides Gomez and the IAP classification (Refer Chapter 3, Tables 3.1 and 3.2), two more classifications have been proposed:

- **Jelliffe's classification:** Proposed in 1965, it has been categorized into 4 classes as shown in Table 23.1.[4]
- **Wellcome Trust or International Classification:** This is based on clinical assessment as suggested by Wellcome Trust in 1970. Besides weight for age, it also considers presence or absence of edema as seen in Table 23.2.[5]

Spectrum of PEM

There are three forms of PEM recognized, based on the clinical presentations:

- Kwashiorkor
- Marasmus
- Marasmic Kwashiorkor.

A picture of the various features of PEM can be had from Table 23.3.

TABLE 23.1: Jelliffe's classification of PEM

Nutritional status (PEM)	Wt. for age (Harvard) % of expected
Normal	> 90
First degree	80–90
Second degree	70–80
Third degree	60–70
Fourth degree	< 60

TABLE 23.2: Wellcome Trust classification

Weight for age (Boston) % of expected	Edema	Clinical type of PEM
60–80	+	Kwashiorkor
60–80	–	Underweight
< 60	–	Marasmus
< 60	+	Marasmic Kwashiorkor

TABLE 23.3: Clinical features of PEM

Spectrum	Clinical Symptoms	
	Always present	Sometimes present
Marasmus	Wasting	Hunger, Wizened appearance
Kwashiorkor	Edema	Mental changes: Irritability, poor appetite Skin changes: Flaky paint dermatosis Hair: Sparse, loose, straight
Marasmic Kwashiorkor	Wasting + Edema	Any of the above symptoms and signs

Kwashiorkor

The word 'kwashiorkor' was first described by Dr Cicely Williams in 1933. The word originates from the African language—*Ga* of Ghana, meaning the 'red boy' due to the characteristic pigmentation.[6] Other workers from the West Indies described this as 'sugar baby' due to the characteristic 'prominent cheeks' and edema. This deficiency is known to occur with the coming of the second sib, when the child is displaced from the breast by another child. This condition is seen mostly in children in their second year of life, following abrupt weaning. They appear to be apathetic, irritable, weak and inactive, with the presence of edema and fatty liver. The edema is detected by the production of a definite pit on exerting moderate pressure for 3 seconds with the thumb over the lower end of the tibia and dorsum of the foot.

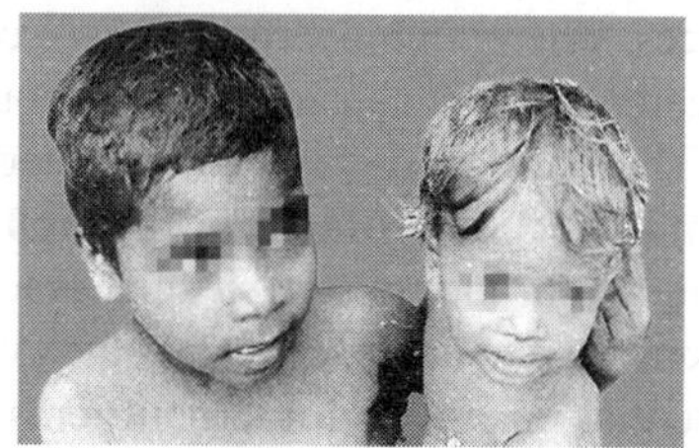

FIGURE 23.1A: Child with sparse hair

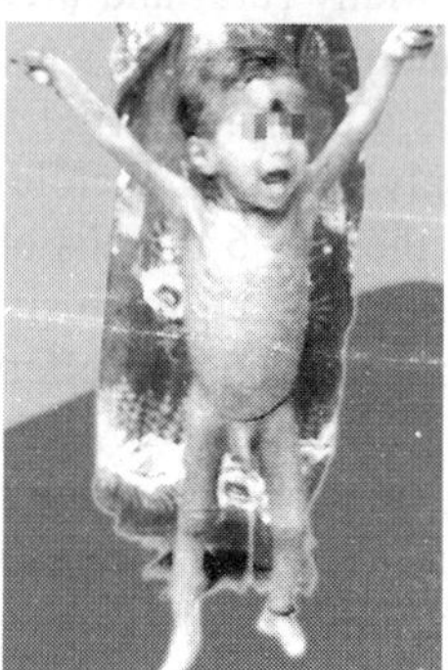

FIGURE 23.1B: Child with pot belly

Initially, parents may miss these features and on the contrary be satisfied by the false image of a 'fatty child' but what is not generally realized by the lay person is that this fat appears typically on the belly and is commonly referred to as 'pot belly', but from his buttocks would be flat and give a wasted appearance (Figs 23.1A and 23.1B).

The typical signs of PEM are described by the following associated abnormalities:

- *Body:* All body parts, especially buttocks, arms and legs have decreased subcutanous fat layer.
- *Skin:* The skin appears dry and flaky (flaky paint dermatosis). Hyper pigmented plaques may be visible over areas of trauma.
- *Hair*: It becomes thin, sparse and brittle. It also turns dull brown or red, giving an appearance of a 'flag sign'.
- *Nails:* There will be fissures or ridges and increased fragility.
- *Abdomen*: The presence of edema due to accumulation of ascetic fluid and also hepatomegaly (fatty liver), makes the abdomen appear distended.

- *Mouth:* Signs of vitamin B group deficiency-cheilosis, angular stomatitis and papillary atrophy are commonly present.
- *Behavior:* The child neither appears irritable and avoids social interaction, nor responds socially. They have a poor appetite and refuse to eat.
- *Deficiencies:* It is common to observe deficiency signs of vitamins, like, vitamin A, D and B group and minerals like iron and iodine.

Marasmus

The term marasmus is derived from the Greek 'marasms' which means wasting. In this condition, there is gross wasting of muscle and subcutanous tissues, marked stunting but no edema. This picture can be seen in early infancy unlike in kwashiorkor (Fig. 23.2).

The marasmic condition is typical of sequel to prolonged starvation, chronic or recurrent infections and limited food intake. Marasmus represents an *adaptive* response to starvation, unlike kwashiorkor which represents *maladaptive* response to starvation. In marasmus, the body utilizes all fat stores before using muscles. It is commonly seen in the first year of life due to lack of breastfeeding and the use of diluted animal milk. Poverty or famine like conditions and presence of diarrhea besides ignorance and poor maternal nutrition, are the precipitating factors. There is severe wasting of the shoulders, arms, buttocks and thighs with no visible rib outlines. The typical appearance of a marasmic child is described as:

- A 'thin old' man.
- Baggy pants (the loose skin of the buttocks hanging down).

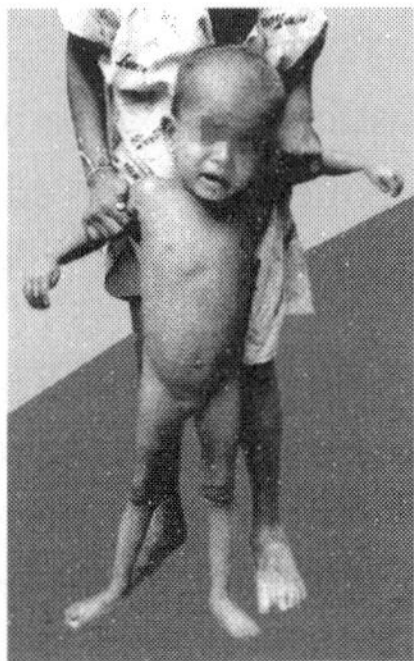

Figure 23.2: Marasmic child

- Child may be alert despite his condition.
- Absence of edema on the lower extremities.
- Prominent ribs.
- Large head with sunken eyes.
- A hungry child.
- Associated diarrhea or dehydration.

In marasmus there is a marked deficit of weight but not as much in height. The marasmic infant has a good appetite but may also appear irritable, fretful and apathetic as in cases of kwashiorkor. Though the skin might appear dry, the typical characteristic peeling or patchy hypopigmentation may not be there.

It is worth mentioning here that during the past decade or so, the profile of PEM presenting in our hospitals has gradually changed. Frank cases of kwashiorkor are rarely encountered, but the marasmic type of picture is frequently observed. The prevalence of clinical form of malnutrition has been reduced to less than 1%. Hospital statistics also show that in recent years, admissions due to severe PEM have come down significantly.[7]

Marasmic Kwashiorkar

This condition is intermediary between marasmus and kwashiorkor, since such children present with a mixed picture. The body weight is less than 60% of the expected along with the presence of edema. The degree of stunting seems greater in marasmic kwashiorkor, indicating that duration of illness in this condition is greater than in kwashiorkor.

Management of PEM

Treatment of severe malnutrition is a challenging task and involves multipronged approach. Most of the cases of severe malnutrition are not without complications on presentation. Severe infection is one major complication to be tackled. Management of these children involves hospitalization in majority of the cases. Noncomplicated cases can be managed on outpatient basis in a hospital or any primary health care centre. But children presenting with complications can be managed in a hospital setting alone. Initial approach involves treating the complications first which may be:

Resuscitation

This involves tackling the life threatening medical emergencies on priority, which may include:

a. *Hypothermia/Hypoglycemia*: These are generally found together. The child is managed by keeping him warm and 'bedding in' with the mother is encouraged. Feeding if possible may be initiated. For hypoglycemia, the child is put on IV glucose10%, if immediate feeding is not possible. Child is treated for sepsis.
b. *Infections*: Infections are a major cause of mortality in PEM. Appropriate antibiotic therapy is initiated.
c. *Anemia*: If not managed appropriately, severe anemia may lead to heart failure. If required blood transfusion is resorted to.

Deydration/Electrolyte Imbalance

Most often such children present with diarrhea. Depending upon the severity of stooling, ORS should be initiated. In moderate dehydration 70–100 ml/kg ORS in 4 hours is given by sips. In severe dehydration, 100 ml/kg normal saline or ringer lactate is given over 3–6 hours. Mostly hypokalemia is present which can be managed by potassium supplement.

Congestive Heart Failure

In case of presence of heart failure, fluid intake is restricted and kept on maintenance dose. Diuretics may be given to prevent fluid overload.

Vitamin Deficiencies

Deficiency of vitamins is a common feature among children with PEM. Vitamin A can be supplemented in all cases. Vitamin K also is given to those with florid PEM and accompanied by diarrhea. All B complex vitamins, vitamin C, E and D too are administered along with calcium and zinc. Magnesium also needs to be supplemented if seizures, tetany or apathy are present.

Dietary Management

Different workers have laid down special formulae for achieving high energy intakes and to fulfill protein requirements for maximum catch up growth rates.

The general pattern followed by them was of providing first class protein, in the form of milk protein powder, oil for energy along with sugar for flavor as well as extra-energy. Oil is used to increase the density of the feed without increasing the bulk. Medium chain triglycerides are more desirable to enhance absorption and metabolism.

Almost all workers advocated regimens providing calories of around 150–200 per kg/d for maximum catch up growth. The protein requirements have been suggested around 3–4 g/kg/d. But certain workers preferred to maintain calories at around100 cal/kg/d initially and gradually increased over a week till the full volume is tolerated. This is specially so in children with kwashiorkor until the edema disappeared.

World Health Organization (WHO) in 1999,[8] laid down guidelines for routine treatment of severe malnutrition where the nutrition component was also stressed as follows:

Stabilization Phase: Initiate Refeeding

Feeding should be initiated gradually as soon as possible after admission. It should be formulated to provide just sufficient calories and proteins to maintain basic physiological functions. The main features include:

- Small frequent feeds of low osmalarity (< 350) mosm/L and low lactose (< 2–3 g/kg/d)
- Oral or nasogastric feeds
- 100 cal./kg/d—(not to exceed in initial phase)
- 1.0–1.5 g prot./kg/d
- 130 ml/kg/d of liquid (may begin with 100 ml/kg/d if edema present)
- Feed should be of low viscosity, easy to prepare and socially acceptable
- Continue breastfeeding if already doing so.

The above regimen is achieved using the F-75 formula which is designed to provide 75 cals./100 ml and 0.9 g pot. /100 ml of the feed. (Table 23.4) These should be fed by cup and spoon. The recommended schedule suggested is as shown in Table 23.5.

For children with good appetite, without edema, the schedule can be completed in 2–3 days. Careful monitoring should be done for

TABLE 23.4: Recipes and composition of starter formulae and catch up formula

Ingredients	Starter formula (F 75)	Starter formula with cereal (F75)	Catch up formula (F 100)
Dried skim milk (g)	25	25	80
Sugar (g)	100	70	50
Cereal flour (g)	–	35	–
Vegetable oil (ml)	27	27	60
Electrolyte mineral solution (ml)	20	20	20
Water: To make up to final soln (ml)	1000	1000	1000
Contents per 100 ml			
Calories (kcal)	75	75	100
Protein (g)	0.9	1.1	2.9
Lactose (g)	1.3	1.3	4.2
Potassium (mmol)	4.0	4.2	6.3
Sodium (mmol)	0.6	0.6	1.9
Magnesium (mmol)	0.43	0.46	0.73
Zinc (mg)	2.0	2.0	2.3
Copper (mg)	0.25	0.25	0.25
%energy from protein	5	6	12
%energy from fat	32	32	53
Osmolality (mOsm/l)	413	334	419

(WHO 2000)

TABLE 23.5: Feeding schedule for children with severe malnutrition

Days	Frequency (hrly)	Vol/kg/feed (ml)	Vol/kg/d (ml)
1–2	2	11	130
3–5	3	16	130
6–7+	4	22	130

- Amounts offered and left over
- Vomiting
- Stool frequency and consistency
- Daily body weight.

There may be accompanying diarrhea in some children, in which case milk based feeds can be replaced with soya based or any lactose free feeds till such time the stools settle down. Gradually low lactose feeds like curd may be initiated, and if tolerated, the amounts increased, and even milk based cereal feeds can be initiated.

In both types of PEM, basal energy expenditure increases gradually during refeeding. As the child loses weight, total body water as percentage of body weight increases and the child becomes relatively over hydrated. In children with edema, initiation of nutritional recovery is characterized by a progressive loss of extra-cellular fluid resulting in an initial loss of weight, followed by stabilization for 10–12 days and again followed by weight gain.[9]

Methods of feeding should be ideally from a cup and spoon along with continuation of breast feeds. Even when breastfeeds are inadequate, non-nutritive sucking should be encouraged which itself can enhance lactation. In case oral feeds are difficult to achieve, tube feeding can be resorted to for a few days till such time oral feeding is restored adequately.

A weight gain of 0.5 kg/week in children and 70

TABLE 23.6: Starter diets F 75

Diet contents (per 100 ml)	F-75 starter	F-75 cereal based-(1)	F-75 Cereal based-(2)
Cow's milk (ml)	30	30	25
Sugar (g)	9	6	3
Cereal puffed rice (g)	–	2.5	6
Vegetable Oil (ml)	2	2.5	3
Water- to make up to 100 ml	100	100	100
Calories (Kcal)	75	75	75
Proteins (g)	0.9	1.1	1.2
Lactose (g)	1.2	1.2	1.2

Source: IAP 2006[11]

TABLE 23.7: Catch up diets F 100

Diets contents (per 100 ml)	F-100 Catchup	F-100 catchup (cereal based) Example 1
Cows milk/toned dairy milk (ml)	95	75
Sugar (g)	5	2.5
Cereal: Puffed rice (g)	–	7
Vegetable oil (g)	2	2
Water to make (ml)	101	100
Energy (kcal)	100	100
Protein (g)	2.9	2.9
Lactose (g)	3.8	3

Source: IAP 2006[11]

gms/kg/week in infants is the goal. With recurrent infections this goal may be difficult; therefore control of infections is very important.

Catch up Growth

This is the rehabilitation phase, when the appetite of the child is restored within 8–10 days, return of social smile and the child begins to take interest in the surroundings. These are the first signs of recovery in a child with PEM. The increase in the feeds should be done gradually at this point to avoid risk of heart failure. To achieve the catch up growth the transition made is as follows:

- Replace F-75 by F100 which contains 100 cal. and 2.9 g protein per 100 ml. This can be achieved by incorporating oil and sugar with milk or using milk cereal based preparations (Table 23.6).
- Subsequently, the feeds are increased by 10–20 ml and finally 25–30 ml/kg/ feed. This can provide up till 200 cal/kg/d.
- Monitoring for respiration and pulse rates are done regularly. The volume of feeds needs to be decreased as also the frequency (4 hourly) in case increase in respiration is observed. Once stabilized:
- Increased amounts of F100 formula at least 3–4 hourly can be started
- Calories given—150–200 kg/d
- Proteins increased—4–6 g/kg/d
- Continue breast feeding
- Ensure administration of 6 monthly vitamin A dose.

The Indian Academy of Pediatrics in 2006 formed a working committee to bring out a revised consensus on the management of severely malnourished children in the Indian context,[10] which were adapted from the WHO guidelines of 2000 mentioned earlier. These guidelines are based on the hospital management of such children.

The modified formulae recommended for F 75 and the catch up formula F 100 are as given in Tables 23.6 and 23.7.

- Egg white can be replaced by 3 g of chicken or commercially available casein
- Powdered puffed rice can be replaced by commercial rice or pre-cooked rice (in same amounts).

The cereal-based low lactose (lower osmolarity) diets are recommended as starter diets for those with persistent diarrhea.[11] Lactose free diets are rarely needed for persistent diarrhea as most children do well on the above mentioned, low lactose F-75 diets. Children with persistent diarrhea, who continue to have diarrhea on the low lactose diets, should be given lactose (milk) free starter diets, as shown in Table 23.8.[12] They can be followed on to lactose free catch up diets as shown in Table 23.9.

The low lactose catch up diets F100, can be started at the rehabilitation phase as shown in Table 23.10.

Complementary foods should be added as soon as possible to prepare the child for home foods at discharge. They should have comparable energy and protein concentrations once the catchup diets are well tolerated. Khichdi, dalia, banana, curd-rice and other

TABLE 23.8: Starter lactose free diet

Egg white *(g)	5
Glucose (g)	3.5
Cereal flour: Powdered puffed rice** (g)	7
Vegetable oil (g)	4
Water to make (ml)	100
Energy (kcal)	75
Protein (g)	1
Lactose	–

*Egg white may be replaced by 3 g of chicken or commercially available pure protein like casein.

**Powdered puffed rice may be replaced by commercial pre-cooked rice preparations (in same amounts).

(*Source*: IAP, 2006)

TABLE 23.9: Catchup lactose free diet

Egg white *(g)	20
Glucose or sugar (g)	4
Cereal Flour: Puffed rice** (g)	12
Vegetable oil (g)	4
Water to make (ml)	100
Energy (kcal)	100
Protein (g)	3
Lactose (g)	–

*Egg white may be replaced by 3 g of chicken or commercially available pure protein like casein.

**Powdered puffed rice may be replaced by commercial pre-cooked rice preparations (in same amounts).

(*Source*: IAP, 2006)

Table 23.10: Low lactose catch up diets (F 100)

Catchup low lactose diets	Example 1	Example 2
Milk (cow's milk or toned dairy milk)	25 ml	25 ml
Egg white *(g)	12	–
Roasted powdered groundnut	–	5 g
Vegetable oil (g)	4	
Cereal flour: Powdered puffed rice** (g)	12	12
Energy (kcal)	100	100
Protein (g)	2.9	2.9
Lactose (g)	1	1

*Egg white may be replaced by 3 g of chicken or commercially available pure protein like casein.

**Powdered puffed rice may be replaced by commercial pre-cooked rice preparations (in same amounts). Jaggery could be used instead of glucose/sugar.

(*Source*: IAP, 2006)

culturally acceptable and locally available diets can also be offered liberally.

Nutrition recovery syndrome is a condition encountered generally during the rehabilitation phase of a child with severe PEM. It is marked by hepatomegaly, gynecomastia, abdominal distension, ascites, splenomegaly, etc. This is attributed to sudden increase in energy and protein intake by these children. It is mostly self limiting and might also be associated with tremors (kwashi shake) during treatment. Protein restriction during this period was generally advocated. But recently it has also been thought to result of excess hormones secreted during recovery phase.

REFERENCES

1. WHO/FAO Expert Committee. WHO Tech. Rep. Ser. No. 522. 1973.
2. Gopalan C. In: Calorie deficiencies and protein deficiencies, (RA Mc Cance and EM Widdowson, Editors. Edinburgh and London: Churchill. Livingtone. 1968.p.49
3. Alleyne GAO, Hay RW, Picou DI, Stanfield JP, Whitehead RG, Jaypee Brothers New Delhi. 1988.
4. Jelliffe DB. WHO Monog Ser. No.53. 1966.
5. Wellcome Trust Working party. Lancet (ii), 302. 1970.
6. Vinodini Reddy, In: Textbook of Human Nutrtition, Ed. Mahtab S Bamji, N Prahalad Rao, Vinodini Reddy. 1996.p.252.
7. Elizabeth KE. Protein energy malnutrition. In: Nutrition and Child Development. 3rd Ed. Paras Medical Publishers. 2004.p.133-7
8. WHO. Management of the child with a serious infection or severe malnutrition. Guidelines for the care at the first referral level in developing countries; Geneva: WHO. 2000.

9. Fernando E Viteri. Protein Energy Malnutrition; In: Textbook of Pediatric Nutrition, Ed. Suskind RM, New York Raven Press. 1981.pp.189-213.
10. Bhatnagar S, Lodha R, Chowdhary P. Sachdeva HPS etal IAP guidelines 2006 on hospital based management of severely malnourished children (Adapted from WHO guidelines) Ind Pediatr. 2007;44:443-61.
11. Bhatnagar S, Bhan MK, Singh KD, et al. Efficiency of milk based diets in persistent diarrhea: A randomized controlled trial. Pediatrics. 1996;98:1122-6.
12. Bhan MK, Bhandari N, Bhal R. Management of the severely malnourished child: Perspective from developing countries. BMJ. 2003 Jan 18;326: 146-51.

24 Childhood Obesity

"One should strive to maintain good health by taking balanced diet and exercising regularly"

Atharva Veda

At one time the term childhood obesity was rarely seen in our country. The main nutritional problems in children focused around malnutrition which was in the form of undernutrition, anemia and vitamin A deficiency. However, gradually, over a period of a decade or two, the other aspect of malnutrition, that of over nutrition in the form of childhood obesity has emerged as a major health problem in India too. In the USA childhood obesity has increased at least by 50% since 1976. It is well known that 80% of obese adolescents become obese adults. Over weight in adolescence predicts a broad range of adverse health affects that are independent of adult weight after 55 years of follow-up.[1]

Effective treatment and prevention of obesity must begin in childhood. However, studies indicate that care providers recommend initiation of treatment for only less than 20% of obese children.

The causes of higher rates of fatness in developing countries are poorly studied, but likely to include the extreme and rapid changes in lifestyle, physical activity and diet that accompany urbanization and rapid economic development. The results of such lifestyle are already being seen. Most cardiovascular disease deaths, generally associated only with Western industrialized countries now occur in developing countries.[2]

Common childhood and adolescent medical consequences of obesity include increased growth, then stunting, increased fat free mass, early menarche, hyperlipidemia, increased heart rate and cardiac output, hepatic steatosis with elevated transaminases and abnormal glucose metabolism.[3,4,5]

The various causative factors attributed to the increasing prevalence of obesity in the Indian scenario may perhaps be attributed to the lifestyle changes of the families. Increased purchasing power, better and comfortable living thanks to the improving technology, increased variety and availability of food products in the market and increased hours of inactivity have all been blamed for the changing trends. Television, video games and computers have replaced the hours of outdoor games and other activities leading to childhood obesity.

It is thought that the tendency of adults becoming obese is determined by genetic, intrauterine, childhood and adolescent condition. Critical periods for the development of obesity and its sequel have been postulated, including period of gestation, the period of adiposity rebound (between 5–6 years) and adolescence. Studies have also demonstrated that an active lifestyle in childhood is more likely to be reflected in more active adolescents and adults. Although 10% weight loss in adults can improve the co-morbidities of obesity, most co-morbidities are irreversible.[6]

DEFINITION OF CHILDHOOD OBESITY

Obesity actually can be viewed as the energy balance of any individual. Energy expended should be equal to that of energy expended. Therefore, basically it can be defined as energy expended to be equivalent to energy consumed. In other words it means that the energy balance should not be tilted. A positive energy balance will probably lead to overweight and finally obesity.

Overweight and obesity are both labels for ranges of weight that are greater than what is generally considered healthy for a given height. The terms also identify ranges of weight that have been shown to increase the likelihood of certain diseases and other health problems.

For adults overweight and obesity ranges are determined by using weight and height to calculate a number called the Body Mass Index (BMI). BMI is used because, for most people it correlates with their amount of body fat.

- An adult who has a BMI between 25–29.9 is considered overweight
- An adult who has a BMI of 30 or higher is considered obese.

What is BMI

Body mass index (BMI) is a number calculated from a child's weight and height. It does not measure fat directly, but research has shown that BMI correlates to direct measures of body fat. Moreover it is a simple and inexpensive method of screening for weight categories that may lead to health problems. For children and teens, BMI is age and sex specific and is often referred to as BMI for age.[7]

What is a BMI Percentile

After BMI is calculated for children and teens, the BMI number is plotted on the CDC BMI-for-age growth charts, either for boys or girls, to obtain a percentile ranking (Refer Chapter 3, Figs 3.7, 3.8). The percentile indicates the relative position of the child's BMI number among children of the same sex and age. The growth charts show the weight status categories used with children and teens (underweight, healthy weight, a risk of over weight and over weight).

Body mass index (BMI) for age weight status categories and the corresponding percentiles are shown in Table 24.1.

TABLE 24.1: BMI for status categories and percentile

Weight status category	Percentile range
Underweight	Less than the 5th percentile
Healthy weight	5th percentile to less than the 85th percentile
At risk of overweight	85th to less than the 95th percentile
Overweight	Equal to or greater than the 95th percentile

Refer. 7

Body mass index (BMI) is used as a screening tool to identify possible weight problems for children. CDC and the American Academy of Pediatrics (AAP) recommend the use of BMI to screen for overweight beginning at 2 years of age. It is used to screen for overweight, at risk of overweight, or underweight. But it definitely is not a diagnostic tool. High BMI for age and sex in a child may not necessary determine if excess fat is a problem. For this some other parameters like skinfold thickness measurements, evaluation of diet, physical activity, family histories, etc. are also required.

The BMI for age percentile is used to interpret the BMI number because BMI is both age and sex specific for children and teens. These criteria are different from those used to interpret BMI for adults, which do not take into account age or sex. Age and sex are considered because.

- The amount of body fat changes with age
- The amount of body fat differs between girls and boys.

The CDC BMI-for-age growth charts for girls and boys take into account these differences and allow translation of a BMI number into a percentile for a child's or teen's sex and age.[7]

Body mass index (BMI) is now a universally accepted standard to measure childhood obesity. A consensus proposed the use of a BMI above the 85th percentile as a screening index for overweight and a BMI above the 95th percentile as an index of excess adiposity in adolescents.[8,9] In other words, when the weight exceeds 110% of the standard weight or when the skin fold thickness is more than 30 mm. Obesity is considered when the weight exceeds 120% of the standard weight. Super obesity has been described when the weight for height above the 95th percentile on the growth charts from NCHS, and weight in excess of 140% of the median weight for a given height.[10] (See Chapter 3 for IAP Guidelines on BMI for children).

Measuring skin fold thickness (SFT) can help distinguish patients who are over fat from those who are over weight due to increased muscle and bone. SFT provides direct measure of body fat. It can be measured at several sites, including triceps, biceps axilla, mid-abdominal, subscapular and suprailiac. SFT above 85th percentile for age and sex suggests obesity and above 95th percentile for age suggests super obesity. The trunk skinfold measurement, subscapular, axilla, suprailiac and abdominal may be suitable indicators of abdominal adipose tissue in children.[11,12]

However, at the workshop on childhood obesity in 1999, views from participants were presented, where the use of SFT for measuring obesity in children was debated. It was remarked that the validity of SFT measurement in different populations has not been carefully explored. Further no evidence suggests that SFT measurements predict hyperinsulinemia, hypertension or other illness in children better than does BMI. Results from several data suggest that childhood BMI remains stable into adulthood, better than does SFT. This observation may reflect measurement error in SFT changes in fat distribution.

The group noted that circumference (e.g. waist or hip) may reflect morbidity in adults, but the relation between visceral fat and morbidity in children and adolescents has not been clarified.[13]

Pathogenesis of Childhood Obesity

Genetic Factors

Hereditary or genetic factor also has been recognized for obesity. It considers expression of a complex interaction between genetic and environmental factors including food intake. Parental obesity has been considered as a strong predictor, especially when both parents are obese. The resting energy expenditure (REE) and metabolic rate are known to be based on heredity.

Genetic factors have also been linked to birth weight in the pathogenesis of obesity. This has now been recognized as the Barker's theory.[14] This theory is supported by studies suggesting that a low birth weight is adversely associated with a greater risk of cardiovascular disease and type II diabetes in adult life. The relationship between birth weight and adult fatness is affected by many confounding factors, such as gestational age, parental factors and socioeconomic classes.[15]

Many studies have observed that familial aggregation of obesity can be traced through three generations as shown by a report indicating that the grandparents' obesity is related to that of the parents' BMI and also to obesity indices in grand children.[16] It has also been shown that familial factors with regard to eating habits also influence the children's eating behavior and consequently obesity. Similarly, a strong relationship was also found between the level of parental physical activity and that of their preschool children.[17]

Early Feeding vs. Obesity Risk

Scientists have shown that perinatal nutrition is related to obesity risk in young adulthood. In a study during the Dutch famine of 1944–45, significantly lower obesity rates were observed in young adults exposed to famine conditions in the last trimester of gestation and the first months of postnatal life, compared to controls that were not exposed perinatally to the famine.[18]

The feeding of children during the early infancy on breast or formula milk has been found to influence overweight or obesity in them. Previously breastfed children are less likely to be overweight or obese at school entry than children who were previously formula fed. Breastfeeding for at least 6 months was found to be associated with a risk reduction for overweight and obesity of > 30% and > 40% respectively.[19]

Metabolic Factors

There can be syndromic obesity which basically is due to certain metabolic diseases. Such obesities are commonly found in children, e.g. Praden Willi syndrome, Beckwith-Wiedemann syndrome, Laurence-Moon-Biedl-Bardet syndrome, etc.

Environmental/Lifestyle Factors

The most commonly observed form of childhood obesity is due to environmental factors, which are linked to high fat, high sugar foods, junk foods, aerated sweetened beverages, long hours of television viewing or computer/video games and above all sedentary lifestyle.

Other Factors

Constitutional obesity is known in children and perhaps the commonest type. This is basically a result of excess caloric intake.

Endocrine disorders is also known to cause obesity in children, e.g. in Cushings syndrome or Turner syndrome. Hypothyroidism and growth hormone deficiency can also lead to obesity.

Polycystic ovarian syndrome is one typical example of obesity in adolescent girls and this is considered to be lined with excess calorie intake also.

There are certain conditions related to neuro-psychiatric disorders which can result in obesity. These include bulimia nervosa and other conditions like hypothalamic, pituitary and other brain lesions like craniopharyngioma. The mechanism involved is thought to be of disregulating appetite.

Assessment of Obesity

The general approach to assess obesity involves:

History

A detailed history is of utmost importance to evaluate obesity. This includes:

- Family history
- Lifestyle pattern
- Dietary history
- Anthropometry
- Laboratory investigations.

Family history: It is generally observed that parents of overweight or obese children are also inclined to be overweight or obese. Heredity or genetic factors might have some role in contributing towards obesity in children, as mentioned earlier in this chapter.

Lifestyle pattern: This is a major contributing factor in the etiology of obesity. Therefore a detailed history of the complete daily routine of the child is essential which includes hours of sleeping, waking, time spent in commuting to school and mode of transport, outdoor activities involving aerobic games, etc. and number of hours of television viewing or involvement in video games. Besides this, frequency of dining out, type of meals taken at school, frequency of celebrations/feasts at home involving food and in between munching are also significant indicators to ascertain their lifestyle

Dietary history: This involves a detailed dietary intake of the child / adolescent for the whole day (See Chapter 3)

Anthropometry: Assessing BMI of these children and evaluating them on the growth charts is used to determine them on the growth charts is used to determine the extent of obesity (See Chapter 3)

Clinical/laboratory investigations: These involve bone age which is suggestive of hypothyroidism and may be confirmed by T3, T4 and TSH estimation in serum. A detailed clinical examination can be done which include checking of blood pressure, sugar and lipid profile.

Management of Childhood Obesity

Management of childhood obesity involves multipronged intervention which includes dietary, physical activity, behavioral/psychotherapy, drug therapy and ultimately may be surgical approaches. The factors responsible for the etiology of obesity are also the ones which can be influenced in the treatment or even prevention of obesity. Therefore, exploring the impact of the home environment is crucial to design effective programs to help children establish healthy eating patterns and lifestyle.

Socio Economic Status (SES)

Socio economic status is thought to influence management of obesity indirectly. It is known that adults of lower SES and lower educational qualifications have less healthy diets and are les likely to participate in physical activities like sports. Hence, their children if predisposed to adiposity are likely to live in environments that promote obesity. According to Epstein,[20] if socio economic levels are related to parent management success, then families with fewer children also may be of higher SES and may benefit more from parent than do larger families in lower socio economic levels. Effective programs emphasize parental attention as an important motivational factor for weight loss. Therefore parental availability is the key to successful management.

Food Consumption and Eating Pattern

It has been worked out that increasing energy intake by as 150 calories per day above the RDA for weight maintenance would result in a significant weight gain over one year.[21]

Besides our social interaction in any sphere of work or area, encourages and facilitates a way of life that promotes weight gain gradually leading to obesity. This imposes a great challenge on the part of the individual to resist or adapt to a criteria of eating behavior to enable them to maintain the required energy balance. Food composition varies from place to place and from family to family. This may also influence adiposity. High fat/sugar diets are generally energy dense and palatable. Therefore it is important to effectively maintain the energy balance. Food choices need to be strictly monitored. Changes in the recipes can be effected at the same time retaining the palatability. In case of children, care needs to be taken that emphasis is laid on home based diets. This can be facilitated by encouraging home environments to suit the needs of the child's requirements in terms of optimal growth without tilting the positive energy balance. Social events can incorporate home based foods with a variety of food choices and preferences. The increasing culture of dining out in the younger age groups is setting a negative trend with regard to eating behavior. School canteens can be supervised to ensure healthy foods and stress should be made on children getting home packed tiffin. These too can be supervised and monitored by the authorities. Parent teacher meets can be made more meaningful by involving parents in activities like competitions etc. on healthy packed tiffin. Current dietary recommendations according to American Academy of Pediatrics advocate reducing fat intake and increasing consumption of complex carbohydrates and fiber containing foods including vegetables and fruits.[22]

The early exposure that children have to fruits and vegetables and to foods high in energy, sugar and fats, may play an important role in establishing an hierarchy of preferences and selection. It was shown that children consumed more fruits and vegetables at schools where more of these items were served and the extent to which these are made available and accessible to children may shape their liking for and consumption of these foods.[23]

Food Availability

Generally the access to food is controlled by parents and older siblings. The types of food that are stored at home by them influence the younger child's food consumption and preferences. Therefore parents and elders can be instrumental in providing and facilitating the right type of healthy foods. Junk foods or other energy dense foods should be in restricted access and portion size of such foods if available may be suitably divided. However when storing the month's ration one should take care to avoid storage of such food which are calorie dense and likely to be a source of temptation for youngsters, and easy susceptibility to obesity.

Food Preferences and Child Feeding Practices

Observations from familial eating patterns suggest that it is the parents who are more likely to over indulge and prompt eating in obese children, compared to the lean ones whose parents are more selective in choosing food varieties for them. Most authors are of the view that children should be allowed to choose from foods that they are offered and control the amounts they choose to eat.[24,25,26]

It has been seen that children are quite responsive to parental attempts to control their intakes. However, it is also established that on the contrary, stringent parental control can exert a negative impact also. They (children) tend to make just the opposite choices and prefer high fat, high calorie foods. Children have also been known to learn to dislike foods when they are encouraged to eat for rewards or when they are bribed into eating. It has been suggested that parental and child feeding practices play a crucial role in the development of individual food preferences and control of food intake.

Social Learning Environment/Early Learning

It is well accepted that the family plays a pivotal role in providing a social learning environment. Certain behaviors, meal patterns and leisure activities that are associated with the development and persistence of obesity are often modeled and reinforced by parents and older siblings at home. Parents who over eat or eat very fast or ignore their internal satiety cue, set a poor example to the children. The onus lies on the parents to present healthy eating styles at home, as well as in external social environments where the family interacts and to model a healthy selection and consumption of foods and regular physical activity. It is a common observation that obese families appear to store more food in all the targeted areas of the home. Since children tend to influence parental habits and even modify them, they can play an active role in the transmission of messages in the home which focus on healthy eating patterns.

The first choice of flavor in a child's diet is either breast milk or formula milk. The perception of flavor in milk also is one of human infant's earliest sensory experiences; and there is evidence to show that this early experience with flavors has an effect on milk intake and later on food acceptance.[27] It has been reported that flavors in breast milk influence infant's consumption. Early experience with a variety of flavors leads to more ready acceptance of new foods later. Studies in rats have shown that because of repeated early experiences with flavors of the maternal diet present in the mother's milk, rat pups learn to prefer their mother's diet. In humans, formula fed infants have experience with only a single flavor, whereas breast fed babies are exposed to a variety of flavors from maternal diet that are transmitted to the milk. It is postulated that varied flavor experience of breast fed infants can facilitate accepted of solid foods during the weaning period, with breast fed infants showing greater initial acceptance of new foods than formula fed infants.[27] Infants and children do not accept new flavors instantly with the exception of sweet or salty foods; but after repeated exposures to new foods, preferences for new foods generally increases, providing increased intakes, although 5–10 exposures may be required.[28]

Physical Activity

Sedentary life style with low activity levels is known to promote childhood obesity. Therefore, increasing physical activity preferably the aerobic type can prove very beneficial in the treatment of obesity in children. Exercise showed a beneficial effect when combined with reduced energy intake programs, dietary and behavioral management techniques or as part of a multicomponent program.[29] Targeting either sedentary behavior or promoting increased physical activity was associated with significant decrease in percent overweight and body fat and improves erobic fitness. The American Academy of Pediatrics has recommended limiting television viewing to 1–2 hours a day. Limiting television watching and playing video and computer games appears to compel the choice of other pastimes. The couch potato culture among young children and adolescents, if curtailed can give more options and time for them to go for outdoor activities.

Parental Role

The role of parents in making the food choices is also significant. When parents participate actively in their child's weight program, they are expected to modify their own behaviors that contribute to the child's condition and to model eating and exercise behaviors in ways that promote weight loss. They are also expected to work towards accepting new habits and lifestyles. When parents are targeted and provided with reinforcing intervention to promote weight loss, the results are more effective. When parents involved in such programs are supportive and the child motivated enough, long-term success is more likely. Therefore for effective weight loss programs, it is the whole family that should be targeted, rather than just the child alone.

Some authors have found greater success with involving just the parents and excluding the obese child. According to them, this strategy also inculcates healthy eating behavior in the child rather than the conventional dietary interventions that target the child alone.[30,31]

In this model, change is delivered through the parents instead of the obese child. This approach is basically to target a healthy lifestyle and not just weight reduction. This approach seems more rational, since parents are the ones who can play authoritative role models, at the same time provide a family environment, which provides healthy practices related to weight control issues. Moreover it was observed that this approach was more suitable for the young children as compared to the older ones, since the former seem to be more receptive.

Parental involvement without the obese child is thought to help by prompting change in two areas. Firstly, parental cognition and behavior is involved by increasing nutrition/health skills, regular exercise and improved parenting skills. They are encouraged to provide company at meal times and promote participation of all family members in meals. Secondly they are involved to follow regular meal times and scheduled snacks, thereby setting standards for day to day eating practice.

Parents are advised to serve meals to the members individually rather than self helping, teach portion sizes and provide alternate leisure time activities. The second area involves environmental changes so designed to facilitate a healthy lifestyle, rather than relying in individual self control in eating. They are encouraged to create opportunities for physical activities. Healthy eating is encouraged and inappropriate foods are kept out of reach or sight. At the same time restriction on the amount of food eaten by the child is avoided. The instructions given to parents are:

1. To avoid mixed messages and unintentionally reinforce undesired behavior.
2. To use praise and corrective actions that are directed to the child's behavior rather than pinpointing at his personal attributes.
3. To identify ways to help children develop independence and initiative,
4. To regulate and empower children to make decisions about selected issues and to cultivate friends and outlets in the community.
5. To promote positive attitudes and self acceptance and to strengthen self confidence and self esteem.

CONCLUSION

- Obesity has been recognized as a major public health problem by WHO, but childhood obesity also has posed a equally challenging role for nutritionists and pediatricians. Obese children are at an increased risk of becoming obese adults and the risk is higher if both parents are obese.
- Exclusive breastfeeding in the early months may have a protective role against childhood obesity. Early introduction to a variety of flavors introduced through breast milk can indicate healthy food preferences in the child.
- Education regarding choice of healthy foods i.e. low fat, low sugars and high fiber foods like fruits and vegetables needs to be imparted from early years of childhood. This can help instill healthy food preferences.
- Management of obesity in children should be with the involvement of the family without focusing on the child in isolation.
- Behavioral and lifestyle modifications with the help of the dietician, ped iatrician and a counselor in collaboration with the family can give encouraging results.

REFERENCES

1. Popkin BM. The nutritional transition in low income countries: An emerging crisis. Nutr Rev. 52:285-98.
2. Pearson TA. Cardiovascular disease as a growing health problem in developing countries. The role of nutrition in the epidemiological transition. Public Health Rev. 1996;24:131-46.
3. Gidding SS, Bao W, Srinivasan et al. Effects of secular trends in obesity on coronary risk factors in children. The Bogalusa Heart study. J Pediatrics. 1995;127:868.
4. Arab M. Diabetes mellitus in Egypt World Health Stat. Q.1992;45:334-7.
5. Burns TL, Moll PP, Lanner RM; Increased familial mortality in obese school children: The Muscatine Ponderosity, Family Study, Pediatrics. 1992;39:262.
6. Schonfeld-Warden N, Warden CH. Pediatric Obesity. An overview of etiology and treatment. Ped Clinics of N America Apr. 1997;44(20):339-61.
7. National Center for Chronic Disease Prevention and Health Promotion, Division of Nutrition, Physical Activity and Obesity. 2000.
8. Himes JH, Dietz WH. Guidelines for overweight in adolescent prevalence services: recommendations

from an expert committee. Am J Clin Nutr. 1994;59: 307-16.

9. Must A, Dallal GE, Dietz WH. Reference data for adiposity: 85th and 95th percentiles of body mass index wt/ht^2 and triceps skinfold thickness. Am J Clin Nutr. 1999;53:839-46.
10. Kanders BS. Weighing the options. Criteria for evaluating weight management programs. In TPR (Ed):Pediatric Obesity, Washington DC, Academy Press. 1995.p.210.
11. Brambilla P, Mauzoni P, Simon S, et al. Peripheral abdominal adiposity in childhood obesity. Int J Obe Adol Metab Disord. 1994;18:793.
12. Goen MI, Kaskaun M, Shiman WP. Intra-abdominal adipose tissue in young children. Int J Obes Relat Metab Disord. 1995;19:279.
13. Mary C, Bellizi, Williams H Dietz. Workshop on Childhood Obesity: summary of the discussion. Am J Clin Nutr. 1999;70:1735-55.
14. Barker DJ. Fetal origin of cardiovascular disease. Ann Med. 1999;31(Suppl.1):3-6.
15. ParsonsTJ, Powen C, Logan S, Summerbell CD. Childhood predictors of adult obesity: a systematic review. Int J Obes. 1999;23(suppl8):S1-107.
16. Guillaume M, Lapidus L, Beckers F, et al. Familial trends of obesity through three generations, the Belgian-Luxembourg child study. Int J Obes. 1995;19:55-59.
17. Moore LL, Lombardi DA White MJ, et al. Influence of parents' physical activity levels or activity levels of young children. J Pediatr. 1991;118:215-19.
18. Ravelli ACJ, van der Meulex JHP, Osmond C, et al. Obesity in young men after famine exposure in utero and early infancy. N Engl J Med. 1976;295:349-53.
19. von Kries R, Koletzko B, Saurerwald T, et al. Breast feeding and obesity: cross sectional study. BMJ. 1999;319:147-50.
20. Epstein LH, Koeske R, Wing RR, et al. The effect of family variables on child weight change. Health Psychol. 1986;5:1-11.
21. Rosenbaun M, Leibel RL. The physiology of body weight regulation: relevance to the etiology of obesity in children. Pediatrics. 1998;101:525-39.
22. American Academy of Pediatrics. Committee on Nutrition Statement on cholesterol. Pediatrics. 1992; 90:469-73.
23. Hearn MD, Baranowski T, Baranowski J, et al. Environmental influences on dietary behavior among children: availability and accessibility of fruits and vegetables enable consumption. J Health Educ. 1998.
24. Evers C. Empower children to develop healthful eating habits. J Am Diet Assoc. 1997;97(suppl 2):S116-18.
25. Birch LL. Development of food acceptance in first years of life. Proc Nutr Soc. 1998;57:617-24.
26. Birch LL, Fischer Lo. Development of eating behaviors among children and adolescents. Pediatrics. 1998;101:539-49.
27. Sulivan SA, Birch LL. Infant dietary experience and acceptance of solid foods. Pediatrics. 1994;93:271-7.
28. Carpretta PI, Petersik IT, Steward AI. Acceptance of novel flavors is increased after early experience of diverse tastes. Nature. 1975;254:689-91.
29. Epstein LH, Valoski AM, Vara LS, et al. Effects of decreasing sedentary behavior and increasing activity on weight change in obese children. Health Psychol. 1995;14:109-15.
30. Golan M, Weizman A, Apter A, et al. Parents as the exclusive agents of change in the treatment of childhood obesity. Am J Clin Nutr. 1998;67:1130-8.
31. Golan M; Fainaru M, Weizman A. Role of behavior modification in the treatment of childhood obesity, with parents as the exclusive agents of change. Int J Obes. 1998;22:1217-24.

25 Management of Severe Acute Malnutrition

Severe acute malnutrition (SAM) in children is termed to describe a state of acute malnutrition, with a very low weight for height, below-3 Z score for the median WHO child growth standards (or < 70% or more below the median), a mid arm circumference (MUAC) of < 110 mms or by the presence of nutritional or pitting edema. It is considered as a killer disease among children between 6 months to 60 months of age.[1] The incidence is estimated to be to the tune of 26 million children under 5 years globally, the maximum being in Saharan. Africa and in the sub Saharan Africa. In India approximately 8,104,00 children under 5 are known to be affected by SAM, which amounts to about 31.2% of the world's severely wasted children. Mortality rates in SAM children are 9 times higher than in well nourished children.[2] Severe wasting has been observed to be one of the leading causes of death among < 5 years, with a high incidence, long duration of episodes and high case fatality rates.[3]

New approaches for the management of SAM, like community based therapeutic care, complement the existing WHO inpatient protocols. These programs use ready to use therapeutic foods (RUTF) to treat most children suffering from SAM as outpatients, reserving the inpatient treatment for those with complications. The goal of these programs is to decrease barriers to access, encourage earlier presentation, reduced costs associated with treatment and encourage compliance by patients. Treatment of patients with SAM as outpatients reduces inpatient case loads to more manageable levels, helps decongest crowded inpatient units, decrease the risk of nosocomial infections and increase the time available to devote to sick children. These new approaches have greatly reduced case fatality rates and increased coverage rates, besides being cost effective.[4]

DIAGNOSIS OF SAM

Diagnosing and establishing SAM involves a combination of the following 3 criteria:

- Anthropometric measurement techniques
- Interpretation of anthropometric indicators
- Decision making at a glance.

A. Anthropometric Measurement Techniques

These include:

1. ***Weight for height (W/H) or weight for length (W/L):*** The first step involves identification and referral of children with malnutrition from primary health care centers. This is done by the use of growth monitoring chart.

   The weight for height table is used to calculate the weight for height/length percentage (W/H/L %) or standard deviation (Z score). This reference table helps in the interpretation of anthropometric measurement through the Wt for Ht/Lth % or SD (Z score).

   Another reference used is the Wall Chart for calculating the weight for height/length percentage or standard deviation (Z score). This chart helps in the interpretation of anthropometric measurements through a color coding system which corresponds to the equivalent of for W/H/L % or SD.

But this chart is not commonly used. (See Chapter 3 for Growth Charts).

2. ***Mid upper arm circumference (MUCA):*** This involves screening for children with length > 65 cm. It was observed that MUAC < 110 mm, with presence of bipedal edema, is the best indicator for screening and case detection of child malnutrition in the community.[5] MUAC is measured using a tape around the left arm (hanging down on the side and relaxed) and measured to the nearest 1 mm).

   MUAC is an indicator of acute malnutrition that reflects mortality risk[6] and has been endorsed as an independent criterion for admission into therapeutic feeding program by an informal consultation of WHO.[7]

3. ***Bipedal pitting edema***: Edema is diagnosed by using thumb pressure to the top of the feet for about 3 seconds. An impression left on the feet at the pressure point indicates edema. Nutritional edema starts from the feet and extends upwards to other parts of the body.

B. Interpretation of anthropometric indicators

Then follows the interpretation of good or bad growth based on the curve pattern on the chart. A flat curve indicates static growth, which is a dangerous sign and needs further investigations. Children are referred for suspected acute malnutrition if:

- They do not gain weight for > 2 months
- They are losing weight
- They are falling below the bottom line.

However, these criteria are not recognized by international standards as diagnostic criteria for admission in acute malnutrition treatment program.

The MUAC value obtained is measured using a 3 color tape and interpreted as follows:

- A measurement in the green zone indicates normal or good nutrition.
- A measurement in the yellow zone indicates the child is at risk of malnutrition.
- A measurement in the red zone indicates that the child is acutely malnourished.

Moderate acute malnutrition

A child may be considered to fall under the category 'moderate acute malnutrition' if:

- Wt/ht/lth is < 80% or less than—2SD of the median of the reference population (NCHS/WHO)

  Or
- MUAC is < 125 mm

  And
- There is no bilateral pedal edema evident.

Severe acute malnutrition

The child is interpreted to have SAM if:

- Wt/ht/lth is < 70% or < -3 SD (marasmus) of the NCHS

  Or
- Bilateral pedal edema is evident

  Or
- MUAC < 110 mm.

Clinical Signs of marasmus/kwashiorkor (see Chapter 23).

C. Decision making at a glance/implementation

Once the child is screened and diagnosed as SAM, the next step is to decide the course of action for management. Based on their degree of severity, decision is made regarding managing them from the outpatient treatment unit or to admit them in Therapeutic feeding unit (TFU). The criteria used for this decision making is summarized as follows:

a. Child with SAM with medical complications and no appetite needs to be admitted for inpatient care. The medical complications may be:
   - Edema (+++)
   - Fever
   - Acute or prolonged respiratory infections
   - Watery diarrhea/vomiting
   - Extensive oral thrush
   - Severe anemia.

b. Child with SAM and no medical complications and good appetite may be admitted as an outpatient with RUTF.

c. Child with moderate acute malnutrition (MAM) may be referred to a Supplementary Feeding Program (if available).

Figure 25.1 summarizes the decision making criteria at a glance.[6]

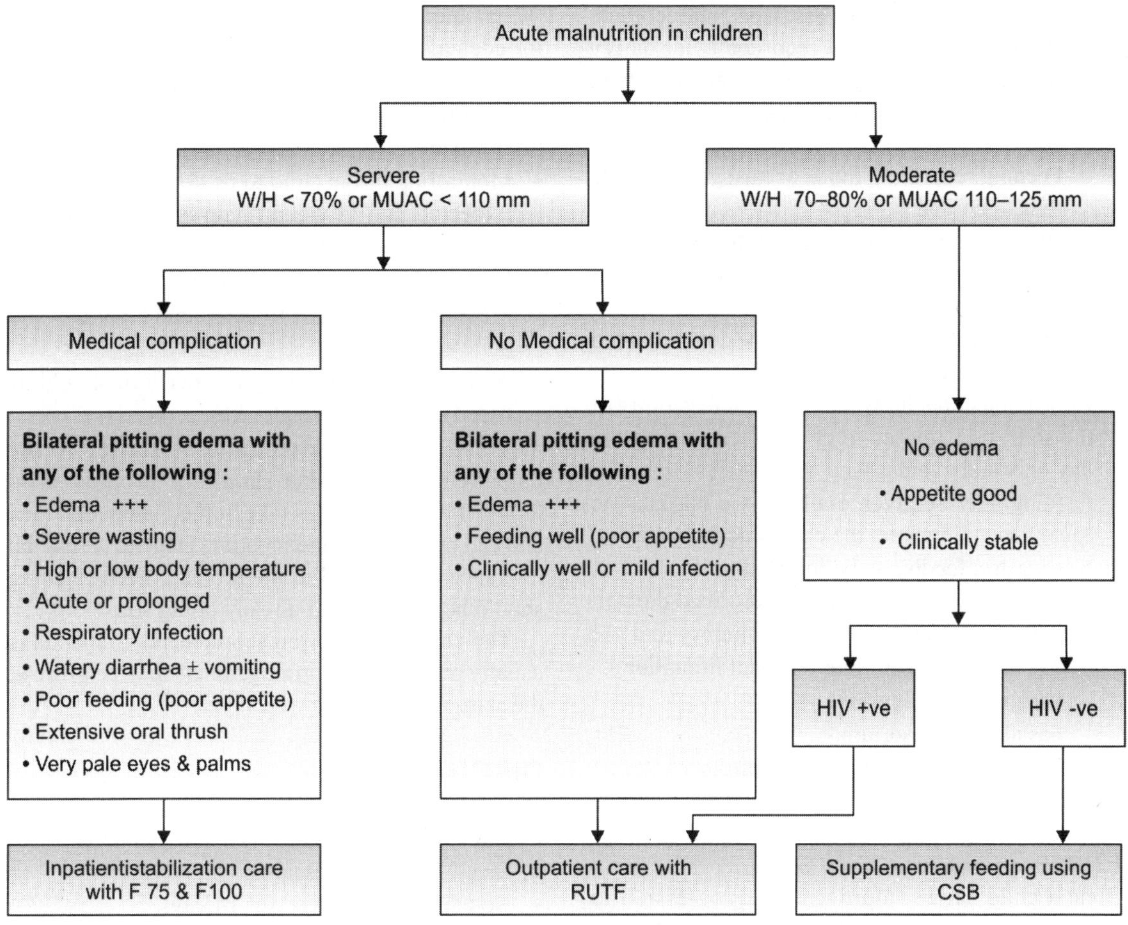

FIGURE 25.1: Decision making criteria at a glance

Refer. 6

ADMISSION

Once the child is referred for admission

- Child is offered sugar water (10 g of sugar in 100 ml water).
- Anthropometric measurements are checked.
  - W/H or W/l < 70% (WHO/NCHS chart)
  - MUAC > 110 mm with length of > 65 cm or
  - Presence of bilateral pedal edema.
- The mother is explained about the nutritional status of the child and its implications.

In Patient Treatment

Phase 1

Treatment in Phase 1 is always given in an inpatient setting. It is preferable that the child in this phase of treatment should never be kept in an emergency or general ward, but always in a therapeutic feeding unit.

At this stage F-75 formula is initiated, which is a starter formula so designed to provide low protein and sodium and high in carbohydrates. Severely malnourished children are not able to tolerate a very high protein or sodium diet at the initial stage and at the same time they need reasonably high amount of carbohydrates. It is for this purpose that F-75 is designed (see Chapter 23, Table 23.6). The use of this formula is known to prevent deaths.[8]

a. At this phase the children should be monitored daily:
   - Weight to be recorded and plotted on the growth chart

  - Degree of edema to be assessed and recorded
  - Body temperature to be recorded twice daily
  - Standard clinical signs assessed and recorded (stool, vomiting, cough, respiration and liver size)
  - Feeding record, IV fluids or nasogastric feeds to be recorded.

b. Breastfeeding to continue if already feeding.
c. If signs of dehydration evident, to give ORS accordingly.
d. Amount and frequency of F-75 to be decided based on the weight of the child.
e. Depending upon the availability and feasibility of the staff, it is advised to give 6 feeds during the day only and avoid giving at night.
f. Feeding may be given orally or via nasogastric route depending upon the child's acceptance.
g. Nasogastric feeding to be resorted to if
  - oral intake is < 75% of the prescribed diet.
  - has pneumonia with rapid respiratory rate.
  - has cleft palate or other physical limitation.
  - has painful oral lesions.
  - has altered sensorium.
  - has pneumonia with rapid respiratory rate.

h. Medical complications to be treated accordingly.

Phase 2 (Transition Phase)

Once a child shows improvement, progression to Transition phase is initiated based on the following criteria:

a. Return of appetite.
b. Loss of edema as assessed by weight loss.

In this phase feed is progressed to F-100 formula (See Chapter 23. Table 23.7).

- Frequency of feeding to be maintained at 6 per day.
- Routine medical treatment to be continued.

The child might be required to shift back to phase 1 if:

- There is too rapid weight gain (>10 g/kg/d).
- Increasing edema or sudden onset of edema seen.
- Hepatomegaly present.
- Signs of fluid overload evident.
- Abdomen distension observed.

The child can be restarted on F-100 if appetite returns to normal and edema disappears entirely. Weight monitoring to be done 3/week and also assess for edema. F-100 should never be given for home use.

During the Transition phase, the main steps involved are:

- Monitoring of the child to be done as in Phase 1. Expected rate of weight gain is 6 g/kg/d, if the child accepts the food and is well tolerated.
- Breastfeeding to be continued as in Phase 1.
- Frequency of feeding to be around 6 per day and none at night.
- Amount of F-100 to be given per feed should be based on class of weight (kg).

When the child is ready to be shifted to the outpatient unit, the diet should be progressed to RUTF. It can be used as take home therapeutic feed and can be started at the inpatient stage to assess the tolerance of the child to the product. Breastfeeding should be continued, if already doing so.

The child is given iron supplements if anemia is usually present. De worming tablets may be given at the start of Phase 2 for over a year.

DISCHARGE

The child is considered fit for discharge if:

- w/h or w/l is > 85% of WHO/NCHS tables on at least 2 weighing sessions.
- No edema is observed for 14 days.

FOLLOW-UP

Follow-up of these patients is equally important. Therefore, they need to be enrolled with a nutritional support program or nearest health center for 4–6 months on monthly basis.

FAILURE TO RESPOND

Some children may not respond to the above management, either in inpatient or outpatient setting. Some common causes for this failure may be attributed to various factors as listed in Table 25.1.[8]

Problems of Individual Children

- Insufficient food given
- Food shared by siblings
- Vitamin/mineral deficiency

TABLE 25.1: Common causes of failure to respond to treatment

Problems with treatment facility	
In patient	**Outpatient**
• Poor environment for malnourished children • Failure to treat children in a separate area • Failure to complete the multichart completely • Insufficient staff (especially at night) • Poorly trained staff • Inaccurate weighing scale • Food prepared or given incorrectly	• Inappropriate selection of patients to go directly to outpatient unit • Poorly conducted appetite test • Inadequate instructions give to care takers • Wrong amount of RUTF dispensed to children • Sharing within families • Sibling sharing the food • Sharing a common plate • Unwilling care taker or caretaker too busy to fulfill responsibilities

Refer. 8

- Malabsorption
- Psychological trauma (in case of refugee situations or families).

CRITERIA TO ASSESS FAILURE TO RESPOND

To assess whether the child has failed to respond to the management, a set of criteria has been laid down based on the time taken for various parameters as shown in Table 25.2.[9]

Failure to respond should be tacked based on the causes determined on assessment.

Every 'primary failure' to respond should be checked for infections.

'Secondary failure' to respond may occur after the child has progressed satisfactorily to Phase 2 with a good appetite and weight gain in Transition phase for in patients and deteriorated after an initial response in outpatient unit. This may be due to either aspiration of the feed/diet into the lungs caused by faulty feeding technique like:

- Forced feeding.
- Feeding while laying the child flat on the bed.
- An acute infection contracted at the center (nosocomial).
- Reactivation of infection after recovery, e.g. during onset of malaria/tuberculosis.

TABLE 25.2: Criteria to assess failure to respond to treatment

In patients	
Criteria for patients to respond	Time after admission
Primary Failure (Phase 1)	
Failure to regain appetite	Day 4
Failure to begin to lose edema	Day 4
Edema still present	Day 10
Failure to enter phase 2 and gain > 5 g/kg/d	Day 10
Secondary Failure to Respond	
Failure to gain > 5 g/kg/d for 3 successive days	During phase 2
Outpatients	
Primary Failure to respond	
Failure to gain weight (nonedematous children)	21 days
Failure to begin to lose edema	14 days
Edema still present	14 days
Weight loss since admission to program (nonedematous)	14 days
Secondary Failure to Respond	
Failure to gain appetite at any visit	
Weight loss of 5% of body weight	at any visit
Weight loss at 2 successive visits	during outpatient care
Failure to gain > 2.5 g/kg/d for 21 days	during outpatient care
After loss of edema (kwashiorkor) or after	
14 days (marasmus)	

Refer. 9

- Introduction of 'family plate', slows the rate of recovery of a malnourished child.
- With outpatient traditional medicines, other treatments and change in home circumstances can significantly affect the recovery of malnourished child.

  For out patients the following points need to be considered:
- Follow-up through home visits to determine whether the child needs to be referred back to in patient facility between visits.
- Discuss with mother/care giver, factors that may be affecting the child's progress.

A follow-up or home visit is required when.

- Mother/care giver has refused admission to in patient care.
- Patient fails to attend appointments at the outpatient program.

RUTF (Ready to use Therapeutic Feed)

RUTF is an energy dense food enriched with minerals and vitamins, with a similar nutrient profile but greater energy and nutrient density than F-100, the diet recommended by WHO in recovery phase of the treatment of SAM. In contrast to the water based F-100, RUTF is an oil based paste with an extremely low water activity.[10]

The food is made uncooked, thereby making the heat labile vitamins available besides reducing the burden of labor, fuel and water demands on poor households. The production process is simple and ready to use, made from local crops with basic technology available in the developing countries.[11]

REFERENCES

1. WHO. Management of severe malnutrition: a manual for physicians and other senior health workers. Geneva, WHO. 1999.
2. Kapil U. Management of children with severe acute malnutrition (SAM) is a National Priority to Achieve Reduction in Under Five Mortality, SAM Expert Group India, Indmedica - http:/cyberlaectures.indmedica.com/show/246/1.
3. Garenme M, Willie D, Marie B, Fontaine O, et al. Incidence and duration of severe wasting in two African populations. Public Health Nutrition. 2009;12(ii):1974-82.
4. Steve Collins, Nicky Dent, Paul Binns, et al. Management of severe acute malnutrition in children. Review Lancet. 2006;368:1992-2000.
5. Myatt M, Khara T, Collins S. A review of methods to detect cases of severely malnourished children in the community for their admission into community based therapeutic care programs. Food and Nutr Bull. 2006; 27(3 suppl):S7-S23.
6. WHO. Report of an informal discussion on the community based management of severe malnutrition in children. http//: www.who.int/child adolescent. health/publications/NUTRITION/CBSM htm.accessed Sep. 10, 2006.
7. Briend A, Garenne M, Maire B, Fontainne O, et al. Nutritional status, age and survival: the muscle mass hypothesis. Eur J Clin Nutr. 1989;43:715-26.
8. Michael Golden and Yvonne Grellety, 2006, Guidelines for the management of the severely malnourished http://motherchildnutrition.org/resiurces/pdfmcn.
9. Michael Golden and Yvonne, Protocol for the management of severe acute malnutrition, Ethiopia Federal ministry of Health 2007, (based on the Guidelines for management of the severely malnourished).
10. Briend A. Treatment of severe malnutrition with a therapeutic spread. Field Exchange. 1997;2:15.
11. Sandige H, Ndekka MJ, Briend A, Ashorn P, et al. Home based treatment of malnourished Malawian children with locally produced or imported ready to use food. J Pedatr Gastroenterol Nutr. 2004;39: 141-46.

26 Nutrition in Diarrheal Diseases

Diarrheal diseases have been recognized as a major public health problem in the developing world. According to WHO estimate, every child under the age of 5 years in the developing world suffers from, on average 2–3 episodes of diarrhea per year. In the first two years of life as many as 20 per 1000 children may die from diarrhea.[1]

This means that the acute diarrheal diseases cause an estimated 750–1000 million episodes of illness and some 4–5 million episodes of death per year in children under the age of 5 years. This gravity of the problem assumes more significance in the light of the fact that repeated attacks of diarrhea expose children to the diarrhea-malnutrition cycle, which can have long lasting effects on the quality of life of the child.

Diarrhea is a prominent clinical feature of childhood malnutrition and is mostly associated with infections and infestations. These are generally a result of multiple pathogens which may be associated with other systemic infections especially the respiratory tract.

INTERACTION BETWEEN DIARRHEAL DISEASES AND MALNUTRITION

Mechanisms causing diarrhea in malnourished children can be grouped into those associated with structural damage to the intestinal mucosa and those due to changes in the intra-luminal environment. Structural damage occurs characteristically with entero-invasive bacteria or enteric viruses, e.g. *E. coli*, which cause intestinal fluid secretion, stimulated by entero-toxins and mediated my enzymatic processes within the enterocytes. Microbial contamination of the upper intestinal secretions is a feature of childhood malnutrition and has damaging effects on intestinal digestion and absorption. The intestinal mucosa itself is extremely damage in children with malnutrition and this contributes to the diarrhea-malnutrition cycle.

The adverse affects of diarrhea are:

- *Reduced food consumption:* Most often diarrheal disease affects the appetite which may be due to presence of vomiting, dehydration, fever and discomfort. To add to this, it is the prevailing food myths and false beliefs regarding different foods and their affects on digestion and absorption, which prevents the intake of adequate food intake, during acute attacks of diarrhea.
- *Reduced absorption of nutrients:* Besides inadequate food intake, there is reduced absorption of macronutrients. The entero-toxins released by adhesion of bacteria to the mucosa, damage the enterocyte and crypt cells which results in diminished capacity of absorption of macro and micronutrients. The recovery, of the mucosa takes almost 6–8 weeks to recover, only after which some absorption can gradually begin to occur.
- *Increased secretion*: The damage to the villous tips and the immature crypt cells left due to replacement of absorptive surfaces, results in increased secretion of water from the infected segment of the small intestine into the lumen. This

hypersecretory state results in important deficits in sodium, potassium, chloride and water and also certain minerals and vitamins.

- *Nutrient losses:* Most often in the diarrheal state due to the rota virus, shigella and campylobacter, there is an increased loss of proteins from the mucosa which can lead to a protein deficient state like in kwashiorkor. Other metabolic alterations like negative nitrogen balance, decreased magnesium, potassium and phosphorous also are found to occur.
- *Effect on growth and development*: Diarrhea induces acute weight loss and arrests in linear growth just like in any other infection. But a negative affect of diarrhea on growth has been described in a number of studies. The wasting and stunting have been found to be more pronounced in children who have had marked fetal retardation. They are prone to suffer from a more severe course of diarrhea and also have a higher risk of mortality. Therefore diarrhea, be it due to any cause has a malnourishing effect, which in turn enhances the risk of dying from infection, thus causing a vicious cycle.

Diarrheas may broadly be looked into from two aspects:

- The Acute Diarrheas (AD)
- The Persistent/Protracted diarrhea (PD).

Acute diarrheas (AD): Acute diarrheas can be a result of acute infections as mentioned earlier in this chapter and is likely to resolve within a few days. But repeated episodes of AD can result in poor appetite, reduced intake and hence reduced absorption of nutrients. Nutritional management therefore is of prime importance to prevent the child from slipping into the cycle of infection and malnutrition.

Nutritional management of AD: A common practice observed in the developing countries during acute episodes of diarrhea is to withhold feeding. This leads to increased losses which are not able to be met. It also delays the repair of the intestinal mucosa and reversal of digestive enzymes, besides malabsorption of important micronutrients. The concept that feeding increases the stool volume and length of illness is totally unfounded. A number of studies have demonstrated the beneficial effects of early feeding during the course of the illness and the resulting shorter duration of hospital stay.[2,3]

Oral Rehydration Therapy (ORT)

The first step to consider in the management of AD is to tackle the dehydration if existing. ORT is the mainstay of the initial treatment. The oral rehydration solution (ORS) recommended by WHO contains 20 g glucose, sodium chloride, 3.5 g, sodium bicarbonate 2.5 g or sodium citrate *2*.9 g and potassium chloride 1.5 g to be mixed in 1 liter of water.[4] However it was found that this composition of ORS proved to be hyperosmolar most of the time since the electrolyte content of noncholera stool is such that it contains only about 56 mmol/lt of sodium and potassium of about 25 mmol. By using this ORS, a state of hyperosmolarity may be achieved which can only worsen the diarrhea. Some authors have also termed this solution as oral dehydration solution (ODS) instead of ORS.[5] Therefore, it would be prudent to assess the type of diarrhea before choosing the type of ORS. A more user friendly ORS has been formulated the hypoosmolar ORS and the super ORS, which is rice based.

Among the hypo osmolar solutions available, two are more common:

a. with sodium 75 and glucose 75 mmol/Lt
b. with sodium 60 and glucose 24 mmol/Lt.

The super ORS solution contains starch 40 g instead of 20 g of glucose per packet.[5] The advantage of using super ORS is that it decreases the stool output by 25%, besides avoiding nutrient compromise in the child during the diarrheal episode. Normal feeding is otherwise affected during acute episodes, resulting in significant nutrient losses. By using super ORS which is rice based, some amount of feeding can be ensured. This has been aptly demonstrated by various studies, where a decrease in stool output too was reported by 28% and ORS consumption too decreased by 27%.[6]

Dietary Management

Adequate feeding during the episodes of diarrhea can not be over emphasized. Anorexia is a common feature observed during any illness but may vary on the type of illness. Febrile illnesses are more prone to lead to decreased intake especially in children. In diarrheal episodes, though there may not be frank anorexia, children and even mothers themselves, prefer to feed only plain liquids more than solids, e.g. weak tea, milk or even fruit juice. Infants on breast feeds must be allowed to continue on the same. In fact, it has been demonstrated that infants fed on breast milk during AD, gain weight better and are prevented from going into a state of malnutrition. Moreover, cessation of breastfeeds is known to exert a deleterious effect on the nutritional status of the child, besides increasing the risk of dehydration 5 times as compared to breastfed infants.[7]

In the acute diarrheal episode most children may be lactose tolerant, therefore, withdrawing of milk from their diet should be avoided, unless and until the child has had a history of lactose intolerance earlier. Bhan and his team have had a vast experience on the management of such children and have recommended a calorie intake of at least 125% of the normal required with nutrient dense foods and should be continued till the child achieves the pre-illness weight and normal nutritional status.[8]

The WHO has formulated some guidelines for the feeding schedule of infants and children during AD episodes, which is tabulated as in Table 26.1.[9,10]

TABLE 26.1: Feeding during acute diarrhea

Stage of hydration and feeding pattern	Recommended schedule of feeding
A. During rehydration phase	
• Breastfed infants • Non-breastfed infants • In severely malnourished children	Continue breastfeeds preferably give ORS till re hydration. Beyond 4 hours, animal milk/food offer some food as soon as possible
B. After rehydration phase	
Breastfed infants	continue breastfeeds more frequently
Non-breastfed infants	offer undiluted animal milk/ formula as before
Infants 4–6 months	add energy dense cereal /pulse supplements
Older children	give energy dense thick ened feeds with oil-pulse (K rich) and green leafy vegetables, carrots, etc. encourage feeding 6 times a day

(WHO, 1991)

As evident from this table, stress has been laid on continuation of breastfeeds in young infants. This also helps maintenance of lactation in the mother for a longer duration and also ensures better milk production due to the sucking stimulus. For older children or the non-breastfed infants, animal milk can be offered but, it should be full strength, as soon as dehydration is corrected, as has been advocated by numerous authors.[10,11]

Older children can be fed on a mixed diet of cereal, pulse and vegetables, with addition of oil/ghee/butter for increasing the density without increasing the bulk. Milk cereal combinations are also well tolerated even among the slightly lactose intolerant children. Amylase rich factor (ARF) can be made use of to reduce the viscosity of the feeds. (Refer Chapter 5).

Nutritional Management of Persistent Diarrhea

Persistent diarrhea (PD) or protracted diarrhea is defined when the duration of passage of stools exceeds 14 days. The state of hydration may or may not be preserved. Growth faltering and severe malnutrition are characteristic features in this condition. This is due mainly to inadequate intake and in most cases with malabsorption.

Pathogenesis of Persistent Diarrhea

The pathogenesis in PD may involve digestion and absorption of all the nutrients—carbohydrates, proteins and fats.

In carbohydrate malabsorption usually there is disaccharide deficiency due to the decreased luminal amylase resulting in impaired exocrine pancreatic function. Lactose enzyme is the one which is mostly affected, leading to secondary lactose intolerance. This condition is frequently encountered following rota viral diarrheas where the villous tip cells are partially damaged. Lactose enzyme being the first to be affected is also the last to be restored for adequate absorption of lactose.

Sucrase enzyme too can be affected leading to malabsorption of sucrose in protracted diarrheas. These can lead to ineffective villous repair or prolonged mucosal injury in malnourished children. This in fact also can be the cause of PD.

Steatorrhea is often associated in PD due to insufficient pancreatic lipase or due to the defect in bile acid metabolism. Similarly protease activity in the pancreatic secretion may also be compromised, especially in children with PD.

Cow's milk protein intolerance (CMPI) is sometimes associated with PD and can be seen in children below 6 months of life. The β lactoglobulin fraction in cow's milk is the cause for CMPI in such children. Milk antibody and IgE are increased in the mucosa in this condition, and this itself can lead to PD also. Such children may also be known to be intolerant to soya protein and may present with blood and mucus.

Finally, PD can also result from abnormal bacterial colonization in any part of the gastro-intestinal tract. Breastfed babies are however prone to be protected from such attacks. It is mostly the older children who are on mixed diet or formula feds, who may be affected by such over growth of bacteria. Common examples are the clostridium difficle and bacteriodes.

TABLE 26.2: Low lactose diets for infants (milk with rice) (4–12 months)

Ingredients	Amount	Calories (%)	Proteins (g%)
Milk	75 ml	52	2.6
Rice	5 g	17	0.4
Sugar	2.5 g	10	–
Water	100 ml		
Total		79	3

Lactose content-4.5 g%

(IAP, 2006)

TABLE 26.3: Curd with rice feed

Ingredients	Amount	Calories (%)	Protein (g %)
Curd	75 ml	45	2.3
Rice	5 g	17	–
Sugar	2.5 g	10 ml	–
Water	100 ml		
		72	2.7

DIETARY MANAGEMENT

As emphasized earlier, infants below 6 months already on breastfeeds should be continued on the same. Older infants will however not be satisfied with breast milk alone nor will their nutritional needs be met with only breast milk.

Dietary manipulation in older children presenting with diarrhea depends upon the malabsorptive state of the child. They may be partially lactose intolerant to sucrose besides lactose. Children presenting with PD generally might already have been fed on milk based diets for the first week or ten days. In such children the lactose load cabe decreased by substituting curd for milk or buttermilk too can be offered also. For older infants beyond 6 months, cereal and milk based formulae can be used where the total quality of milk used is quite less. Rice is the most preferred cereal used. Rice can be made into flour which makes it easier to cook into porridge or gruel form. Some of the formulae used have been recommended by the Indian Academy of Pediatrics as shown in Tables 26.2 and 26.3. These provide approximately 80 cals/100 ml and about 2.5 g/100 ml of protein.

These feeds can be given by nasogastric route also in cases where oral feeding is difficult to achieve. It is generally observed that children who are difficult to feed and are put on tube feeding, generally regain their appetite within 5–6 days and if oral feeding is restored over a period of time naso-gastric feeds can be stopped.

At this stage, the feeds can be made slightly thicker, to make them more calorie dense, by either increasing the amount of cereal or addition of oil proportionately. Coconut oil, a good source of medium chain triglyceride (MCT), can be used successfully to avoid further deterioration of malabsorption. Older children can be given a mixed cereal pulse based family diet, e.g. 'khichdi', which is traditionally used even otherwise in Indian families. Banana is a good calorie dense supplement and also potassium rich, and hence can be used for most children.

There are also a considerable percentage of children who may not tolerate lactose based diets and may need to be taken off milk/curd completely. This is evident from the perianal excoriation seen in children with continuous purging. In such cases, a total milk/curd free feed is advised, where in cereal pulse based diets like blenderised khichdi can be fed. Some of these feeds are shown in Tables 26.4 and 26.5.

TABLE 26.4: Lactose free diets
Cereal pulse based feeds (Sweet)

Ingredients	Amount	Calories (%)	Protein (g %)
Rice	15	48	1.2
Moong dal	5	17	1.1
Sugar	2.5	10	–
Oil	2.5	22	–
Water	100		
		97	2.3

TABLE 26.5: Cereal pulse based feeds (salty)

Ingredients	Amount	Calories (%)	Proteins (g %)
Rice	4.0 g	13.8	2.7
Moong dal	6.0 g	21.0	14.7
Oil	5.0 ml	45.0	–
Water	100 ml		
		80	1.7

TABLE 26.6: Rice gruel (sweet)

Ingredients	Amount	Calories (%)	Proteins (%)
Rice	5.0 g	17	0.3 g
Sugar	4.5 g	18	-
Oil	3.0 g	27	-
Water	100 ml		
		62	0.3

TABLE 26.7: Comminuted chicken feed

Ingredients	Amount (g)	Calories	Proteins (g)
Chicken	100	110	26
Glucose	50	200	–
Coconut oil	50	440	–
Water	1000		
		750	26

(Per 100 ml of feed contains 75 cal. and 2.6 g of protein)

Egg white based feeds along with rice powder, glucose and oil has also been formulated by WHO,[10] but in the Indian context, due to certain religious and cultural constraints, it may not be well accepted.

Only rice based formulae can be used for infants below 6 months of age at this stage. The gut malnutrition in terms of enzymes is more efficient after the age of 6 months and secondly too early introduction of variable proteins may also lead to hyper sensitization in some cases. Rice is considered the least allergenic among the cereals, therefore, it is better to begin first with rice based feed alone and then gradually add other protein sources. An example of rice based formula is given in Table 26.6. This formula is slightly low in calories and also in proteins, but the energy can be increased by addition of more oil, preferably MCT, and the protein content can be enhanced by addition of any commercially available protein supplement like protinex. Most of the supplements available are skim milk based, therefore care should be taken to read the labels before using them in such feeds. Other lactose free commercial supplements available are soyal, prosoyal, zerolac nusobee and Simyl MCT. These contain in addition some essential micronutrients, like vitamins and minerals and varying amounts of taurine, carnitine and MCT.

It has been observed that some children, who are lactose intolerant, are also intolerant to soya protein, and therefore these children can not be offered such feeds. In such situations, the only option left is to use rice based feeds and pulses can be added in older infants.

A small percentage of infants may not respond to even lactose free diets as they may be intolerant to sucrose also. In such cases, lactose and sucrose free formulae have to be used which are available commercially. These have been tried successfully in many centers.

Some centers also use comminuted chicken for lactose and sucrose free diets (Table 26.7), but due to religious issues, these are not very commonly popular.

Once the child is put on any of the above mentioned feeds, the quantity can be gradually increased. Small frequent feeding, about 5–6 times a day helps ensure adequate nutrient intake and also in faster recovery. Older children can be fed with the home based solid diets without including lactose. It may be borne in mind, that once the child slips into a state of PD, the recovery also is a slow process. The lactose enzyme which is the first to be affected is also the last to return to normalcy. It is usually about 4–6 weeks by the time lactose foods can be reintroduced successfully. Therefore, low lactose diets may first be introduced, like curd, which can be tried initially and gradually milk based porridge or gruels can be initiated. The amounts may be small first and gradually increased as tolerance improves.

In case if a child with chronic or intractable diarrhea fails to respond to the above regimen, parenteral nutrition (PN) needs to be considered. The major part of energy is provided by the fat emulsion mixture, containing essential fatty acids. However, PN has its own disadvantages, if used over a prolonged period. Hence, it should be given only till the oral intake is restored.

REFERENCES

1. Synder JD, Merson MH. The magnitude of the global problem of acute diarrheal disease: a review of acute surveillance data. Bull WHO. 1982;60:605-13.
2. BrownKH, Gastanaduy AS, Saavedra JM, et al. Effect of continued oral feeding on clinical and nutritional outcomes of acute diarrhea in children. J Pediatr. 1998;112:191-200.
3. Ornestein SR. Enteral vs. parenteral therapy for intractable diarrhea of infancy. A prospective randomized trial. J Pediatr. 1981;99:360-1.
4. Mahalanbis D, Bhan MK. Development of an improved oral rehydretion solution, Ind J Pediatr. 1991; 58:757-61.
5. KE Elizabeth. Diet in various diseases, In: Nutrition and Child Development. 3rd Ed. Paras Medical Publishers. p.224-230.
6. Molla AM, Ahmed SM, Greenough WB III. Rice based oral rehydation solution decrease the stool volume in acute diarrhea. Bull WHO. 1985;63(4):751-6.
7. Faraque AS, Mahalanabis D, Islam A, Hoque SS, Hasnat A. Breastfeeding and oral rehydration at home during diarrhea to prevent dehydration. Arch Dis Child. 1992;67:1027-29.
8. Arora NK, Bhan MK. Nutritional management of acute diarrhea. Ind J Pediatr. 1991;58:763-67.
9. Jelliffe DR, Jelliffe EFP. Dietary management of young children with acute diarrhea, 2nd Ed. Geneva, WHO. 1991.pp.3-26.
10. World Health Organisation. The management and prevention of diarrhea. Practical Guidelines. 3rd Ed. Geneva, WHO. 1993.pp.1-4.
11. Bhan MK, Arora NK Khoshoo V, et al. Comparison of a lactose free cereal based formula and cow's milk in infants and children with acute gastroenteritis. J Pediatr Gastroenterol Nut. 1998;7:208-13.

27 Diet in Constipation

Constipation in children is a very common disorder and is responsible for up to 25% of all pediatric gastroenterological consultations and up to 3% of all pediatric outpatient visits. It is estimate that in 90% of the cases, the problem is functional in origin while about 10% of them might have some latent organic cause.[1]

A systematic review of literature reveals a prevalence of constipation ranging from 7%–29.6% both in Western and non-Western countries.[2] According to Baker,[3] most of the time there does not seem to be any obvious anatomic, biochemical or physiologic abnormalities. A majority of them seem to be associated with functional factors resulting due to probable improper toilet training. Children usually have a tendency to with hold stool, either due to laziness, or preoccupation with playing or even after a painful experience of stool passage on earlier occasions.

Parents generally keep a keen track of the stooling pattern of their child, since this reflects his status of well being, rather a healthy digestive system. This is particularly true for most mothers with children especially in their first 2 years of life.

The normal frequency of bowel movements varies with age. Infants pass a mean of 4 stools per day, which progressively decreases on an average, to 2 stools per day at 1 year and 1 stool every 2–3 days. But as long as the stools are soft and passage is painless, it cannot be termed as constipation. It may be defined as a delay or difficulty in defecation present for 2 or more weeks or as passing less than 3 stools per week.

Based on the type of presentation of symptoms,[4] etiology of constipation can be broadly divided into:

- Medical cause
- Surgical cause.

IDIOPATHIC/FUNCTIONAL CONSTIPATION

This is perhaps the most common causes of constipation observed among children. The gastrointestinal tract undergoes changes in its physiological forms as the child grows from infancy to older age. The frequency of stool passage can be as frequent as one stool after every feed to almost 1–2 stools every 2–3 days in a breastfed child. As the child is introduced to complementary cereal based diet, the frequency and the consistency of the child also alters to 1–2 stools per day. To a large extent this may depend on how effective is the toilet training received by the child from the first year of his life. To term constipation as functional, certain criteria need to be fulfilled.[5] These are:

a. Two stools or less per week.
b. At least one episode of incontinence per week.
c. History of stool with holding behavior.
d. Abdominal pain.
e. Fecaloma in the rectum.
f. Presence of bulky stools tending to clog toilets.

MANAGEMENT

Children with such type of constipation require timely and prompt action on the part of the parents and the health care givers. Proper toilet training at an age when the child is able to sit without support can help prevent such situations. A great deal of patience may be required to deal with toddlers as they tend to be restless and easily distractible. Training from an early age can help the child form a habit, so that by the time he reaches the school going stage, he is completely habituated to a set time to pass stool.

It is equally important to maintain a fixed routine for the child regarding his eating and sleeping pattern. Erratic timings of waking and sleeping also influence the gastrointestinal reflex to conform to a regular normal cycle of evacuation.

Stress is another factor which could cause functional constipation. It could be pressure on the child to get ready for school or in older children, the fear of an approaching examination or just disinterest in attending school.

The key to management lies in disciplining the child's routine in such a way that it does not impact the normal physiological functions like sleep hours, meal timings and bowel functions. Waking up late and consequently rising late can affect the eating pattern of the child thus disturbing the normal physiological cycle. An adequate diet with a good amount of fiber and residue can help maintain the normal bowel movements. Encouraging consumption of green leafy vegetables and liberal amounts of fruits, whole grain cereals and pulses from the early years will help them develop taste for these foods, and thus develop healthy eating habits. Excess consumption of milk and milk products, processed or tinned foods need to be curtailed in the schedule of the child's diet. Excess of milk in the diet also should be avoided as it can compensate for the solid cereal based food intake, thereby depriving adequate fiber in the diet. Apart from this cow's milk allergy has also been reported to present like features of Hirschsprung's disease.[4,5] Plenty of fluids in the form of water are equally important to maintain hydration, thus helping in maintaining the motility of the gut and softening of stools.

Medical Causes of Constipation

Apart from functional factors, occasionally certain other factors can affect the normal bowel movement of children. Among them hypothyroidism is a well known cause.

At times just electrolyte imbalance can also alter the normal functioning as in case of hyper calcemia. Dehydration is an important nonfunctional factor affecting bowel functioning.

Some other factors like medicines used for any other problems can cause constipation like anticholinergics, antispasmodics and certain resins (cholestyramine).

Finally, dietary factors as already mentioned earlier have a definitive role in causing constipation. These may be summed up as:

- Malnutrition
- Anorexia
- Dehydration[6]
- Excess cow's milk intake
- Residue insufficiency (especially in older children)
- Celiac disease
- Cystic fibrosis (pancreatic enzyme related)
- Meconium ileus (at birth).

Surgical Causes of Constipation

Certain infrequent causes of constipation could be:

- Hirschsprung's disease
- Colonic or ileal atresia
- Meconium ileus related to cystic fibrosis
- Chronic intestinal pseudo-obstruction syndrome
- Anorectal malformations
- Medullar and sacral malformations.

All of the above require surgical interventions where dietary support can help post-surgery

Management of Constipation

Management of constipation in a child calls for prompt dietary intervention and education of the parents. The primary goal of dietary management is aimed at:

- Providing relief to the child
- Modifying diet as per the age and requirement of the child
- Education of the parents
- Behavioral therapy and lifestyle modifications.

Most of the problems of constipation among children are a chronic one thus requiring long-term management. Approximately 30% of the children even beyond puberty continue to struggle with symptoms of constipation like infrequent and partial stool evacuation and fecal incontinence.[7]

This can have a long-term debilitating affect on the overall growth and development of the patient, besides affecting his morale. It is therefore important to focus on the management in terms of diet and lifestyle to prevent significant morbidity.[8]

Treatment of chronic constipation involves 4 phases as recommended by NAPSGHAN (North American Society for Pediatric Gastroenterology, Hepatology and Nutrition.[1] These are:

1. Education
2. Dissipation
3. Prevention of reaccumulation of feces
4. Follow-up.

Parents need to be educated, reassured and counseled regarding the normal stooling pattern of children which varies from that at birth or early infancy when the child is exclusively breastfed to older children when they are weaned off to a full 'family pot' diet.

They should be advised to refrain from blaming the child for his/her bowel habits. On the contrary, they should try to inculcate prompt toilet training, so that the child is accustomed in terms of his eating and sleeping habits.

Adequate and the right type of diet is no doubt one factor which can influence the bowel habits by a good proportion of dietary fiber, but it may not always be the sole cause for chronic constipation in certain children. Dietary fiber given in therapeutic doses may not always be acceptable by the child due to the high bulk form and difficulty in consuming it, besides not being very palatable. Therefore it would be wise if parents do not insist or pressurize the child to consume fiber in this form. Rather the use of laxatives will help the child in passage of soft stools besides regulating the intestinal motility. Fears of side effects of prolonged or recurrent use of laxatives are unfounded since studies have not revealed any such evidence against them.[9]

Parents need to be reassured about the safety of such medicines used as laxatives in prescribed doses offered. The myth of osmotic laxatives having long-term side effects is in fact unfounded. However, a balanced diet with a good helping of whole cereals, pulses, green leafy vegetables and fruits still need to be complied with for long-term healthy gut motility, but of course without forceful implementation of fiber in the diet.[1]

Another factor commonly recommended is a liberal intake of fluids or water to improve bowel function with a view that increased amounts will help in smoother stool output. Actually, this again is another myth as indicated by various studies.[10,11] It is in fact the solutes and not the water which contributes to ileal effluents; therefore minor increase in liquid intake will not help in altering stool consistency. Hence it is recommended that unless there is evidence of dehydration, children with constipation should not be forced to drink more than normal amounts of water.

DISIMPACTION

This is done to remove large fecal mass present usually in children with constipation, to relieve the child of pain and discomfort. Rectal disimpaction is done with phosphate soda enemas, saline enemas or mineral oil enemas.

Recently use of PEG (polyurethane glycol) at the doses of 1–1.5 kg/d has been found to be very effective and acceptable by both children and parents.

MAINTENANCE THERAPY

Use of laxatives to maintain soft stools and prevent constipation is usually recommended initially to prevent recurrence of impaction. Osmotic laxatives and PRG are used intermittently to prevent constipation.

BEHAVIORAL THERAPY

Along with maintenance therapy, behavioral therapy also is initiated for long-term results and maintaining regular bowel movements. Toilet training is encouraged by allowing the child to get on the toilet for 5–10 minutes daily if a fixed time after every meal. This stimulates the gastrocolic reflex allowing for an attempt to defecate. The child is asked to strain actively while placing his feet on the footrest, thus avoiding holding back the urge to defecate. Children failing to respond to any of the combined above therapies are then referred to for psychological counseling.

FOLLOW-UP

Studies have shown that even after successful intervention in a child with constipation, relapse within the first 5 years was found in 50% of the treated children, while 30%–50% of them persisted to have symptoms after 5 years of follow-up, even beyond age 18 years.[7]

To summarize successful management of children with constipation lies in:

- Education of parents and children about normal bowel habits and long-term adherence to treatment program.
- Use of PEG as first line drug in childhood constipation close and long term follow-up in children with constipation to monitor relapse or persistence of symptoms.

REFERENCES

1. Constiption Guidelines Committee of the North American Society for Pediatric Gastoenterology, Hepatology and Nutrition: Evaluation and treatment of constipation in infants and children: recommendations of the North American Society for Pediatric gastroenterology, Hepatology and Nutrition 2006;43: el-e13.
2. Van den Berg MM, Benning MA, Di Lorenzo C: Epidemiology of childhood constipation: a systematic review. Am J Gastroenterol. 2006;101:2401-09.
3. Baker SS, Liptak GS, Colletti RB, et al. A medical position statement of the North American Society for Pediatric Gastroenterogy, Hepatology and Nutrition. J Pediatr Gastroenterol Nutr. 1999;29:612-26.
4. Singh SJ, Arbuckle S, Little D, et al. Mortality due to constipation and short segment Hirschprung's disease. Pediatr Surg Int. 2004;20:289-91.
5. Kawai M, Kubota A, Ida S, et al. Cow's milk allergy presenting as Hirschprung's disease mimicking symptoms. Pediatr Surg Int. 2005;21:850-52.
6. Manz F, Weatz A: The importance of good hydration for prevention of chronic diseases. Nutr Rev. 2005;63:S2-S5.
7. Van Ginkel R, Reitsma JB, Buller HA, et al. Childhood constipation: longitudinal follow up beyond puberty. Gastroenterology. 2003;125:357-63.
8. Loening-Baucke V: Constipation in early childhood: patient characteristics, treatment and long-term follow up. Gut. 1993;34;1400-04
9. Muller-Lissner SA, Kamn MA, Scarpignato C, Wald A: Myths and misconceptions about chronic constipation. Am J Gastroenterol. 2005;100:232-42.
10. Schlessinger M, Fordtran JS (eds) Gastroenterology,ed 6. Phiadelphia, Saunders. 1998.pp.1451-71.
11. Debongnie JC, Phillips SF: Capacity of the human colon to absorb fluid. Gastroenterolgy. 1978;74:698-703.

28 Diet in Inflammatory Bowel Disease

Inflammatory bowel disease (IBD) comprises two main entities:

CROHN'S DISEASE (CD)

Ulcerative Colitis (UC)

The characteristic features of inflammatory bowel disease are weight loss and nutritional deficiencies. Crohn's disease can involve any part of the Gastrointestinal tract (GIT), while ulcerative colitis is mostly confined to the colon with minimal involvement of the terminal ileum.[1]

Both CD and UC may present with overlapping signs and symptoms like diarrhea, GI bleed, protein loss, abdominal pain, weight loss, anemia and growth failure. Abdominal pain accounts for almost 72% of IBD diarrhea and weight loss presents in about 56% and 58% of the children while only 25% of the cases may present with growth failure. As CD involves mainly the terminal ileum, it was described as ileitis. But recent reports also give evidence of Crohn's involving the gastroduodenal section in about 50% of the cases and about 20% involving the jejunum.[2]

INCIDENCE

Inflammatory bowel disease (IBD) is now emerging as a major challenge for pediatricians, especially so in the industrialized countries and it is believed that childhood IBD accounts for about 30% of the total cases reported. The reason for this has been attributed to partly certain environmental factors like hygiene, diet, breastfeeding, smoking (ante natal period), oral contraceptive pills and infectious agents like mumps, measles, etc.[3]

In the Pediatric Inflammatory Bowel disease Clinic at St. Bartholomew's Hospital from 1978–1995, and then from 1995–99 at the Free Hospital at London, there were reported to be about 30–40 new children referred each year. In the UK, estimates put the incidence of CD per 100,000 children as 10.7, while in Japan it has been indicated to be only 0.6%.[4]

Although IBD has extensively been reported from the Western countries, the incidence is not uncommon in India also. Estimates from Indian observations report about 5% of the total admissions for colonic disorders as UC in children.[5] Similar observations have been reported from other parts of India.[6,7] In fact there seems to be an increasing trend mainly for CD in childhood. A recent study from Chennai reported the clinical manifestations of CD in children and adolescents. The youngest child reported from South India is 4 years and 6 months who presented unusually with palatal ulcer.[8]

According to an epidemiological review by Sood from North India,[9] there is convincing evidence of rising trend of IBD in Asian countries and India probably heads the list, sadly catching up with the West. In his words, 'ulcerative colitis is already here and we have to brace ourselves to face the onslaught of Crohn's disease in coming years.' The same may hold true in the case of pediatric age group too.

AGE OF ONSET OF INFLAMMATORY BOWEL DISEASE

Varied reports on age of onset of IBD in children are available but it is observed that children less than 5 years of age comprise about 4% of the pediatric Crohn's disease, while the modern age of presentation of CD is 7.9 years.[10] Though IBD can manifest at any age, it is rarely seen in infancy. Only1% of IBD children are diagnosed before one year of age.[11] Armitage observed an association of CD with affluence. It was suggested that this may be due to low level/delayed exposure to common childhood infectious agents due to improved domestic hygiene resulting in altered immune response in genetically susceptible host the so called 'hygiene hypothesis'.[12]

Recent data from the British Isles have shown that significantly greater proportion of children of Asian origin feature among under 5 with IBD (25% vs 6%) with a relative risk of 3:9.[2] The first national prospective survey of childhood IBD from the British Isles documented an incidence of 5.2/100,000 children and less than 16 years per year.[13] It is believed that the incidence increases steadily with age during childhood and adolescence peaking at about 14 years of age. Unlike in adults pediatric onset CD has clear male preponderance. In the UK study, 62% of pediatric CD in a cohort of 379 children were males.[2]

PATHOGENESIS

As mentioned earlier Crohn's disease and ulcerative colitis both have many features in common like diarrhea, GI bleed, abdominal pain, weight loss, anemia and a number of nutritional deficiencies. Approximately 30% of children with CD are have growth failure and children with CD are three times as likely to have permanent growth stunting than are patients with UC.[14]

The onset is often insidious and may remain undiagnosed for long. By the time the diagnosis is pinpointed, the child has possibly lost his precious years of growth resulting in considerable failure to thrive due to inadequate intake, besides nutritional losses associated with the disease.[15] At times extraintestinal manifestations may be observed which could comprise 25%–30% of children with IBD and these may remain undiagnosed for many years.[16] Recurrent apthous ulcers is the most common manifestation of IBD and a frequent finding in Crohn's disease. Other disease specific manifestations include the oral cavity like mucosal tags, lip swelling, fissures, buccal swelling or cobble stoning, deep linear ulcerations and localised mucogingivitis[17] Unusual manifestations like just oral lesions in the form of a palatal ulcer has been reported without the presence of any other reported symptoms in a child from South India who was perhaps the youngest reported from India.[18]

NUTRITIONAL IMPLICATIONS OF IBD IN CHILDREN

The range of nutritional problems developing in IBD as given in Table 28.1 may have the following implications.[19]

a. Immunologic impairment and increased incidence of infection
b. Poor wound and fistula healing
c. Decreased tolerance to blood loss
d. Increased morbidity and mortality following surgical intervention.

TABLE 28.1: Frequency of nutritional deficiencies reported in patients with IBD

Nutritional deficiencies	Percentage
Weight loss	65%–75%
Growth Retardation	15%–30%
Hypoalbumenimia	25%–80%
Anemia	60%–80%
Iron deficiency	48%
Vitamin B_{12}	36%–54%
Calcium deficiency	13%
Magnesium deficiency	14%–33%
Potassium deficiency	6%–20%
Vitamin A deficiency	11%
Vitamin C deficiency	*
Vitamin D deficiency	75%
Vitamin K deficiency	40%–50%
Copper deficiency	*
Vitamin E deficiency	*
Metabolic bone disease	*

Refer. 19

*Reported but prevalence not described[19]

TABLE 28.2: Causative factors of malnutrition in IBD

Inadequate Intake
Anorexia, altered taste
Abdominal pain, diarrhea, nausea, vomiting
Restrictive diet
Malabsorption
Diminished digestive function secondary to decreased bile salts
Diminished absorptive surface area secondary to extensive disease and /or previous bowel resection
Drug induced malabsorption, e.g. steroid/calcium
Increased GI losses
Protein losing enteropathy
GI bleed
Electrolyte and mineral loss
Increased Nutritional Requirements
Fever, fistula, infection
Repletion of body stores

Refer. 19

NUTRITIONAL MANAGEMENT OF IBD

For management of IBD it is important to know the factors which predispose to malnutrition in such children. Table 28.2 gives a brief picture of the possible causes:

GOALS OF MANAGEMENT OF CROHN'S DISEASE AND ULCERATIVE COLITIS

1. To induce remission
2. To maintain remission
3. To maintain optimal growth and development
4. To optimize nutritional support and prevent deficiency state.

Crohn's Disease

As mentioned earlier, Crohn's disease is more prevalent in the pediatric age group and therefore the main implication in them is growth failure due to the reasons cited in Table 28.2. It has been demonstrated that introduction of nutritional repletion reverses growth failure along with induction of remission.[20,21] Nutritional support for children with Crohn's disease involves either enteral in the form of elemental diet or parenteral nutrition. At times a combination of the two may also be used. Elemental diets have been used with success in most centers.

Elemental Diets

Elemental diets can be described as a chemically defined diet with amino acids or short chain peptides as the protein source along with short chain carbohydrates and added fat, minerals and vitamins. It is observed that almost 50%–60% of the children with CD when treated with enteral nutrition in clinical trials achieve clinical remission.[22] It has been recommended that enteral nutrition should be the sole source of nutrition as offering regular food may compromise efficiency,[23] since the child tends to get full sooner and thereby may not tolerate the formulated feed. However, oral sips of water or clear fluids may be allowed. Nasogastric feeding tubes have been recommended for night feeding to compensate any deficit intake during day time. Enteral nutrition is thought to bring about some extensive changes within the gut, some of them being:

- Bowel rest
- Reduction in antigenic load
- Low resilience diet
- Correction of nutritional deficit
- Alteration of gut flora.

The enteral nutrition formula should be such that it provides 100% of the child's estimated requirements for energy and proteins. The volume should be increased gradually as per individual tolerance. Polymeric peptide based and amino acid based diets have also been used to treat active CD, and if a child can drink orally, a polymeric liquid diet can be encouraged due to its greater palatability.

The duration of exclusive enteral feeding has been recommended to continue for a minimum of 4 weeks or longer if the child has not attained the desired weight and height. Gradual introduction of semi solids to solids is done, preferably with a low fiber diet as shown in Table 28.3.

Observations have pointed out that almost 60%–70% of the patients experience a relapse within 1 year of stopping enteral nutrition, therefore two nutritional strategies have been considered to maintain remission—

TABLE 28.3: Dietary regimen for introduction of solid foods

Day of introduction	Type of foods	Example
1–4	Low fiber cereals	white bread, rice, biscuits plain cereal pulse(khichdi)
5–9	Pulses washed/fish/ eggs	washed dals, fish(low fat), eggs, chicken tender, tofu
10–14	Low fiber vegetables/	raw fruits without skin, membrane fruits tender cooked vegetable without skin seeds, plain soup, noodles
15–17	Low fat dairy products	toned/skimmed milk, yogurt, cottage cheese
18	Regular diet as per tolerance	Increase fat and fiber gradually

1. Cyclical exclusive enteral nutrition in which nocturnal feeding is continued without regular food, once in 4 months.[24]
2. Supplementary enteral nutrition in which nocturnal nasogastric feeding is continued 4–5 times weekly as a supplement to unrestricted daytime diet.[25]

The success of the therapy is marked by normal and catch up linear growth of children treated for CD. If a child does not show linear growth velocity despite weight gain, it is an indicator that the inflamed intestine has not healed completely and might call for other methods of treatment. Inappropriate use of corticosteroids are known to impede catch up height velocity due to the contributory growth inhibiting effects of proinflammatory cytokines produced by the inflamed intestine.

NUTRITIONAL DEFICIENCIES

Most of the children with CD suffer from multiple vitamin and mineral deficiencies due to the malabsorptive state of the gut, poor intake and intestinal losses some of which are discussed as under:

Vitamins and minerals: Most Indian children on vegetarian diets may not be able to get the folic acid sources like animal foods and hence supplements need to be provided. Even if they are non vegetarians, due to poor absorption it may be deficient in them.

TABLE 28.4: Vitamin and mineral supplements for children with IBD

Nutrients	Dose
Multivitamin with mineral	1 tablet daily
Iron	4–6 mg/kg (3 doses)
Folate (for sulfasalazine therapy)	1 mg/d
Vitamin B_{12}	1 mg (q 3 months)
Calcium	1200 mg
Zinc	50–100 mg
Magnesium	200–400 mg

Refer. 26

Davis AM, etal. Pediatric Gastrointestinal Disorders, In: The ASPEN Nutrition Support Practice Manual. R. Meeritt ed. 27:12-13.

Use of certain medications like sulfasalazine inhibit folic acid absorption too. And hence supplementing this becomes essential.

Other nutrients like vitamins B_{12}, magnesium and vitamin E are also known to be deficient in them which need supplementation (Table 28.4).[26] Foods like banana and potatoes are good sources of magnesium and including them in the diet of such children can be beneficial. But large doses of oral supplements may exert a laxative effect and hence needs to be given inmoderation or monitored as per requirement.

Iron, calcium and vitamin D may also be deficient in children with IBD (Crohn's disease). Iron can interfere with calcium if taken together and may also be a gastric irritant, therefore iron supplements need to be appropriately selected and advised. Encouraging foods rich in iron like green leafy vegetables, banana and cooking in iron pans can enhance the iron content of diets of such children. Use of ascorbic acid in food in the form of lemon or other citrus fruits if tolerated can enhance absorption of iron.

Small frequent feeding would be a better way to feed children and the preparations can be formulated such that the caloric density of the feeds can be enhanced. Larger bolus feeds tend to put off children from eating besides triggering abdominal pain and bloating, therefore best avoided.

Fluid requirements also need to be kept in mind to avoid dehydration in the presence of frequent stooling.

Probiotics: The role of probiotics in minimizing gastrointestinal symptoms in children with IBD has been considered by some authors. Usually the lactobacillus or the acidophilus forms available in capsule form can perhaps help normalize intestinal function by restoring a healthy balance. Children who are intolerant to milk, may benefit by curd which is a natural probiotic. The role of prebiotics like psyllium has also been suggested in the healing process.

Marine food: The use of fish oil and flaxseed oil has been considered by various authors in patients with IBD. Fish oil therapy in the form of enteric coated capsules is known to be effective in preventing relapses in patients with Crohn's disease in remission.[27] Patients with ulcerative colitis too have been shown to demonstrate positive results by use of fish oil and supplements. It was speculated that the EPA in the fish oil interferes with the symptoms of the highly inflammatory leukotriene B_4 in the lining of the colon and that effect accounts for the improvement.[28] It was suggested that fish oil may work by reducing existing inflammation but that it may not necessarily be effective in preventing inflammation. Further research needs to confirm these observations.

Ulcerative Colitis

In ulcerative colitis (UC) the aim is to maintain remission as in case of CD. The principle of nutritional management is same as that applied in case of CD where growth failure along with the nutritional deficiencies coexists. Corticosteroids are usually recommended in children having extensive involvement of the colon. Fluid and electrolyte needs to be balanced along with blood and albumin transfusion if excess blood loss occurs. Most of the children may require surgery in which case nutritional rehabilitation (with appropriate nutrients) is an important component of the treatment.

Summary of Dietary Support for IBD in Children

- Maintain hydration of the patient by ensuring a good fluid intake which will also prevent constipation.
- A high fiber diet when child is in remission.
- During a flare up, limit fiber in the diet as also a low residue diet should be encouraged. This gives rest to the bowels and minimize symptoms.
- Avoid lactose containing foods (milk and other milk concentrated foods).
- Small frequent feeding should be encouraged rather than 2–3 bolus feeds.
- The diet should be high in protein and calories. Fats should be moderate and MCT (medium chain triglycerides) might be a good option as these are better tolerated as compared to the polyunsaturated or saturated fats. Coconut oil is an example of MCT which can be used as a cooking medium. Fried foods or other high fat foods need to be avoided.
- Tea and coffee should be avoided as there can irritate the bowel and exacerbate symptoms.
- Restrict gas producing foods like cabbage, cauliflower, sprouts and gram, dried peas, onions pepper and carbonated drinks.
- Use of fish and fish oil and flaxseeds can be beneficial for such patients due to their high omega 3 contents which exert an anti-inflammatory effect.
- Probiotics especially with live culture like curd can also prove beneficial for such patients.

Sample Menu for Children with IBD

Early morning	Water—1–2 glasses
Breakfast	Cereal—1 serving (Suji/dalia sewain) Curd—1 serving Egg (optional)—1 serving
Mid morning	Brown bread/Cereal (poha/dalia, etc.) Buttermilk (if tolerated)/ vegetable soup
Lunch	Cereal (Rice/Chapatti) Pulses (washed)—1 serving Soft green vegetables—1 serving Curd (if tolerated) —1serving
Evening	Herbal tea Biscuits/Rusk—1–2
Dinner	Cereal (as for lunch) Pulse/Chicken/Fish—1 serving Soft vegetables —1 serving Salad (if in remission)—as desired

REFERENCES

1. Motil KJ, Grand RJ. Inflammatory Bowel disease. In: Walker WA, Watkins JB, (eds) Nutrition in Pediatrics: Basic science and Clinical Applications. Hamilton, Ontarrio; BC Decka. 1997:516.
2. Saweczenko A, Sandhu BK. Presenting features of IBD in Great Britain and Ireland. Arch Dis Child. 2003;88:995-1000.
3. Buller H, Chin S, Kirschnen B, et al. Inflammatory Bowel Disease I children and adolescents: Working Group Report of First World Congress of Pediatric Gastroenterology Hepatology and Nutrition, J Pediatr Gastroenterol Nutr 2002;35:Suppl 2 S 151-58.
4. Robert B Heuschkel, John A Walker Smith, Enteral Nutrition in IBD of Childhood. J Enter Parenteral Nutr. 1999;23(5):529-532.
5. Mehta S. Inflammatory Bowel Diseases in Children: Indian perspective. Ind J Pediatr. 1999;587-88.
6. R Ganesh, N Singh, S ezhilarasis, et al. Crohn's disease presenting as Palatal Ulcer. Ind J Pediatr. 2006; 73(3):229-331.
7. Vikrant Khana, Abhinav Sharma, Harsh Deep Sahni, et al. Inflamatory Bowel Disease: Clinical Spectrum in North India. Prdgastro 2005- Conference abstracts, Pediatric on Call, http://www.pediatric on call.com/for doctor/ conference_abstracts.
8. Malathi S, Bhaskar Raju B, Shivbalan So, et al. Disease in South India. Indian Pediatrics. 2005;42:459-63.
9. Sood A, Midha V. Epidemiology of bowel disease in Asia. Indian J Gastroenterol . 2007;26:285-9.
10. Baldaasson RN, Piccoli DA. Inflammatory bowel disease in pediatric and adolescent patients. Gastroenterol Clin N Am. 1999;28:445-55.
11. Armitage EL, Alhdous MC, Anderson N, et al. Incidence of juvenile onset of Crohn's disease in Scotland: association with Northern latitude and affluence. Gastroenetrology. 2004;127:1051-57.
12. Montogomery SM, Pounder RE, Wakefield AJ. Infant mortality and the incidence of inflammatory bowel disease. Lancet. 1997;349:427-73.
13. Sawczenko A, Sandhu BK, Logan RF, et al. Prospective survey of childhood inflammatory disease. Lancet. 2001;357:1093-94.
14. Motil KJ, Grand RJ. Inflammatory bowel disease. In: Basic Sciences and Clinical Applications. Walker WA, Watkins JB eds. Hamilton, Ontario: BC Decker. 1997:516.
15. Walker Smith JA. Disease of the Small Intestine in Childhood. 2nd Ed. London Pitman Meical. 1979.
16. Pittock S, Drumm B, Fleming P, et al. The oral cavity in Crohn's disease. J Pediatr. 2002;138(5):767-71.
17. Ganesh R, Suresh N, Ezhilarari S, et al. Crohn's Disease presenting as palatal ulcer. Ind J Ped. 2006;73; 3:229-31.
18. Melissa F, Perkell, John H, Seashore. Nutrition and IBD. Gastroenterology Clinics of North America. 1989; 183:567-77.
19. Melissa F, Perkell, John H, Seashore. Nutrition and Inflammatory Bowel Disease, Gastroenterology Clinics of North America. 1989;183:567-77.
20. Kirschner BS, Klich JR, Kalman SS, et al. Reversal of growth retardation in Crohn's disease with therapy emphasizing oral nutrition restitution. Gastroenterology. 1981;80:10-15.
21. O'Moran CA, Segal AW and Levi AJ. Elemental diets in the treatment of acute Crohn's disease: a controlled study. Gut. 23;891.
22. Griffiths AM, Ohlsson A, Sherman PM, et al. Meta analysis of enteral nutrition as a primary treatment of active Crohn's disease. Gastroenetrology. 1995;108:1056-67.
23. Johnson T, Mac Donald S, Hill SM, et al. Treatment of active Crohn's disease in children using partial enteral nutrition with liquid formula: a randomized control trial. Gut. 2006;55:356-61.
24. Belli DC, Seidman E, Bouthillier F, et al. Chronic intermittent diet improves growth failure in children with Crohn's disease. Gastroenterology. 1988;94: 603-10.
25. Wilschanski M, Sherman P, Pencharz P, et al. Supplementary enteral nutrition maintains remission in pediatric Crohn's Disease Gut. 1996;38:543-48.
26. Davis AM, etal. Pediatric Gastrointestinal Disorders, In: The ASPEN Nutrition Support Practice Manual. R. Meeritt ed. 27:12-13.
27. Belluzz I A, Brignola C, Campieri M, et al. Effects of an enteric coated fish oil preparation on relapses in Crohn's disease. The N Eng J Med 1996, Vol 334, No.24, June 13, 1996 pp.1557-60.
28. Salomon, Pete, et al. The treatment of ulcerative colitis with fish oil in n-3 omega fatty acid: an open trial. J Clin Gastroenterol. 1990;12;2:157-61.

29 Nutrition Support in Short Bowel Syndrome

Short bowel syndrome (SBS) is a complex condition which usually occurs following massive surgical resection of the small intestinal tract. The subsequent management of a child with SBS depends on a number of factors which determine the overall clinical course and nutritional outcome. These are the length of the remaining intestine, the site of resection, presence of colon and functional differences between small and large intestine.

ETIOLOGY

Short bowel syndrome (SBS) generally presents in infants by birth due to a congenital anomaly or can also present later in older children consequent to any trauma. Intestinal atresia is the most common cause occurring along the portion of the small intestine within an isolated area or along multiple segments. These can cause obstruction leading to GI ischemia, necrosis and resection.[1] Gastroschiasis due to some abdominal wall defect can also lead to necrosis resulting in resection.[1,2]

In preterm infants, necrotizing enterocolitis leading to injury of the small intestine may also lead to SBS. Other factors like presence of pathogenic bacteria, aggressive feeding with hyperosmolar formulae may also lead to SBS.[3]

Malrotation of the GI leading to volvulus, is another cause of SBS in older infants and children resulting in occlusion of the mesenteric artery and ischemia.[1,2] Hernias and intussusception leading to intestinal hypoxic injury can necessitate resection leading to SBS.[1]

PATHOPHYSIOLOGY

In a condition of SBS, it is assumed that post surgery, the patient is left with < 200 cm of functional small intestine. The absorption is related to the amount of residual small intestine. It has been demonstrated that with as little as 15 cm of the jejunum and ileum with the presence of ileoceacal valve, a good outcome can be expected clinically in terms of meeting the nutritional needs of the infant. However, without the valve, about 40 cm of the jejunum is minimally required.[4]

The site of resection of the intestine also determines the degree and extent of malabsorption. The duodenum and jejunum being the major sites for absorption of proteins, fats and certain minerals, cannot take on the functions of the ileum which is the only site for absorption of B_{12} and bile salts. On the other hand, the ileum can adapt and compensate for jejunal loss. Therefore resection of the ileal portion can result in decreased enterohepatic circulation and malabsorption of vitamin B_{12} and bile salts and also the fat soluble vitamins due to impaired micelle formation.

There is malabsorption of the carbohydrates in condition of jejunal resection due to the loss of mucosa containing brush border hydrolases. Nonabsorbed sugars produce an osmotic diarrhea. The risk of small bowel overgrowth is increased, resulting in deconjugation of bile acids, mucosal inflammation and further compromising digestion and absorption. Reduced levels of cholecystokinin and secretion along with loss of jejunum contribute to impaired pancreatic and biliary secretion. There is evidence of N deficiency as a result of malabsorption and peptides and amino acids which further leads to impaired pancreatic exocrine secretion.

The proximal small bowel absorbs minerals like iron, calcium and magnesium and in the absence of this part of the bowel calcium and fat malabsorption combined leads to formation of insoluble soaps. This could result in increased absorption of dietary oxalates. Patients with colon in continuity with shortened bowel may be inclined to have hyperoxaluria and are at risk of forming renal oxalate stones.

In children with high stoma and fluid stools, there is excessive loss of micronutrients like magnesium, zinc, copper and selenium. Iron deficiency can result from loss of the duodenal jejunal area or from complications of ileocecal anstomosis.

Water soluble vitamin deficiencies like B_{12} and other B group vitamins occur in conditions of extensive loss of jejunum and ileum. Vitamin D absorption may also be affected in the event of loss of ileum. Unabsorbed fatty acids are converted to hydroxyl fatty acids by colonic bacteria and together with unabsorbed bile acids, induce colonic secretion exacerbating diarrhea.

Overall gut adaptation and functional prognosis is more of a challenge following ileal resection compared to jejuna resection. Ileal resection and the length of the remaining colon also can impact the course of the nutritional management and overall clinical outcome of SBS. Fluid and electrolyte losses are also increased due to rapid transit time. These can be better maintained if the colon is relatively preserved. Energy balance is also known to improve through colonic preservation as short chain fatty acids, a byproduct of bacterial carbohydrate fermentation in the colon, can provide up to an additional 500 calories per day.[5]

Nutritional Management in Short Bowel Syndrome

Nutritional management is the most important aspect of medical management of SBS the goals of which being:

Promote adaptation
Maintain normal growth
Avoid complications.

After resection of the small bowel, there follows a process of adaptation by the remaining intestine by the process of cell hyperplasia, leading to increased mucosal surface area. Besides, there is increase in bowel circumference length and bowel wall thickness, villous height, crypt depth, cell proliferation and role of cell migration up the villous.[6] For these adaptive processes to take place, good luminal nutrition is essential and should begin as early as possible.

The foremost consideration while managing a child with SBS is to maintain or provide adequate macro- and micronutrients and fluid to prevent energy protein malnutrition and correction of acid base disturbances.

Ideally the nutritional management of a child with SBS is done in 3 stages although it may vary from one child to another depending upon a number of factors, clinical and physiological.[2,7]

The three stages are based on the requirements and physiological condition of the infants to be able to tolerate and assimilate the nutrients administered without any adverse affects. It begins with initially starting with parenteral nutrition (PN), which generally takes care of electrolyte and initial hydration. Gradually, the child is weaned on to enteral nutrition (EN), after initial stabilization and improved intestinal adaptation. In the final stage, which takes a time period of a few months to a year, the child is able to tolerate feeds and begins to accept orally well.

Stage 1

Parenteral nutrition: In the case of pediatric SBS, central venous route is used to administer PN which can take care of the macronutrients requirements in the initial phase. Carbohydrates, proteins and amino acids are used in a balanced ratio suitable to the individual requirements to achieve optimal growth.

Parenteral lipids are infused at 1 g/kg/d and gradually increased by 1 g/kg/d. These should be maintained at around 30%–40% of the total calories. This ratio helps to minimize the risk of hyperlipidemia, especially in small for date or stressed neonates.[6]

Carbohydrates are provided by infusion of dextrose at 5–7 mg glucose/kg/min. and increased gradually by 1–3 mg glucose/kg/min to a maximum of 12–14 mg glucose/kg/min.[7] This way there is minimum risk of hyperglycemia due to gradual response of endogenous insulin. Excess carbohydrate provision can also lead to risk of excess carbon dioxide production and retention, besides preventing immune dysfunction.[6]

Amino acids are infused parenterally about 1.5–2 g/kg/d and increased to the required goal gradually. Neonates generally tolerate amino acids well in progressive doses.

The requirement of electrolytes and minerals for a child with SBS is met by supplementing them with the PN. Pediatric multivitamin solutions are available which can be supplemented with the PN. Most children tend to have high ostomy output and diarrhea for which electrolytes and fluid need to be replaced in addition to the normal requirements.

STAGE 2

Enteral nutrition: Once the child is stable on PN therapy in terms of fluids and electrolytes, gradual initiation of EN should be encouraged. In new borns, EN is generally introduced as a lactose free based formula, preferably having protein hydrolysate. In the Western Market products like 'Pregestimil' from Mead and Johnson are tailor made and readily available. In the Indian setting in the absence of such formulae, there are a few commercially available formulae (like protinex, containing protein hyrolysate containing 56.6% protein hydrolysate or Nova source peptide containing proteins in peptide forms) which can be used as a protein source. Mostly the formula used in feeding, in infants and children with SBS are elemental, semi-elemental or peptide based, as in contrast to adult patients, where complex proteins are preferred due to their better promotion of intestinal adaptation. The reason is that infants and children are more prone to allergenic reactions if exposed to complex macro- or micromolecules. Moreover, this can predispose to bacterial overgrowth and GI allergies.[8]

Initially the feeds are given as a continuous nasogastric form with a flow rate of 1 ml/hr, and slowly increased over weeks or months as PN is gradually reduced and tapered off. The advantage of giving continuous feedings is that the risk of emesis, abdomen distension and high ostomy output are greatly reduced. The rate of increasing the flow of EN would depend upon the nature and length of the residual bowel. The ideal mucosa is better able to absorb solutes against a concentration gradient than jejuna mucosa. Therefore in children with ileal resection there is increased likelihood of fluid and electrolyte losses. The earlier the EN is initiated, sooner is the likelihood of greater intestinal adaptation which refers to the process of cellular hyperplasia, villous hypertrophy, intestinal lengthening and enhanced hormonal response, thus facilitating greater absorptive surface area.[5] It has been shown that the process of intestinal adaptation can occur anywhere from 24–48 hours post resection, the entire process can take up to over a year to occur depending on the course of EN therapy and clinical response based on numerous physiological and metabolic factors.[1,2,9] With gradually increasing the strength of the EN, there is better intestinal adaptation, which can allow for further reduction in dependence on PN. But, in some infants, if there is evidence of increased diarrhea or ostomy output by about 50%, the increase in EN is usually contra-indicated.

The preferred lipids are generally long chain fatty acids, since as compared to medium chain triglycerides (MCT), they have a greater potential for exerting trophic effect and promoting intestinal adaptation. Though MCT are more water soluble and hence have improved absorption, they have a higher osmotic load and lower trophic affect.[10,11]

Carbohydrates should comprise about 40% of the total calories since excess levels can exert significant osmotic effects, thereby exacerbating diarrheas. It has been recommended that if the colon is absent, the diet should include 40%–50% of calories from complex carbohydrates, 20%–30% of calories from protein and 30%–40% from fats. If the colon is intact, the diet, the diet should be higher in complex carbohydrates and contain approximately 20%–30% of calories as fat. The lower fat diet is useful for patients who have a colon, and especially for those who have had significant ileal resection, because malabsorbed fat causes steatorrhea and further fluid losses. In children with intact colon, higher carbohydrate diets are beneficial, as these can be converted into short chain fatty acids by colonic bacterial fermentation and utilized for energy. Lactose restriction is not necessary unless the patient is lactose intolerant.[12,13] Avoiding simple sugars is the most important part of dietary modification in SBS as these tend to increase the osmolar load to the GIT, resulting in secretory diarrhea. Therefore it may be summarized that in children with SBS, where EN is to be initiated, it would be prudent to use either a protein hydrolysate or occasionally if indicated amino acid based formula, with a high percentage of fat of the long chain triglyceride type (LCT) as the optimal enteral fed formula. However depending on the site and extent of resection and the remaining functional gut, some infants and children may also be managed very well with standard polymeric infant formula, as demonstrated by some workers.[14]

Role of Breast Milk

The role of breast milk in enteral formula has been considered due to evidence of increased GI tolerance and reduced duration of PN as compared to protein hydrolysate formula.[6,15] It was inferred that the advantage of breast milk could be due to its good source of immunoglobulins and growth factor, which could enhance intestinal adaptation.

Electrolytes, Vitamins and Mineral Supplementation

Infants require about 4–8 mEq/kg/d of sodium to achieve normal growth,[1,7,8] and as per estimates there is usually excess sodium loss from high output ostomy or diarrhea. Therefore, supplementation of sodium in adequate doses is recommended. Liberal use of salt and salty foods has been recommended for patients with an end jejunostomy or ileostomy, as losses of sodium range from 90–140 mEq/l.[13]

There are also excessive losses of fat soluble vitamins, A, D and E and minerals due to reduced absorptive surface area and steatorrhea, therefore pediatric multivitamin preparations may also be considered for supplementation.[7] However, due to the porential toxicity of fat soluble vitamins, monitoring of serum levels would be advisable before supplementation. In children with ileal resection vitamin B_{12} injections are recommended on a monthly basis to maintain adequate levels.

Role of Fiber and Glutamine

Fiber has been used with success in infants and children with an intact colon in the management of short bowel syndrome. The explanation given is that pectin and polysaccharides which are soluble fibers can help lengthen the transit time, thereby facilitating enhanced nutrient absorption, due to a longer contact time with the intestinal mucosa.[7]

Secondly it is believed that short chain fatty acids which are produced as metabolites of undigested fiber, can induce a trophic effect on the colon and serve as a primary energy source for the colon cells. For patients without a colon, soluble fiber can be beneficial to thicken the ostomy effluent and prolong transit time.[14] Addition of 1%–3% pectin to the semi-solid elemental formula of preterm infants following bowel resection resulted in a reduction of reducing substances in stools and reduced fecal fat loss from 21% to 10%, besides resolving metabolic acidosis within 2 weeks.[16]

Glutamine, a nonessential amino acid in the body is considered to play an important role in enhancing intestinal adaptation in infants with intestinal immaturity or with short bowel syndrome.[7]

Stage 3

Introduction of solid foods: Oral semi-solid foods may be initiated in children with SBS as early as possible coinciding with the recommended age for weaning in any normal child. To begin with, high osmotic foods or those with very high carbohydrates should be avoided. A high protein, low to moderate fat foods are generally recommended.[8] They are encouraged to take small frequent meals during the day and it should be chewed well. The deficit calories and other nutrients can be given as nocturnal EN in proportions as per their requirements. Children with an intact colon are known to develop oxalate and renal stones as oxalate are bound to calcium which restricts its absorption by the colon and is excreted in the urine, leading to stone formation.[2,14] High oxalate foods are colas, tea, chocolate, nuts, black tea, green leafy, vegetables and strawberries. Fluids should be adequate enough to prevent dehydration.

The management of a child with SBS, may be summarized as follows:[17]

Stage 1: PN

- Stabilise fluid and electrolytes
- Initiate PN
- Increase gradually macronutrients to the desired goal.

Carbohydrates:

- Dextrose starting at 5–7 mg/kg/min
- Increase by 1–3 mg/kg/min
- Adjust calorie level as per requirement in older infants and children.

Protein:

- Begin at 1–2 g/kg/d
- *Increase to goal by day 2 of PN.*

Lipids:

- Begin at 1 g/kg/d
- Increase by 1 g/kg/d–3 g/kg/d (infants < 2 years and
- 1.5–2.0 g/kg/d (children >2 years).

Stage 2: EN

- Initiate continuous enteral feeds with appropriate optimize gut trophic stimulation
- Gradually wean PN
- Begin small intermittent feedings by mouth and proceed to nocturnal continuous feeding
- Begin appropriate electrolyte, vitamins and mineral supplement.

Stage 3: Semi Solids

- Begin semi solids as for weaning by 5–6 months.
- Before introducing carbohydrates, stress on high protein, low to moderate fats
- Supplementation of semi elemental or polymeric formula orally with increase in take
- Feeding evaluation by speech or occupational therapist.

Nutritional Complications in SBS

Constipation could be one complication of SBS after cessation of diarrhea, especially in children with cerebral palsy. Excessive use of refined enteral feeds and inadequate fluid intake can also cause constipation.

Anemia can be another follow through in such patients due to excessive blood loss probably from the gastrostomy site, mechanical erosion from enteric catheters or associated stress ulcers.

There could be a risk of protein sensitive enteropathy, as due to anastomatic inflammation and bacterial overgrowth, absorption of intact proteins occurs across the gut. Secondary anemia could also result due to inadequate gut length for absorption of iron, folic acid, vitamin B_{12} and copper.

REFERENCES

1. Vanderhoff JA. Short bowel syndrome. In: Walker WA, Watkins JB (ed) Nutrition in Pediatrics: Basic Science and Clinical Applications, BC. Decker Inc Hamilton. 1997;609-18.
2. Jojnson MD. Management of short bowel syndrome- a review, Support Line. 2000;22(6):11-23.
3. Price PT. Necrotising eneterocolitis, In: Grok-Wargo, S Thompson M, Hovasi Cox J (ed) Nutritional Care of High Risk Newborns, Precept press, Chicago, IL. 2000;425-28.
4. Sibert JR. Small intestine length in infants and children. Am J Dis Child. 1980;18:513-96.
5. Vandrehoff JA, Matyr SM. Enteral and Parenteral nutrition in patients with short bowel syndrome. Eur J Pediatr Surg. 1999;9:214-19.
6. Hughes CA. Intestinal adaptation. In: Tanna MS, Stocks RJ, ed. Neonatal Gastroenetrology: contemporary issues. London: Intercept. 1984:69-91.
7. Serrano MS, Schmidt-Sommerfeld E. Nutritional support of infants with short bowel syndrome. Nutrition. 2002;18(11-12):966-70.
8. Warner BW, Vanderhoff JA, Reyes JD. What's new in the management of short bowel syndrome in children. JACS. 2000;190(6):725-36.

9. Wessel JJ. Short Bowel Syndrome, IN: Groh-Wargo S, Thompson M, Howasi Cox J (ed). Nutritional care of high risk new borns, Precept Press, Chicago, IL. 2000;469-87.
10. Vanderhoff JA, Grandjean CJ, Kaufman SS, et al. Effect of high percentage MCT diet on mucosal adaptation following massive bowel resection in rats. JPEN. 1984;8:685-89.
11. Vanderhofff JA, Blackwood DA, Mohammadpur H, et al. Effect of dietary menhaden oil on normal growth and development and on ameliorating mucosal injury in the rat. ACJN. 1991;54(2):346-50.
12. Matarese LE, O'Keef SJD, Kandil HM, et al. Short bowel syndrome. Clinical guidelines for nutritional management. Nutr Clin Pract. 2005;20(5): 493-502.
13. Parrish CR. The Clinician's Guide to short bowel syndrome. Pract Gastroeneterol. 2005;XXIX (9):67-106.
14. Ksiazyk J, Piena M, Kierkus J, et al. Hydrolysed *vs* non hydrolysed protein diet in short bowel syndrome in children. J Pediatr Gastr Nutr. 2002;35(5):615-18.
15. Andorsky DJ, Lund DP, Lillehei CW, et al. Nutritional and other post operative management of new borns of neonates with short bowel syndrome co relates with clinical outcomes. J Pediatr. 2001;139(1):27-33.
16. Hawkins R, et al. Pectin supplemented enteral feeding in the treatment of short bowel syndrome in two infants. J Am Diet Assoc. 1995;96(5):1010-22.
17. Sinden AA and Sutphen J. Nutritional management of pediatric short bowel syndrome. Nutr Issues In: Gastroeneterolgy, Series 12, pp 29-48.

30 Nutritional Management in Celiac Disease

Celiac disease (CD) was first described in 1950 by Dicke in Holland[1] by chance observation that during the German occupation when food availability was scarce and nutrition poor, children kept better health. Subsequently, with improved nutrition, when wheat was more liberally available, children actually deteriorated in health. This set him to infer that perhaps it was the wheat which was the culprit, the introduction of which could cause features of malabsorption. The classical histopathological description of the disease was given by Paulley in 1954.[2] Other cereals like barley wheat and rye were also identified around the same period to cause CD. By 1960 it was also identified in India and perhaps for the first time reported by Walia et al.[3] In 1979, Walker- Smith described it as a disease of the proximal small intestine characterized by an abnormal small intestine mucosa and associated with permanent intolerance to gluten. Removal of gluten from the diet leads to a full clinical and pathological remission.[4]

INCIDENCE

Celiac disease (CD) was earlier known to occur in the predominantly wheat eating areas like Europe, Australia and North America. It was first thought to be around 1 in 3000 in England but over a period of time, it was observed by Mylotte in the West Ireland that the incidence could be as high as 1 in 300.[5]

However, Asian countries like India too are not spared of this entity, and there are reports from the Middle East in Arab children as well. Reports of CD from the Northern India have shown a remarkable steady increase over a time period. His could be partly attributed to the fact that there is growing awareness regarding the existence of this entity among the clinicians as compared to what was true about a couple of decades ago. Genetic factors are also known to predispose to gluten hypersensitivity as the disease is also known as. The condition may occur in one or member of the same family. Reports of concordance for CD in monozygotic twins are also available.[6]

PATHOGENESIS—*WHAT IS GLUTEN?*

Gluten is the protein fraction of found in wheat. It is a large complex molecule that has been divided chemically into four hetrogenous proteins-gliadins, glutenins, albumins and globulins. In CD, it is the gliadin fraction of gluten which is responsible for the pathogenesis. This gliadin itself is a complex protein consisting of 40 different components. The alpha gliadin is the main toxic entity of the gluten, though it has also been associated with a small peptide. The beta gama and omega gliadin are also known to be toxic in nature. Other cereals found to be toxic are rye, barley and oats. But the inclusion of barley and oats as gluten free are controversial with different authors reporting diverse opinions. Barley contains the protein hordein, which is also known to cause mucosal changes when given in highly artificial circumstances.[7]

It was suggested during later years that the amount of gliadin present in the nominally gluten free products may be significant in very sensitive patients. In 1979, WHO proposed a standard for the permitted residual protein in a wheat (or other gluten containing cereal), starch based gluten free product of not more than 0.3% protein in dry matter and the proposed regulations require that the total nitrogen content of wheat, rye or barley, etc. used in gluten free products should not exceed 0.05 g per 10 g of these grains on a dry matter basis and that the nature of the source of the starch should be declared on the label.[8]

The mechanism leading to damage in the intestine is:

- It is caused by an immune response to gluten containing diet
- Factors facilitate the gluten induced injury
- Incomplete digestion of gluten due to deficiency of enzymes results in the accumulation of toxic substances that damage the mucosa
- Toxicity is mediated by a lecithin like interaction between gluten and intestinal epithelial cells.[9,10]

More recently CD is considered as an autoimmune reaction to the tissue transglutaminase in the intestinal mucosa initiated by exposure to dietary gluten in genetically predisposed individuals. It is a symptomatic or symptom free disease, closely associated with risk alleles on the human leukocyte antigen (HLA) class 11 genes and it may develop at any age during childhood or adulthood.[11]

CLINICAL FEATURES OF CD

Diagnosing CD in a child may not always be a straight forward process since there may be variable signs and symptoms. Most of these like recurrent diarrhea or not gaining weight may be overloaded and not given due significance by parents themselves. The former problem may be treated off and on for infections and in a peripheral set up, and the failure to gain weight is often overlooked by parents and hence delaying seeking of medical attention. At times in the absence of diarrhea or failure to thrive, the child may always appear pale and the parents may fail to observe it. The initial signs of mild to moderate anemia are hardly noted by parents and only when he child probably presents with complaints of weakness, fatigue or loss of appetite, do the parents seek medical help. Even if they are in some remote area not accessible to some medical centre, they may be treated with some hematinics or appetite boosters or some multi-vitamin supplememts. Therefore to diagnose CD, it is important that the health care givers think along the lines of features of malabsorption. Only then would an attempt be made to work up for ruling out CD.

The common symptoms suggestive of CD are:

- *Steatorrhea*: Almost 70% of children suffering from CD present with pale bulky, offensive stools. A close look at the stool may also reveal small fat globules sticking around.
- *Failure to thrive*: Often children with CD may present with failure to gain weight despite reasonable intake, and may show features of wasting. At times some may otherwise appear normal but parents may complain of the child appearing smaller for his age as compared to his peers. Pot belly is a typical feature in these children.
- *Anemia*: At times in the absence of any of the above symptoms, parents may just present a child for not eating adequately or loss of appetite, lethargy or easy fatigueability even without much exertion. A routine examination may reveal severe anemia and on further work up for one of the differential diagnosis, the child may prove positive for CD. The anemia in these children is generally of the iron deficiency type rather than the megaloblastic one, though blood folate levels may also be reduced.[12]
- *Skin manifestations*: Some of the children with CD may present with skin manifestations like knuckle pigmentation and skin infections. Dermatitis herpetiformis is commonly observed in such children.
- *Others:* Symptoms like vomiting, pain abdomen, irritability, constipation or rectal prolapse in some may also be found in children with CD.

The European Society for Pediatric Gastroenterology and Nutrition (ESPGHAN) in 1970 evolved definite criteria to label a child with CD.[13]
These include:

a. It is a permanent condition
b. There is a flat mucosa in upper and small intestine
c. There has to be a biochemical evidence of malabsorption, but some of them may be asymptomatic at the time of investigation

d. A gluten free diet (GFD) results in complete restoration of mucosal architecture and tests for malabsorption also become normal.
e. Re introduction of gluten into the diet will be followed by recurrence of the mucosal abnormalities. There may or may not be clinical symptoms for months and years.

DIAGNOSTIC CRITERIA

To diagnose CD a variety of tests are used which can decide further course of management in a child with CD. It should be kept in mind that since the mainstay of management in treating CD is dietary therapy alone, which means withdrawal of gluten from the child's diet and since gluten is the primary component of any diet especially in the Northern India, it can come as a great shock to the parents once diagnosis is confirmed to them and the management explained.

The various diagnostic criteria include:

a. Stool test- a 24 hour fecal fat test is doe to establish the extent of fat malabsorption
b. D-Xylose test
c. Breath hydrogen test
d. Intestinal biopsy challenge tests.

AGE OF PRESENTATION

In an Indian setting the age of presentation of CD in a child is generally after the age of 2 years and more since it is by this age in most communities that the child is more or less totally weaned to a complete solid diet comprising mainly wheat and wheat products. However children between the ages of 10–18 months also are introduced to certain wheat products, mainly in the form of biscuits or suji kheer, but the amount of gluten exposure during this age may be very low and secondly by the time the clinical signs begin to present and parents concerns are aroused, the child may already have reached 2 years or more. As mentioned earlier in the initial stages, recurrent diarrhea or failure to gain weight may be treated as common infections by physicians too. There are reports of CD presenting between ages 1–5 years by some authors.[14]

MANAGEMENT OF GFD

After thorough work up and investigation, if a child is proven to test positive for CD, the next step is the biggest challenge on the part of the clinicians and the dieticians, that of management.

Dietary management is 'the only' management in a child with CD. Gluten withdrawal is the mainstay of management of such children. A typical North Indian diet comprises mainly gluten in all or at least part of the day's diet.

In gluten free diet, i.e. foods totally devoid of wheat and wheat products, rye, barley (jaun) and oats, needs to be excluded from the diet completely. Regarding oats, there are controversies of its being safe to include or exclude. But most dieticians, to be on the safe side and to avoid any benefit of doubt, prefer to advise complete exclusion from the diet. The dictum 'when in doubt discard' holds true in this context. On the face of it, to counsel the parents to stop gluten in the child's diet seems simple enough, but practically when we are faced with such situations, it has been observed that the initial reaction of the parents is that of shock, denial and disbelief. In the predominantly wheat consuming States, like Punjab, Uttar Pradesh, Himachal Pradesh, Haryana and Madhya Pradesh, one cannot even imagine of a day's diet without wheat in some form or the other.

In our day to day life we would observe that wheat and its by products like 'suji', 'dalia', 'sewain' are commonly used in preparations like biscuits, snacks, sweets and even daily meals. There are a host of foods available outside the home which children tend to consume, e.g. breads, biscuits, cakes, pastries or any other bakery products, snacks like 'samosas',' mathi', 'pakoras' and many other savoury products categorized as 'namkeen'. Exclusion of gluten implies a full stop to all these food items. This comes as a rude shock to the parents and a number of times more than the child it is the parents who go into depression and seem visibly upset over the realization of the impact of treatment of their child. Foods that are allowed and restricted are listed in Tables 30.1 and 30.2.

It is here that the dietician's role of counseling comes in and it is indeed a challenge for him or her to convince the parents that there are a host of other alternative foods from which the child has the liberty to choose from, without compromising his growth and development as can be seen from Table 30.2. Soya flour gram flour, rice flour, corn

TABLE 30.1: Foods to be excluded in gluten free diets

• All wheat based products: wheat flour, maida, suji (semolina), oats, barley, rye
• All bakery products like biscuits, rusks, cakes and pastries buns from maida, suji or wheat flour
• Baby foods like cerelac, etc.
• Beverages like horlicks, bournvita, protinex and other products where 'malt' word is shown on the labels of the packings
• All sauces ,creams, pie fillings, chocolates, flavoured milk shakes, yogurt, where gluten may be present in indirect form
• Ready to eat flavored crisps, e.g. Mac Donalds' chips etc.
• Meat products like sausages, hamburgers, tinned meat products, fish fingers, etc. where bread crumbs may be used
• Malt vinegar, soy sauce, spreads, etc.
• Cooking oils (mixed vegetable oil) can contain wheat germ oil, so ensure that oil used is free of it or else sunflower or olive oil can be used safely
• Beer and whisky are made from grain containing gluten but other alcoholic drinks like wine and cider can be used which is gluten free.
• Some medicines contain gluten which needs to be checked with the chemist or clinician
• Vegetable gum
• Noodles and pizza, etc.
• Modified food starch, hydrolysed protein like in 'protinex'

TABLE 30.2: Foods that can be included

• Dairy products like milk (fresh, tinned, powder), butter, cream
• Meat, fish and poultry
• All green vegetables, roots and tubers
• All fruits, dried fruits and nuts
• All pulses and legumes like peas, beans, etc.
• Maize, rice, soya flour, gram flour, jowar, bajra, ragi, waterchestnut('singhara flour')
• Tapioca, sago arrowroot
• Potato flour
• Beverages like tea, coffee, fresh juices, fizzy drinks gelatin, etc.
• Custard powder
• Gluten free flours and cereals available commercially but certified

flour and arrowroot flour are some of the other alternative which can be included into the diets of these children. (See Annexure 1 for GFD receipes).

The parents have to be reassured that excluding gluten from the diet will not be as difficult as may appear to them. On the contrary that should be reassured that this treatment implies restriction of only a particular variety of food item and no other medicine or surgical intervention is required. They have to be explained and impressed upon that dietary modifications is 'the only' treatment for CD and with good compliance the child can lead a healthy normal life just like his peers. Regular follow-up visits are very important for these parents and children and a close rapport between them will help the child understand the significance of dietary restrictions. The parents need to be explained the long-term prognosis of this disease, stressing the importance of such modifications for life without intending to scare them unduly.

Children with CD need not be restricted to go out for social get- togethers where eating is a part of the function, but of course that need to be explained if they are old enough to comprehend, what food can be taken safely, e.g. milk, curd preparations, rice and other rice based recepies, fruits or fruit juices and candies, etc. At the same time it is a good idea if the hostess is aware of such special needs of her guests so that she may be able to include some alternative dish which this child can safely partake. Alternatively they can carry their own tiffins in case they are on a trip outside. Now a days there are some gluten free cereals available in some super markets from where mothers can procure them and plan recopies accordingly. The culinary skills of the mothers with some innovative ideas can help break the monotony of the diet of the child with CD.

GOALS OF NUTRITIONAL THERAPY

1. To achieve the nutritional requirements in terms of macro and micronutrients.
2. To ensure a balanced diet for the desired age.
3. To ensure compliance to GFD.
4. To monitor growth and development periodically-regular follow-up visits.
5. To look for and prevent any associated complications.

The above goals can be achieved as follows:

- The nutritional requirements can be calculated on the basis of age and weight of the child. Most often since these children had been anorexic, their intake would have been very poor. Therefore it would be aimed to begin with a minimum of 100 calories/kg body weight and gradually build up to 200 calories over a period of time. Proteins can be around 1 g/kg body weight since lower than this is not always practical as most of the caloric dense foods in a mixed diet would also be rich in proteins, e.g. cereals, pulses and milk and milk products. It can be gradually increased to 1.5–2 and even 3 g/kg depending upon the appetite of the child as he recovers. Fat content of the diet may vary from 25% to as high as 40% of the total calories, depending upon the need to meet the calorie requirements. Moreover on a gluten free diet there are certain recipes which may require slightly higher ratio of fats in their preparations. Other nutrients may be supplemented as per the requirement based on clinical or biochemical parameters from time to time.
- Having decided upon the requirements, efforts should be made to plan the day's menu such that there is variety and at the same time balanced in terms of all the food groups to be provided.
- Compliance on a gluten free diet is the mainstay in such children. The earliest signs of recovery on GFD are evident by apparent cheerfulness of the child, his appetite returns and looks more alert and takes interest in the surroundings. Weight gain comes much later. It has been noticed that most often where compliance is poor, the parents or other elders in the family have been responsible for it. They might be inclined to give 'a little' of any gluten based diet once in a while, thinking that it will not make much of a difference. This can happen especially in an environment where the literary level of the parents might be low or even in the lower socio-economic strata, where it might be difficult for them to adhere to the restrictions in the absence of availability of alternative foods. Also, it may be due to paucity of time available with the mother to cook separately for this child or due to certain family pressure they may not be able to provide alternative foods to such children. In some cases, despite parental compliance and effort, the child may on the sly share some food with his peers or other siblings. All these factors need to be borne in mind and strict supervision should be maintained for optimum compliance.
- The children are called for regular follow-up visits and monitored for their growth and any other related clinical signs. Initially their visits may be monthly, gradually relaxing to quarterly, six monthly and then annually depending on their progress. This also ensures compliance and reassurance to the parents and the child to maintain on GFD. A good rapport can be built with them and any doubts regarding the choice of foods can be dealt with them from time to time. If required protein supplements may be advised in case of vegetarian children who may also be lactose or milk intolerant.
- In a few cases there may be presence of certain other factors like diabetes or lactose intolerance or cow's milk protein intolerance which could be a part of complications of gluten enteropathy as the disease is also known. Such conditions may have to be tackled accordingly. Careful selection of various food items allowed or disallowed keeping in mind the lactose containing foods or restrictions imposed for the diabetic state also.

COMPLIANCE ON GFD

After counseling sessions on GFD to the parents and the children, the next step is to assess the compliance. This can be done by maintaining regular follow-up records in terms of anthropometry, dietary intake or any other visible signs and symptoms. Failure to gain the desired weight and height can be an alert to suspect noncompliance in any form. This can be assessed by obtaining a detailed dietary history from the parents or a 24 hours dietary recall may be taken regarding the various foods taken in the recent past. Indirect probing from the child regarding his or her activities at home or school or time spent with peer groups may give a clue of the kind of foods he could have access to or would e taking inadvertently. There are a number of food categories which might have gluten in some latent or indirect form which otherwise might be considered gluten free, e.g.

- Sweets made from milk, khoya, paneeer which might have some amount of suji or maida mixed by unscrupulous manufacturers. Products containing malt in any form like chocolates, health supplements, e.g. horlicks, bournvita, protinex, etc.
- Creams, soups and gravies which might have maida or thickening agents.
- Any processed food products when specific labeling is not indicated.
- Inadvertent contamination of gluten free cereals like maize, gram flour or rice flour with residue of wheat products during the processing or milling in a mill.
- Any medicines, gums or toothpaste might have some gluten as a base ingredient.
- Any 'prasad' from religious places even though taken in very minute quantities.
- Social eating especially in outdoor catered foods where one may not be sure of the ingredients used in any unstandardised recipes.

Duration of Treatment/Follow-Up

As per the definition criteria of ESPGAN, GFD needs to be considered for life, i.e. it is usually for life, even though the patient remains asymptomatic. This is because it is expected that on a GFD, chances of complications or late recurrences can be avoided, e.g. chronic deficiencies, infertility, etc. which could be associated with gluten sensitivity. Walker-Smith had laid down criteria for the duration on which to keep a child on GFD (Fig. 30.1),[4] and then give a gluten challenge to determine the response. Based on this response, normal or abnormal mucosa on a biopsy after giving a gluten challenge can help to determine whether GFD needs to be continued or can be stopped safely without chances of relapse.

GLUTEN CHALLENGE

The Working Group of the World Congress of Pediatric Gastroenterology, Hepatology and nutrition in 2002[15] have recommended gluten challenge and subsequent biopsies in children where:

- Initial biopsy was performed before 2 years of age
- Initial diagnosis is doubtful
- Noncompliant patients
- Asymptomatic individuals detected though screening program
- Patient desires a gluten challenge.

However it is opined that gluten challenge should be avoided during the growth period of a child till up to puberty, to avoid the risk of a set back in the velocity of development in the event of exacerbation of symptoms. Challenge may be given by introduction of 10–20 g of gluten in a phased manner or just allowing the child to have a normal diet as the whole family which would include wheat, may be in the form of chapattis, biscuits or any other wheat based preparation.

FACTORS AFFECTING GLUTEN SENSITIVITY

- **Time of gluten introduction:** It is speculated that the timing of exposure of gluten into the child's diet might also have a bearing on the manifestation of symptoms of gluten sensitivity. Norris et al[16] in 2005 have shown links between early infant diet and development of celiac disease. According to their studies in 1560 children it was observed that the initial exposure to gluten in the first 3 months or at 7 months and later significantly increased the risk of CD as compared with exposure at 4–6 months. They had defined CD autoimmunity by the presence of tissue transglutaminase (tTG) auto antibodies or small bowel biopsy evidence of crypt hypoplasia or villous atrophy. Increased risk was defined as having first degree relative with Type I diabetes or the presence of HLA-DR3, alleles, genes that are associated with an increased risk of autoimmune disease. They therefore concluded that the timing of first gluten exposure is associated with the appearance of CD autoimmunity in children at increased risk for the disease.
- **Amount of gluten:** It has been postulated that the amount of gluten ingested could be as important as the timing if gluten introduction. This has been demonstrated by Weile et al[17] where a profound difference in the prevalence of CD exists between Denmark (a very low) and Sweden (high prevalence). The explanation given was a

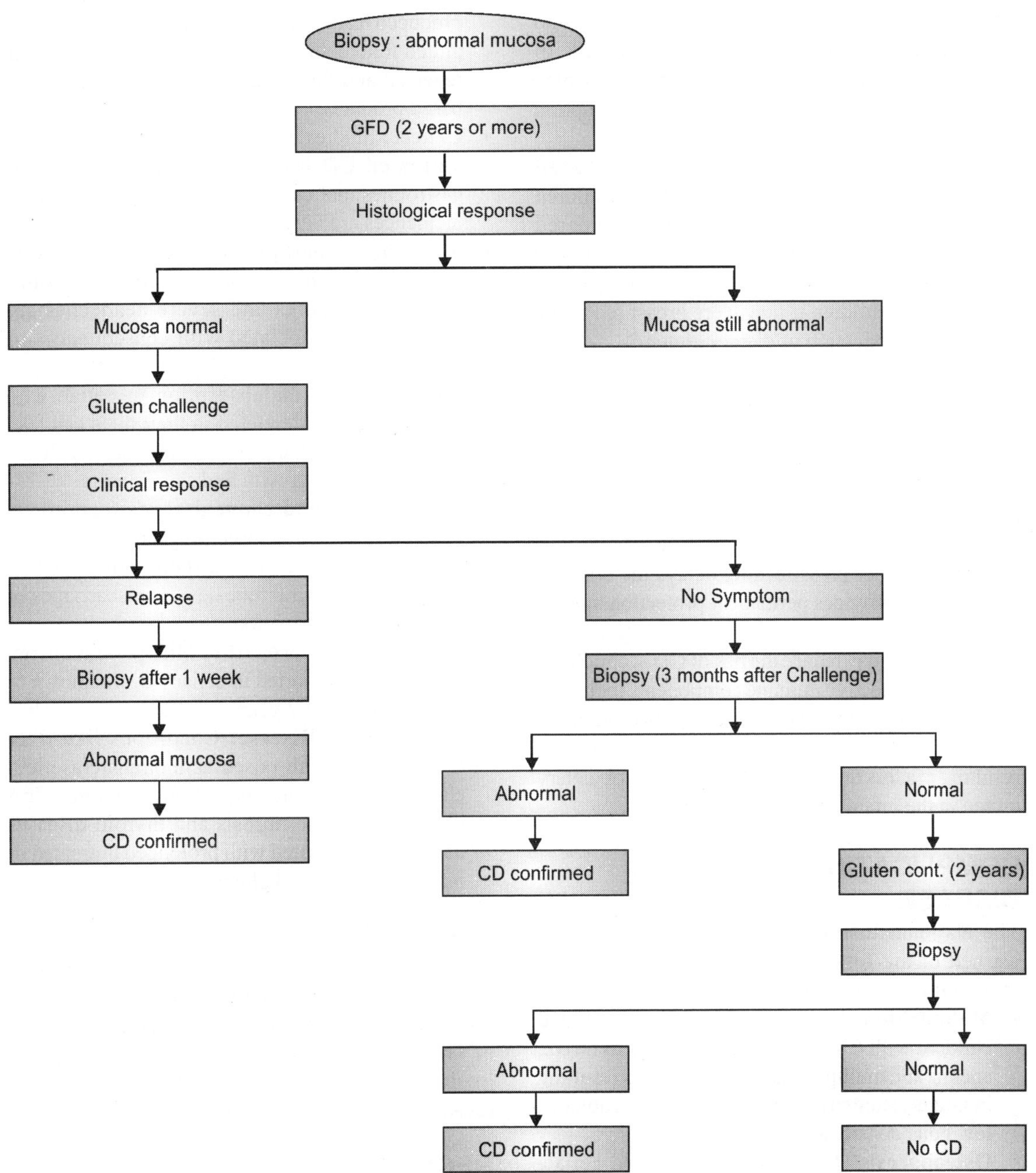

FIGURE 30.1: Diagnostic criteria and investigation for celiac disease (Walker Smith, 1979)[4]

remarkable difference in the diet of infants who actually receive much less gluten in Denmark. In Sweden an epidemic of CD was observed which was related to rapid increase in the consumption of gluten at 6 months of age.[18]

- **Breast feeding and the time of gluten introduction:** In a Swedish study on 627 children with risk of CD exposed to gluten compared to 1254 controls, it was found that the risk of symptomatic CD before 2 years of age was reduced in children if they were breast fed at the time of introduction of dietary gluten.[19]

A systematic review and meta-analysis of observational studies published between 1996 and June 2004,[20] revealed that breastfeeding may offer protection against the development of CD. Breastfeeding during introduction of dietary gluten and duration of breastfeeding were associated with reduced risk of developing CD. However, it was not clear whether breastfeeding delays the onset of symptoms or provides permanent protection against the disease.

Breast milk may reduce the risk of CD in childhood through its protective immune components including secretory IgA. On the other hand, the protective effect of breast milk may modulate gluten introduction, resulting in a less rapid or a reduced amount of dietary gluten in the infant diet.

COMPLICATIONS OF CELIAC DISEASE

The National Institute of Health (NIH) in 2004 warned of the following complications of celiac disease if left untreated:[21]

- **Malnutrition:** If not treated or partially treated children with CD show signs of failure to thrive, anemia and multiple vitamin deficiencies resulting in fatigue, stunted growth, neurological problems, low bone density and malabsorption.
- **Osteoporosis/Ostopenia:** In untreated celiac, there are losses of calcium and vitamin D due to malabsorption, leading to rickets, ostopenia and osteporosis. Reversal of symptoms is observed on gluten withdrawal from the diet.
- **Lactose intolerance:** Due to flattening of the mucosal villi, the lactase enzyme cannot be produced leading to lactose intolerance. Once the gluten free diet is initiated, the lactase enzyme is reversed and the child is able to tolerate lactose based products.
- **Cancer:** Studies have proven that long standing untreated CD leads to an increased risk of gastrointestinal cancer like lymphoma, but such incidences are very rare.
- **Neurological and psychiatric complications:** Symptoms of depression, neuropathy, balance disorders, seizures and severe headaches are known to be associated with consequences of untreated CD.
- **Short stature:** malabsorption in celiac who continue to include gluten in their diets can lead to deprivation of the essential nutrients which can result in stunted growth and short stature.
- **Miscarriages and congenital malformations of the fetus:** Undiagnosed pregnant women who are unaware of their celiac status, not on GFD, have a risk of neural tube defect, miscarriages or congenital malformation
- **Milk protein enteropathy:** Milk protein allergy has also been reported in celiac but are known to resolve by age of 2 years.[22]
- **Autoimmune Disease:** Conditions like liver abnormalities with raised aminotransferase levels, hepatic dysfunction, diabetes mellitus, IgA deficiency, cystic fibrosis and thyroid diseases have been associated with prolonged untreated or inadequately treated gluten enteropathy.

Celiac Crisis

This is a condition manifested by profuse watery diarrhea, dehydration and shock mostly occurring during a gluten challenge or if during the course of GFD, the child suddenly starts gluten either inadverdently or on the sly. This condition is reversible if treated promptly.[1]

RECIPES FOR GLUTEN FREE DIET

Gram Laddoo

Green gram	20 g
Whole corn seeds	20 g
Ground nuts	8 g
Sugar/Jaggery	20 g

- Roast corn whole, green gram and ground nuts and grind them to a powder
- Make jaggery syrup, add the flour mixture
- Mix well and make into balls.

Chidwa Barfi

Pressed rice	25 g
Roasted ground nut	20 g
Jaggery	25 g

- Roast the pressed rice and mix with groundnuts
- Add the pressed rice and nuts and mix quickly
- Spread the above mixture on a greased plate and cut into pieces immediately.

This recipe is extensively used in special nutrition program in Andhra Pradesh.[23]

Chidwa Laddoo

Chidwa	35 g
Roasted ground nuts	20 g
Roasted Bengal gram	25 g
Sugar/Jaggery	25 g

- Powder chidwa, roasted bengal gram dal, groundnuts and sugar and mix the powders.
- Add hot water to make the mixture soft in consistency and make into laddoos.

Dosa

Green gram dal (washed)	25 g
Black gram dal (washed)	25 g
Soyabean	25 g
Salt	to taste
Oil	3 tsp
Water	3–4 tsps

- Soak all the three dals separately overnight
- Remove skin from soyabean by rubbing with hands
- Mix green gram dal, black gram dal, soyabeans and grind to paste
- Add water and prepare the batter. Stir the batter well and keep aside covered for 4 hours to ferment
- Add salt and mix thoroughly
- Grease the pan , heat and pour on to it
- Cook lightly till golden brown using oil on both sides.

Sago Kheer

Sago	100 g
Sugar	30 g
Grated coconut	10 g
Food color	1 drop
Water	for cooking

- Cook sago and sugar in water till soft and the mixture thickens
- Add color and cook till soft and the mixture binds
- Make into balls and dust with grated coconut.

Rice Pura

Rice powder /flour	50 g
Salt	to taste
Curd	20 g
Oil	for frying

- Mix rice powder, curd and salt to make a smooth batter
- Heat the pan and spreadout a little batter to form a thin pura
- Fry lightly on both sides till done.

Idli

Rice	75 g
Black gram dal (washed)	25 g
Salt	to taste

- Soak rice and moong dal separately for 5–6 hours
- Grind both separately and mix together
- Add salt and keep aside overnight, covered, to allow to ferment
- Pour ladel full of mixture on the compartmental stand which are slightly greased
- Place the stand into a pressure cooker filled with water to form steam
- Cover the pressure cooker and remove the done idlis on to a plate

Note: The same batter can be used to make dosa by making it into a pouring consistency and spreading it on a pan to shallow fry on both sides.

SAMPLE MENU FOR GLUTEN FREE DIET

Breakfast

Maize roti/	1–2
Idli/dosa	1–2
Egg	1(optional)
Curd/Milk.	200 ml

Midmorning

Poha/Dhokla/Besan pura/Fruit.

Lunch

Rice	2 serveings
Dal	1 serving
Vegetable	1 serving
Curd	100 g
Salad.	

Evening

Soya porridge/sago kheer/rice kheer (using milk-20 ml).

Dinner

Missi roti/rice	1–2/50–75 g
Paneer/chicken/dal.	30g/100g/1 serving

Bedtime

Milk.	150 ml

REFERENCES

1. Dicke WK. Celiakeie:een onderzoek naar de nadelige involved van sommige graanoorte op de ligder aan coeliake. MD thesis, Utrecht and Transactions of the 6th International Congress of Pediatrics. 1950.pp.117, Zurich.
2. Pauley LW. Observation on the etiology of idiopathic steatorrhea. Br Med J. 1954;2:1318-20.
3. Walia BNS, Sidhu JK, Ghai OP. Celiac Disease in North Indian children. Br Med J. 1966;2:1233-4.
4. Walker Smith JA. Celiac disease, In: Diseases of the Small Intestine in Childhood, 2nd Ed (ed. Walker -Smith JA). London: Pitman Medical. 1979.
5. Myollete M, Egan Mitchelle B, Fottrell PF, et al. Incidence of celiac disease in the west of Ireland. Br Med J. 1973;1:703-5.
6. Thapa BR. Celiac Disese: Indian experience. In: Nutrition in Children, Developing Countries Concerns. Eds. Sachdev HPS and Chaudhary P Dept. of Pediatrics, Maulana Azad Medical College, New Delhi. 1994.
7. Rubin CE, Brandborg LL, Flick AL, et al. Biosy studies on the poathogenesis of celiac sprue. In: Intestinal Biopsy (eds). Wolstenholme GEW and Cameron MP. Edinburgh: Churchill Livingstone. 1962.pp.67.
8. WHO. Proposed draft standard for gluten free products. Codex Alimentarius Commission ALINORM 79/26 Appendix 2 Step 8 1979;pp19-20.
9. Walker-Smith LA. Celiac disease. In: Diseases of the Small Intestine in Childhood, 3rd ed, London, Butterworths. 1988;pp.88-143.
10. Tria JS. Celiac disease. In: Gastrointestinal Disease; Pathophysiology, Diagnosis and Management, 5th ed Eds. Sleisenger M, Fordtran JS Phildelphia, WB Saunders Company. 193.pp.1078-96.
11. Branski D, Fasano A, Trancone R. Latest Developments in the pathogenesis and treatment of celiac disease. J Pediatr. 2006;149:295-300.
12. Cook DM, Evans N, Lloyd A and Strwart JS. Normal serum and red cell folate levels in a child with celiac disease. Lancet. 1970;1:571-2.
13. Meeuwisse GW. Round Table discussion. Diagnostic criteria for celiac disease. Acta Pediatr Scand. 1970; 59:461-68.
14. Sahni A, Thapa BR, Malik AK, et al. Jujunal mucosal histology. Critical appraisal of criteria for diagnosis of CD. Abstracts. 25th Annual Conference of IA, Jodhpur. 24-28 Oct,198.
15. Hill ID, Bhatnagar S, Cameron DJS, et al. Celiac Disease: Working Group Repot of the First World Congress of pediatric Gastroenterology, Hepatology and Nutrition. J Pediatr Gastroenterol Nutr 2002;35: Supplement 2: S78-88.

16. Norris J, Barrriga K, Klingensmith G, et al. Timing of initial cereal exposure in infancy and risk of islet autoimmunity. JAMA. 2003;290:1713-2.
17. Weile B, Cavell B, Nivenius K, et al. Striking differences in the incidence of childhood celiac disease between Denmark and Sweden: a possible explanation. J Pediatr Gastroenterol Nutr. 1995;21:64-8.
18. Carlson A, Agardh D, Borulf S, et al. Prevalence of celiac disease: before and after a national change in feeding recommendations. Scand J Gastroenterol. 2006;41:533-5.
19. Ivarsson A, Hernell O, Stenlud H, et al. Breastfeeding protects against celiac disease. Am J Clin Nutr. 2002; 75:914-21.
20. Akobeng AK, Ramanan AV, Buvhan I, et al. Effect of breastfeeding on risk of CD: a systematic review and meta analysis of observational studies. Arch Dis child. 2006;91:39-43.
21. National Institute of Health. Consensus Development Conference Statement. June 28-30,2004, see website About.com:http://consensus.nik.gov/2004,celiac disease 118 html.htm.
22. Watt J, Pincott JR and harris JT. Combined cow's milk protein and gluten induced enteropathy: commonor rare? Gut 24. 1983;165-70.
23. National Institute of nutrition, ICMR, Hyderabad, India. Low Cost Nutritious Supplements. 1977.

31 Nutritional Support in Cystic Fibrosis

Cystic fibrosis (CF) is the most common autosomal recessive disorder found predominantly in the caucasian population with an incidence of 1:25000 live births[1] and 1 in 25 of the population are carriers.

The disease involves widespread dysfunction of the exocrine glands with disturbances in the ion and fluid movement resulting in abnormally thick and dehydrated secretions. There are multiorgan lesions including:

- Chronic obstructive lung disease with predominant airway obstruction and recurrent, persistent infection.
- Exocrine pancreatic insufficiency with steatorrhea
- Intestinal obstruction in neonates and older patients.
- Abnormally high levels of sodium chloride sweat, resulting from the failure of salt reabsorption in sweat gland ducts.

The basic defect in CF is a mutational change in the gene for chloride conductance channel called cystic fibrosis transmembrane conductance regulator (CFTR). Failure of chloride conductance by epithelial cells leads to dehydration of secretions that are too vivid and difficult to clear.

The prevalence of genetic mutation varies from one population to the other the most common one being the delta 508 which constitutes almost 70% of the total cases. The frequency of this mutation among Asians migrated to UK is almost less than 50%. In view of these figures, CF cannot be considered rare among Indians. The diagnosis is usually delayed due to late suspicion. These patients are mostly treated as tuberculosis, pneumonia and acute exacerbations are labeled as 'bronchopneumonia'. Lack of diagnostic facilities especially a standardized sweat test could be one reason why so few patients have been reported so far.[2]

Gastrointestinal (GI) involvement is present in 85–90% of all cases and symptoms generally appear before age of 2 years but may remain undiagnosed for many years.

CLINICAL PRESENTATION

Children diagnosed with CF may present with features associated with different organs but the most commonly seen are those involving the respiratory and the GI functions (Table 31.1).

Pancreatic Insufficiency

A child usually appears normal in size at birth. There is progressive destruction of exocrine pancreas, leading to impaired intraluminal hydrolysis of dietary lipids and proteins. By age of 2 months the child gradually begins to show signs of protein energy malnutrition with or without diarrhea.[3] GI involvement is present in 85%–95% of all cases. Due to the pancreatic damage involved, the secretion of digestive enzymes and bicarbonate is affected, resulting in malabsorption of fat, proteins, nitrogen, bile, fat soluble vitamins and B_{12}. According to estimates, in 90% of the patients, the enzyme secretion is absent making them pancreatic enzyme dependent. In the rest 10% of the patients, the enzyme secretions are present but in minimal amounts adequate for digestion and

TABLE 31.1: Clinical features of cystic fibrosis

Intestines	Abdominal pain Rectal prolapsed Distal intestinal
Obstruction	Steatorrhea/Diarrhea Abdominal distension Failure to thrive Gastro colic reflux
Pancreas	Pancreatic failure Pancreatitis Glucose intolerance Diabetes mellitus
Gall Bladder	Cholecystitis Cholelithaisis Obstructive jaundice
Lungs infections	Recurrent respiratory Asthma
	Nasal polyps Bronchiectasis Hyperventilation Clubbing of fingers Hemoptysis Pneumothorax
Others deficiencies	Delayed puberty Salt depletion Male sterility Arthritis Fat soluble

absorption of nutrients without the need for enzyme supplementation.

Due to the defect in absorption of nutrients, growth failure is most frequently encountered among these children, ultimately resulting in delayed puberty.

Chronic Respiratory Involvement

The lungs are normal at birth, but may get affected within a few weeks of life. There are abnormal secretions resulting in mucoid production which cause obstruction in the small airways, with secondary infection which is progressive and destructive. The child has persistent cough productive of purulent sputum.

Gastroesophageal Reflux

The GER is a common feature observed among some patients with CF which could be due to inappropriate reaction of the gastroesophageal sphincter. Though it is more frequent among younger age group, the incidence decreases with age.

TABLE 31.2: Definition of nutritional status in patients with cystic fibrosis

Age group	At risk	Nutritional failure
0–2 years	Weight for length 10%–15%	Height percentile < 5% OR Weight for length < 10% OR IBW < 90%
2–20 years	BMI percentile 10th–25th	BMI percentile < 10% OR IBW (< 90%)
Adults	BMI 19–20	BMI < 19 OR Percent IBW < 90%

Refer.6

Growth Failure

The next common problem among children with CF is chronic malnutrition with significant weight loss and failure to thrive. Malnutrition is generally an associated feature observed among most children with CF, which can be prevented or corrected with adequate nutritional measures.

CAUSES OF MALNUTRITION

Nutrition: A Risk Factor

Early detection of nutritional risk is necessary in order to intervene at a time when a proactive approach can make a positive impact on the outcome.[4] Studies have demonstrated that low weight if not corrected can itself pose an independent risk factor of survival.[5]

There is a set criteria defined by the clinical practice guidelines for cystic fibrosis foundation for classifying nutritional status in patients with cystic fibrosis[6] which has been laid down by the Metropolitan Life Insurance company in the USA[7] as presented in Table 31.2.

Nutritional problems in CF are determined by 3 factors:

- Energy Losses
- Increased Energy Expenditure
- Deceased Energy Intake.

Energy Losses

There are significant energy losses due to presence of malabsorption of proteins and fats. It has been estimated that stool energy losses account for 11% of gross energy intake in CF patients, three times higher than normal.[8] Losses also may occur through vomiting following bouts of cough or gastroesophageal reflux which is commonly seen in such children, Nitrogen losses may occur through sputum (rich in aminoacids) during severe acute pulmonary exacerbations.

Increased Energy Expenditure

Abnormal pulmonary mechanisms may increase the resting energy expenditure. Continuous injury to the lungs causing airway obstruction can be associated with increased oxygen cost and breathing.[9]

Low Energy Intake

It is generally seen that the energy intake of most children with CF remains very low resulting in suboptimal growth pattern. This low intake could be due to several factors like:

- Anorexia
- Chronic respiratory infections and other complications of CF like abdominal pain, GER, resulting in vomiting and pain
- Behavior feeding problems in school and preschool children encountered in even normal children
- Depression
- Eating disorders in adolescents
- Dislike of high energy foods
- Poverty, ignorance and food fads.

GOALS OF NUTRITIONAL MANAGEMENT

The three main objectives of nutritional management are:

1. To achieve optimal nutritional status
2. To achieve normal growth and development
3. To maintain normal feeding behavior.

The approach to achieve these goals is 2 pronged:
Nutritional Support
Pancreatic enzyme supplementation

Nutritional Support

Energy

The energy requirements of patients with CF are estimated to be around 120%–150% of the recommended daily allowances (RDA) for age and sex. But usually such patients are unable to meet these standards in the Indian population. As they are already caloric deficit, initially they should be to bring their intake levels to the RDA and then gradually further build up to meet the estimated requirements. The presence of respiratory infections, increased activity and impaired nutritional status makes it difficult to follow a set universal pattern. The best way to monitor the intake is by monitoring their growth velocity. A useful guideline to follow is to assess the existing energy intake and increase this value by a further 20%–30% if weight gain or growth is poor.

Proteins

Protein requirements should be increased to compensate for excessive loss of nitrogen in the stools and sputum and increased protein turnover in malnourished children. About 150%–200% of RDA can be provided by proteins.

Fats

It is widely accepted that fat being the most concentrated source of energy, should be encouraged. Most often it is observed that parents tend to restrict fat content of the diets of their children with CF in view of increased losses in stools, thinking that it will not be digested. This myth needs to be discouraged and parents should be explained the importance of fat sources in the diet. The malabsorption of fats can be dealt with supplementation of pancreatic enzymes as will be discussed further in this chapter. The role of medium chain triglycerides to be substituted for other oils is controversial and not widely accepted, with the view that it may result in deficiency of essential fatty acids and indirectly increase energy requirements as it needs more oxygen than carbohydrates to be oxidized in the liver.[10]

Carbohydrates

About 40%–50% of the energy intake should be provided by carbohydrate sources which are well tolerated. High starch foods like bread, potatoes and pasta as well as simple sugars can be used liberally in the diet of such children. Table 31.3 summarizes the recommendations for nutrient intakes in children with CF.[11,12,13]

TABLE 31.3: Recommendations for nutritional management in cystic fibrosis

Protein	120% of RDA	
Energy average	variable depending on disease status but should be at least 115% of RDA	
Fats EFA	40% of total energy as LCT and 3%–5% as	
Micronutrients	Vitamin A	5000–10,000 IU/d*
	Vitamin D	400–80 IU/d**
	Vitamin E	Infants–50 mg
	Children	100 mg
	Adolescents	200 mg

Refer. 11,12,13

*If serum levels normal, may not require supplements

**Regular exposure to sunlight is adequate in most warm climates.

FEEDING OF INFANTS

Breast Milk

Breastfeeds being high in lipase content in combination with pancreatic enzymes. The advantages of doing so have been highlighted as follows:[14,15]

- It contains long chain fatty acids
- It provides immunological protection against infections
- It contains taurine
- It contains optimal essential amino acids
- It is psychologically better for the mother.

However, as mentioned earlier, due to the increased energy losses in them, breastmilk alone may not be adequate to meet their requirement and hence formula feeds will have to be supplemented. Calorie dense commercial supplements can be incorporated along with formula milk.

For children intolerant to cow's milk or are lactose intolerant, hydrolysed protein formulae are good substitutes. To meet the enhanced caloric requirements of babies with CF in enzyme therapy, extra fats can be used. The deficiency of Essential Fatty Acids (EFA) can be made up with vegetable oils rather than butter.

Feeding of Older Children

As for normal children, by one year of age the child should be fed from the 'family pot', but ensuring to incorporate the feeds such that the enhanced requirements are met with small frequent feeding of high density foods. This could be achieved by 5–6 small but frequent thickened or dense feeds. A bed time snack is a good idea for tiding over the long gap at night time. To ensure adequate intake, regular growth monitoring is the best and simplest way which even parents can record. A suboptimal weight gain or static weight over a prolonged period of time is an indicator of inadequate intake or enzyme dosage. With normal weight gain, the use of supplements (commercial) can be avoided. Even if offered, it should not replace the meals. Standard age related recommendations for the calorie contribution from supplements to the diet of a patient with CF have been laid down as follows.[16]

1–2 years	200 cals/d
3–5 years	400 cals/d
6–11 years	600 cals/d
> 12 years	800 cals/d

- Dietary supplements if indicated need to be given 2–3 times a day after meals or at bed time.
- Care should be taken to avoid excessive supplementation as it can hamper the child's appetite.
- These should not be used as substitutes for meals, but as supplements only.
- High protein supplements indicated for adults should be used with caution as they may not always suit the pediatric patient.
- Supplements with milk shakes require enzymes along with.

An idea of the possible high fat, high carbohydrate and high protein foods can be had from those listed in Table 31.4.

Electrolyte Supplementation

Children with CF are prone to salt depletion with excessive fluid and water losses, leading to hypokalemia, hypochloremia and metabolic acidosis. This problem is aggravated especially in hot tropical weather; therefore it is essential that children should be encouraged to consume plenty of fluids spread over the day along with high salt foods. Significant hyponatremia may be accompanied by vomiting. The doses of salt recommended arbitrarily are as given in Table 31.5.[16] Breast fed babies are prone to get hyponatremic due to its low sodium content, therefore in some centers, routine supplementation of

TABLE 31.4: List of food options for children with cystic fibrosis

High fat foods	High carbohydrate foods	High protein foods
Spreads high in PUFA/MUFA Instead of low spreads (sunflower/olive/ricela), on bread/toasts/potatoes/vegetables Frying foods instead of baking, grilling, and boiling Chocolates, crisps, cream cakes, biscuits, buns, cream added to porridge, drinks, cereals, soups, ice cream, trifle, pastries	Potatoes, bread, cereals, rice, noodles, pizza Breakfast cereals/sandwiches, potatoes, pasta, rice added to salads, fried rice, potato wafers, savoury, biscuits/bread, cheese sandwiches, sweets after meals, sugar in beverages, milk drinks, cereal puddings, kheer, jam, honey, chocolate spreads on bread, roti, squashes, fruits juices, fizz drinks, fruit custard	Beans (rajma), baked or as curry,baked beans with butter toast, nuts, peanuts, dry fruits, fish, wggs, chicken, meat, milk (full cream), cheese sandwiches, grated cheese in vegetables, soups, scrambled eggs, extra cheese on pizza, burgers, cheese slices in between munchies, full cream yoghurt

TABLE 31.5: Guidelines for sodium supplementation in children with cystic fibrosis*

0–1 year	2 mmols/kg (Nacl soln)
1–5 years	1 x 600 mg (10 mmol Na tabs)
6–11 years	2 x 600 mg (20 mmol Na tabs)
> 11 years	3 x 600 mg (30–40 mmol Na tabs)

**Source.* Gavin JE. Nutritional management. In: Pediatric Guidelines for CF Care[16]

salt is practiced. Urinary sodium should be checked if babies show poor weight gain.

One way to ensure that the child is being maintained on adequate nutritional intake as per the desired amounts is to ask the parents or care givers to maintain a food diary of the child. This could include all foods/drinks/beverages consumed throughout the day, which could be recorded date wise with a brief description of the method of preparation or type of food, or source of the food item in terms of any standard household measures, e.g. teaspoons, glass, cups, etc. A record of the enzyme taken along with any specific meal and the dose can also be recorded (Table 31.6). This record can be maintained about 3–4 days before the scheduled follow-up visit with the doctor/dietician. A glance at this diary can help the dietician assess the actual intake of the child and any modification in the dosage of the enzyme or the diet can then be suitably advised.

Vitamin and Mineral Supplements

Although fat soluble vitamin deficiency may be expected in children with CF due to high fat losses in stools, clinical signs of vitamins A, D or K are not commonly seen. However, due to low levels of serum vitamin E levels encountered in such patients, supplementation of vitamin E is recommended (5–10 IU/kg/d).

TABLE 31.6: Food diary of a child with cystic fibrosis

Date: Weight: (kg) Height: (cm)

Time	Food description/ type of preparation	Amount taken (raw measure)	Enzyme (creon)
Early morning			
Breakfast			
Tiffin			
Lunch			
Evening			
Dinner			
Bed Time			
Any other (in between snack/drink)			

Trace Elements

Iron supplementation is known to interfere with pancreatic enzyme supplements; therefore, care should be taken not to administer iron supplements in close proximity to PES.[17]

Absorption of zinc is also known to be affected in patients with CF due to fat malabsorption, due to the formation of zinc forming complexes with fat and phosphorous. Supplementation of 5–10 mg/d of zinc can improve absorption effectively.

Other trace elements like carnitine and taurine are also known to have a beneficial effect on the absorption of fat. Carnitine acts by prevention of toxic accumalation of long chain fatty acids in the cytoplasm and of acyl CoA in the mitochondria. Taurine has been shown to decrease fecal fatty acids and sterol excretion, and also known to decrease the severity of steatorrhea.

Route of Feeding

Enteral feeding or feeding via a nasogastric tube is practiced in many centers in the UK to build up children with CF and even in teenagers reflecting deteriorating nutritional status. However, it is not so aggressively practiced among the Indian Centers where children are diagnosed as CF unless there is acute problem of oral feeding amongst them.

Enteral feeding has shown to improve body fat, height, lean body mass and muscle mass, increase total body, etc. The duration of tube feeding may continue for a period of 1 year to longer depending upon the nutritional status of the child in terms of their nutritional scores.

For children requiring long-term enteral feeding, mostly a percutanous endoscopic gastostomy (PEG) is done which makes it convenient for both the patient and the care giver. In some situations, the child is allowed to have an ad lib diet during the daytime orally and the deficit is made up by giving high energy nocturnal feeds through the gastrostomy. The common practice followed by most CF centers in the UK is feeding for 8–10 hours overnight with 1–2 hours break before the physiotherapy session in the morning.

Pancreatic Enzyme Supplementation

Apart from dietary intervention, the second most crucial aspect of nutritional management of such patients is supplementing their diets with pancreatic enzyme in order to make up the deficit or absent secretion of this enzyme by the pancreas.

Pancreatic enzyme supplements (PES) is available as tablets/capsules of the enzyme which are an extract of the pancreas and is meant to be ingested with meals. These are available in the form of powders or more recently and widely used as enteric coated microsphere enzyme preparations. The powder form was available as pancreatin powder and rarely used today. The main drawback of this powder was

- Unpleasant taste.
- Can cause irritation to the infant's lips if got in touch with the skin as also to the mother's nipples while breastfeeding (the residual granules smeared on the baby's lips can irritate the nipples also while feeding.
- If mixed with formula milk or in a bottle, it may start digesting the milk and also clog the teat of the bottle.

The widely used enteric coated microspheric preparations are available as tablets known as 'creon', which has many advantages over the powdered from. The enteric coating protects the enzymes from inactivation by the acidic medium in the stomach, disintegrating to release the enzyme only when pH rises > 5.5 in the duodenum. The enzyme so administered can achieve 90% fat absorption if given in correct dosage.

The microspheres can be mixed with a little expressed breast milk or formula milk and fed by a spoon or given on a wet finger. There may be some granules left lodged in the oral cavity of the baby, which can be dislodged by using a clean finger and rinsed down with a little milk given along with. The best and easiest way to administer these enzymes is to mix them with a small amount of fruit juice/puree (which will hold the enzyme in a gel form) and give it from a spoon at the beginning of a feed. The commonly used enteric coated microspheres are available in the dose of 10,000 IU of lipase per capsule.

Dosage of PES

The dosage of the enzyme to be given depends on factors like:

- Residual pancreatic enzyme.
- Enzyme supplements properties.
- Amount of fat and protein consumed.
- Pathophysiological factors.
- Stool output (frequency/color/consistency).
- Abdominal pain.
- Fecal fat studies.

Infants

The general acceptable dose for infants, when first diagnosed is approximately 400–800 IU lipase per gram of dietary fat or in other words 1/4–1/3 of the capsule (10,000 IU) mixed with Expressed Breast Milk (EBM) or in some fruit puree and given by spoon directly before the feed. The dose may be increase gradually depending upon the response to clinical symptoms in terms of stool output, absorption and growth. As weaning is initiated, the enzyme can be opened and mixed with any semi-solid food and given before a meal. Parents are encouraged to begin weaning in the normal way by 5–6 months and all home based preparations can be made use of with liberal helpings of fat in them. As for normal children, it is advised that parents should encourage wider variety of foods in the diet of their children in order to get them accustomed to a healthy eating pattern well into their childhood and later.

Older Children

As the children grow, the enzyme dose too has to be mentioned keeping in view their increasing weight and fat intake. Initially 1–2 capsules of standard creon can be recommended with the 3 main meals, depending upon the severity of fat malabsorption. The doses can be titrated based on the response of individual child. Care should be taken to give an additional dose of 1/2-1 capsule with extra fat based food or supplement.[16] Overall, the dose requirements can vary from as low as 500 IU to as high as 2500 IU of lipase per kg body weight. If stools are persistently greasy despite a recent increase in enzyme therapy, the use of antacids should be considered, e.g. omeparazole or ranitidine, which help to make the acidic medium more alkaline, thereby encouraging maximum enzyme activity at the appropriate site in the gut.[16] If the total dietary fat of the child can be assessed accurately, the dose can be fixed as 500 IU lipase of dietary fat. The recommendations made by the Consensus Committee on Cystic Fibrosis[17] have been laid down as given in Table 31.7, based on both fat intake and weight.

The maximum dose of enzyme should never exceed 10,000 IU lipase/kg/meal, due to the risk of fibrosing colonopathy and constipation. Very high doses of lipase in the enzymes containing 22,000–25000 units/capsule have been associated with the development of the above complication. Other adverse reactions noticed are severe acute and chronic reactions.

TABLE 31.7: Recommended dosage of pancreatic enzyme supplements

Age group	Dose	Adjusting dose
Infants	2,000–4000 units lipase/120 ml formula or with each nursing Or 450–900 units lipase/g of fat	Increase by 2000–5000 units lipase/feed as volume increases or if symptoms of malabsorption return
Children < 4 years	1,000–2,000 units lipase/kg/meal Or 500–4,000 units lipase/g of fat	Snacks: ½ meal dose; if dose appears above range, compare unit lipase/g fat.
Adults and children > 4 years	500–2,000 units lipase/kg/meal Or 500–4,000 units lipase/g fat.	Snacks: 2 meal dose. If dose appears above range, compare unit lipase/g fat.

Refer.[18] Consensus Committee, J Pediatr. 1995;127(5): 681-84

Administration of PES

The PES should be administered with all meals and protein and fat containing snacks. It has been recommended that the enzyme should be spread throughout the meal to optimize mixing and minimizing partitioning of the pancreatic enzyme with the liquid phase of the meal, which empties more rapidly than the solid phase.[19]

Younger children should be encouraged to swallow the capsule as a whole at the earliest, usually by 5–6 years of age. But until then, the only option is to open the capsule and add the granules into the feed. Care should be taken that the granules do not come in contact with the oral cavity of the child, inclining to chew them, thus causing ulcers in the mouth. Due to large variation in the amount of food consumed by younger children at every meal, it is a good idea to spread the enzyme throughout the day's meal. However, with certain foods like sugary drinks, fruits, juices or sweets, there is no need to add the enzyme.

General Guidelines for Use of PES

Keeping in view the specific mode of action of PES and its effect on patients, certain guidelines have been formulated which should be kept in mind when recommending them.[20,21]

1. Enzyme should be given with every meal, at the beginning and during the meal, rather than all before or after.
2. An extra fat based snack may require an additional dose of the enzyme, e.g. crisps, chocolate, milk shakes, etc.
3. Creon may be swallowed as a whole by older children but for younger ones, it can be opened and mixed with foods, jam, honey, juice or puree to form a gel.
4. It should never be chewed or crushed to mix it with the food.
5. It should be kept away from hot temperature or left in a parked car outside in the sun to prevent the degradation.
6. The enzyme should not be mixed with very hot food or in food with pH of more than 5.5.
7. The expiry date mentioned on the packing should be strictly adhered to.
8. It is not required to be given with squashes, juices or cold drinks.
9. In case of excess gastric acid secretions, histamine receptor antagonists like cimetidine and ranitidine can help relieve the problem.

COMPLICATIONS OF CYSTIC FBROSIS

Diabetes Mellitus

The most commonly associated complication of CF in children and adolescents is cystic fibrosis related diabetes mellitus (CFRDM). This occurs due to a gradual destruction of glucagons and insulin secreting cells in the pancreas. It is recommended that all children of 10–12 years should be screened for diabetes mellitus, especially when there is evidence of failure to thrive and at times of pulmonary exacerbations requiring IV antibiotics.[21] Management of children with CF having associated diabetes mellitus are managed quite unlike other children with Type I diabetes.

The recommended guidelines for management of such children are laid down as follows.[20]

- Complex carbohydrates should be encouraged.
- Normal sugar containing foods can be allowed.
- Dietary fat content is not restricted.
- Foods like biscuits, chocolates, crisps, etc. are allowed.
- Sugar free drinks can be offered in between meals.
- Regular meal and snack timings should be adhered to.

It is however important to maintain euglycemia which can be done by regulating insulin therapy rather than imposing dietary restrictions. The management should focus on consistent timings and carbohydrate content of meals and snacks, which can be achieved by three main meals and snacks in between. Carbohydrate counting is a good indicator to keep count of the intake. The total fat content of the diet can be up to 40% of the total calories. Monitoring of HbA1c (acylated hemoglobin) every three months is advisable. Early morning (1–3 AM) glucose levels should be checked monthly (Dawn effect) to exclude nocturnal hypoglycemia.[20]

Celiac Disease

Celiac disease is one of the non-pancreatic causes of malabsorption which can contribute to poor growth. Dietary modification in such patients involves excretion of all gluten products from the diet (See chapter 30).

ROLE OF FUNCTIONAL FOODS IN CYSTIC FIBROSIS

Fish Oil

Some recent studies at New South Wales, Australia have shown that fish oil supplementation in the diets of affected children with CF, alleviates many symptoms associated with the disease.[22] It is believed that EPA (eicosapentaenoic acid) acts by modifying the role of leukotriene B4, which is believed to be the main culprit in the excessive inflammatory response to bacteria characterizing CF.[23] Some authors have also advocated the use of IV fish oil supplements in patients with CF. In a study at New York, it was demonstrated that there was improved lung function in children supplemented with IV fish oil emulsion, and no adverse reactions were observed in their subjects.[24]

Turmeric

The role of curcumin an active compound found in the spice turmeric has been recently been studied to observe its effects in correcting the defect in mice. The normal secretion depends upon the function of a protein called CFTR (cystic fibrosis transmembrane conductance regulator) and it is due to some mutation in the gene encoding that is responsible for cystic fibrosis. Curcumin is believed to play a role in correcting this defect at the cellular level and normalizing the secretory mechanism of various organs involved and stimulates CFTR chloride channel activity. It was shown to increase CFTR channel activity in excised inside out membrane patches by reducing channel closed time and prolonging the time channels remained open. Stimulation was found to be dose related, reversible and greater than 'genistein', another functional compound that stimulates CFTR. However, more studies are still required to confirm this hypothesis.[25]

REFERENCES

1. Fitzsimmons S. The changing epidemiology of cystic fibrosis, J Pediatr. 1993;122:1-9.
2. Meenu Singh, Rajender Prasad and Lata Kumar. Cystic fibrosis in North Indian children. Ind J Ped 69. 2002.
3. Sokol RJ, accurse F, Abman SH, et al. Nutritional issues in cystic fibrosis In: Pediatric Gastroenterology and Nutrition In: ASPEN Seminars on Pediatric Disease Vol IV. Ballistresi WF, Vanderhof JA; Eds London: Chapman and Hall Medical. 1990.pp.273-95.
4. Goodin B. Nutrition issues in cystic fibrosis. In: Nutrition issues in Gastroenterology, Series # 27, ed Parrish CR. Practical Gastroenetrology. May 2005. pp.76-93.
5. Berker LR, Russek-Cohen E, et al. Stature as a prognostic factor in survival. J Am Diet Assoc. 2001;101:438-42 Clinical Practice guidelines for cystic fibrosis. Bethesda, MD; Cystic Fibrosis Foundation 1997.
6. Cystic Fibrosis Foundation. Clinical Practice Guidelines for cystic fibrosis. Bethesda, MD: Cystic Fibrosis Foundation. 1997.
7. Metropolitan Life Insurance Company. Statistical Bulletin. 1983;64:2-9.
8. Murphy JL, Wooten SA, Bond SA, Jackson AA. Energy content of stools in normal healthy controls and patients with CF. Arch Dis Childh. 1991;66:495-500.
9. Bell SC, Saunder MJ, Elborn JS, et al. Resting energy expenditure and oxygen cost of breathing in patients with cystic fibrosis. Thorax. 1996;5:126-31.
10. Slesinski MJ, Gloninger MF, Costantino JP, et al. Lipid levels in adults with cystic fibrosis. J Am Diet Assoc. 1994;94:402-8.
11. Peters SA, Rolls CJ. Vitamin therapy in cystic fibrosis- a review and rationale. J Clin Pharm Ther. 1993;18:33-8.
12. Leonard CH, Knox AJ. Pancreatic enzyme supplements and vitamins in cystic fibrosis. J Hum Nutr Diet. 1997;10:3-16.
13. MacDonald A. Nutritional management in cystic fibrosis: personal practice. Arch Dis Childh. 1996;74: 81-7.
14. Green MR, Buchanan E, Weaver LT. Nutritional management with cystic fibrosis. Arch Dis Childh. 1995;72:452-6.
15. Anthony H, Smith A, Phelan P, et al. Current approaches to the nutritional management of children with cystic fibrosis in Australia.J Pediatr Child Health. 1998;34:170-74.
16. Gavin JE. Nutritional management. In: Pediatric Guidelines for cystic fibrosis care. Ed Hill CM; London: Churchill Livingstone. 1998;65-78.
17. Zempsky WT, Rosenstein BJ, Carrol JA, et al. Effect of pancreatic enzyme supplements in iron absorption. Am J Dis Child, 1989;143:962-72.
18. Borwitz DS, Grand RJ, Durie PR. Use of panctratic enzyme supplement for patients with cystic fibrosis in the context of fibrosing colonopathy. Consensus Committee. J Pediatr. 1995;127(5):681-84.
19. Taylor CJ, Hillel PG, Ghosh S, et al. Gastric emptying and intestinal transit of pancreatic supplements in cystic fibrosis. Arch Dis Childh. 1999;80:149-52.
20. Vavessa Shaw and Margaret D Lawson. Cystic fibrosis In: Clinical Pediatric Dietetics, Blackwell Publishers. 2001.
21. Orenstein DM, Rosentein BJ, Stern RC. Gastro-Intestinal System and Pancreas. In: Cystic Fibrosis. Medical Care, Lippincott Williams and Wilkins. Philadelphia. 2000.

22. Beery HK, Kellog FW, Hunt MM, et al. Dietary supplement and nutrition in children with cystic fibrosis. Am J Dis Childh. 1975;129:165-71.
23. Lawrence R and Sorell T. Eicosapentaenoic acid in CF: Evidence of a pathogenic role for leukotrine B4. The Lancet. Vol. 342, Aug 21, 1993 pp 465-69.
24. Katz, David P, et al. The use of IV fish oil emulsion enriched with omega 3-fatty acids in patients with cystic fibrosis. Nutrition. vol.12, No. 5, 1996, pp 324-39.
25. Allan L Berger, Christoph O Randak, Lynda S Ostedgaard, et al. J Biol Chem. 2005, Vol. 280, Issue (7)5221-26.

32 Diet in Liver Diseases

The liver is the largest and most complex organs of the body, involved in multiple functions of nutrient absorption and metabolism like proteins, carbohydrates and lipids besides vitamins and minerals. It is also involved in the detoxification of bacterial decomposition products, mineral poisons and certain drugs and dyes. Any insult on the liver can have direct bearing on the nutritional status of an individual, more so on the child.

When the liver is affected by any infection, it results in the inflammation of the hepatic cells, causing hepatitis. In children, hepatitis is generally infective, caused mainly by infective agents from food and water. Other causes of hepatitis could be metabolic or nutritional, or biliary obstruction. The pathologic changes involved in the liver parenchymal cells are similar regardless of the etiology of the disease.[1]

HEPATITIS

Etiology: Hepatitis in children is generally due to infections, characterized by inflammatory and degenerative changes in the liver. The infective type is mostly due to viral cause, or it may be drug induced due to A, B, C, D, E or any of the numerous types identified. Amongst them hepatitis A is the most commonly identified, which is transmitted through the fecal oral route. Epidemics are generally seen from time to time either by fecal contamination of water or a breakdown in the sanitation system. Serum hepatitis is transmitted only through the parenteral route in blood products containing the specific virus or through faulty sterilization of needles. Drug induced hepatitis may be due to hypersensitivity to certain drugs like sulpha or penicillin or due to a direct toxic affect on the liver by agents like carbon tetrachloride or certain herbal drugs containing alkaloids.

Symptoms: Children with hepatitis A may have symptoms varying from very mild in younger ones to more severe forms in older children. Since the average incubation period could be for about 1 month before the onset of the symptoms, it may appear that the onset has been rather sudden. These include:

- Fatigue
- Vomiting and nausea
- Loss of appetite
- Low grade fever
- High colored urine with stools appearing very pale, giving a clay colored appearance
- Muscle pain
- Itching
- Yellow coloration of the skin and the conjunctiva.

Management

As of now no specific treatment exists for hepatitis A. The main focus is on adequate rest and nutrition and avoids any permanent liver damage. Complete recovery may take a few months.

Dietary modifications: The main objective of dietary treatment is to aid regeneration of the liver tissue and avoid further complications.

Calories: The energy requirement of a child with hepatitis is almost same as that for a normal healthy child. Though the child may be very anorexic or nauseated, it is advisable that small frequent feedings be encouraged to meet the nutritional goal. This could be in the form of any type of diet which the child may prefer. It may be kept in mind that there should be no restrictions on the type of food the child may like. Usually parents tend to impose a lot of restrictions on the type of diet or foods the child should be having. The trend is mostly on highly sweetened foods, e.g. cane sugar juice or radish extract. These may actually cause the child to be more nauseated and deter him from eating at all.

The aim should be to maintain the normal weight of the child and also encourage weight gain if possible in the younger ones. Extremely over weight and obese children with viral hepatitis can add further complications to the liver, such as fatty deposits in the liver and accompanying liver inflammation called nonalcoholic steatohepatitis. An adequate amount of complex carbohydrates, e.g. rice, wholemeal breads, potatoes, sago and whole grain cereals, can provide calories and help maintain weight for those children who are unable to maintain body mass. Adequate rest and moderate activity can also help.

Proteins: Adequate protein intake is important to maintain muscle mass and to regenerate the liver cells. The requirement for such children is as for any other normal child. There is no need for extra proteins nor should it be inadequate which can hinder the regenerative process of the liver.

Carbohydrates: As mentioned earlier, the calorie requirement can be met only if there are adequate complex carbohydrate in the diets of such children. In contrast to the practice of loading children with hepatitis with too much of fruit juices, or cane sugar juice, a mixed carbohydrate diet is more acceptable and better tolerated by such children. This could be in the form of any of the day to day commonly consumed foods, which include sugars and fats. Since in most of these children their appetite is severely compromised, care should be taken not to pressurize the child to eat. On the contrary, they should be given freedom to choose from any of the foods of their choice, be it in the form of sweets, savoury, cakes, pastries or pasta, noodles or pizzas topped with vegetables. The only care to be taken is to ensure the hygiene and safety of the source of the foods to avoid further complications of infections.

Fats: There is no restriction on the amount of fats to be allowed to a child with viral hepatitis. There is a general belief that fats should be restricted in patients suffering from viral hepatitis and hence offered boiled vegetables and other preparations. On the contrary, the appetite of the child is already compromised and in such a condition offering of boiled unpalatable food would only cause more aversion to food. This is the main reason why children affected by viral hepatitis after complete recovery, generally appear very undernourished, weak and fail to gain weight as per the desired velocity. The recommendations are normal fats (not too much or too little), as is advised for any normal child, i.e. 25% of the total calories. Moreover, incorporating small helpings of butter or cream in the preparations served can help increase the density of the food without adding to the bulk of their diet.

Vitamins and minerals: The requirement of all vitamins and minerals remain unchanged as for a normal healthy child. But due to the poor intake by the child, usually certain vitamins and minerals may be compromised and not being met. Care should be taken to avoid iron supplements for such children as it is known to reduce the response rate in patients with hepatitis C virus. It may also cause increased liver enzymes which indicate liver cell damage.[2]

Supplements/alternative medicine: The liver is responsible for the metabolism of medications and drugs. There are certain drugs and medicines, especially the herbal variety which can be toxic to the liver. Therefore parents of children with viral hepatitis must refrain from giving any kind of supplements of herbal origin or any such medicines available over the counter, without discussing with their physician.

Alcohol: Intake of alcohol can precipitate liver toxicity and cause further damage to the liver cells. As children with chronic viral hepatitis approach adolescence, they need to be counseled regarding the dangers of alcohol to their health. The danger is magnified for the affected adolescent or teenager.

It should be kept in mind that viral hepatitis in children can be just like any other infective disease, but the management is quite simple and may not involve too many medications. It is more or less self limiting in duration and may take about 1–2 months for the child to recover completely. A small number of children with hepatitis A may have relapses over 6–9 month period. The mainstays of management involve rest, a healthy balanced unrestricted diet as per the likings of the child and avoid any outdoor or uncooked food likely to be from doubtful source. Fruit juice extracted at home and fruits bought whole, can take care of the vitamins, besides providing carbohydrates and fiber.

Foods that can be offered to a child with viral hepatitis are as follows:

Cereals: Any breakfast cereal like bread, cornflakes, dalia, poha, suji or chapatti/paratha (if the chid demends). Noodles, pasta and macaroni may be included for variety.

Pulses: All dals, washed/whole/dehusked in the form of dals with meals, gram flour in the for of any snacks or sprouts or as per the liking of the child.

Vegetables: All seasonal vegetables including green leafy vegetables can be offered in the form of vegetable cutlets or attractive sandwiches or vegetable soups. Potatoes can be incorporated in a number of dishes in a variety of forms-baked, boiled or mashed.

Fruits: Fruits as a whole are preferable. Fruit juice also can be offered to give a change in the palate. Fruit salad with cream can be an attractive option.

Milk/Milk products: Normal dairy milk used at home is suitable. It can be give as milk shakes, puddings or porridge, curd, cottage cheese in various forms depending upon the child's preference.

Non Vegetarian foods: Eggs, fish and chicken can be offered in any form incorporated with meals or as snacks. Red meat and pork should however be avoided.

Fats: All normal fats used in cooking at home may be used in normal amounts. Cream/butter too may be incorporated in various dishes depending upon the recipe and the child's preference.

Sugars: Simple sugars can be used in normal amounts as per the child's likings or habit. Sweet preparations in any form can add variety in the menu.

Sodium: In infective hepatitis in the absence of ascites, no restriction of sodium is advocated, therefore normal salt as per liking can be used

CIRRHOSIS OF LIVER

Cirrhosis of the liver in children is diagnosed as a waxing and waning course of acute hepatitis. In children cirrhosis is known to occur in those with chronic hepatitis leading to liver cell damage gradually, over a period of more than 8 weeks. It is characterized by jaundice, ascites, hepatomegaly and altered liver function tests. In a few children the condition may lead to fulminant hepatic failure which is characterized by massive necrosis of the liver cells and severe impairment of liver function tests. The child may present with encephalopathy and has a high mortality and morbidity rate.[3]

Nutrition plays an important role in determining the outcome of the disease. The goals of nutritional management of cirrhosis in children are:

- Prevention and treatment of malnutrition by improving growth and development
- Reducing risk of hypoglycemia, infection and encephalopathy
- Avoid potential toxins in specific disorders
- Optimize nutritional status prior to transplant if indicated.

Energy: The energy level of a child with cirrhosis should be as high as 130% of the RDA. If this goal is difficult to achieve, nasogastric feeding may be resorted to.

Proteins: In the presence of hepatic encephalopathy, proteins are reduced in the diet, to not more than 1g/Kg body weight, as drastic restriction can affect the growth and maintenance of the nitrogen (N) balance. Restriction of proteins has been attributed to poor growth and malnutrition. The proteins however should be of high biological value which can be casein based preferably. Vegetable protein source is always advised as these are better tolerated than the animal proteins which are low in branched chain amino acids (BCCA). Moreover, consumption of vegetable proteins can alter the bowel flora with a beneficial effect.

At the same time excess of dietary protein also should be avoided as it can precipitate encephalopathy. A balanced vegetarian diet therefore is the mainstay of dietary management of cirrhosis in children, containing the required amounts of carbohydrates, fats, proteins and calories as per their age.

However, in the absence of encephalopathy, a high protein (casein based), of 2–3 g /kg/d, should be emphasized, which is required for the speedy regeneration of the hepatocytes. This will also help in easing the associated edema and ascites due to hypoproteinemia. High protein supplements with BCCA may prove beneficial at this stage to augment the calorie and protein intake of the child. With BCCA enriched formulae, normal to high protein intakes do not cause encephalopathy. Vegetable proteins are high in BCCA, while animal proteins are not.[4] Studies have shown that enteral feeding with 4g/kg/d of protein and 140% of the RDA of caloric intake in children with chronic liver disease led to improvement of nutritional status without hyperammonuria or any adverse affects.[5]

Carbohydrates: As these children are unable to store glycogen adequately, it is advisable they be fed a high carbohydrate diet which can be spread evenly over the day as it can delay the carbohydrate absorption resulting in its sustained release. Night time feeding of carbohydrates in the form of glucose polymer or uncooked starch can help maintain the glycogen stores and avoid the child going into hypoglycemeia.

Fats: The fat content of the diet during the cirrhotic phase should not be reduced as it can make the food unpalatable for the already anorexic child. Medium chain triglycerides can be given in emulsified form. The concept of low fat is no longer advisable as it was observed that low fat diets, besides reducing the palatability, also lowers the energy density of the diet. Children and adults are known to tolerate fats fairly well, therefore a low fat diet would only compromise the energy intake of the child. Inadequate energy will further affect the protein utilization due to the protein sparing affect. Coconut oil is a good example of MCT fats. Other sources are palm kernel oil and commercial MCT solution available as Simyl MCT. These are rapidly broken down in the small intestine and directly absorbed into the portal circulation being relatively more water soluble. But, since MCT oils are low in essential fatty acids, supplementation of these is required. Using a portion of fat as long chain triglycerides (LCT) in the form of safflower or corn oil can compensate for the deficiency. This is especially applicable to the child with cholestasis. This is applicable in a child with chronic cholestasis also which may be due to primary or secondary biliary cirrhosis, sclerosing cholangitis and biliary atresia.

Fat soluble vitamin supplements like vitamin A, D, E and K also need to be given to such children as they are known to malabsorp these vitamins.

Infants on breastfeeds should be allowed to continue as long as possible or up to a maximum of 2 years along with oral solid feeds.

Sodium: Children with cirrhosis, usually present with ascites too due to fluid retention. The pathogenesis involved may be either low plasma albumin due to defective synthesis, low osmotic pressure of plasma, hepatic venous outflow obstruction, and increased lymph exudation from the liver surface, increased renin aldosterone and low urinary excretion of sodium. All these factors lead to retention of salt and water.[3] It is therefore advisable to restrict dietary sodium to not more than 2g/d, which means not more than approximately 3-4 g per day.

The principles of nutritional therapy in a child with cirrhosis may be summed up as follows.[6]

- *Energy* — *125% 0f RDA (MCT/Glucose polymer)*
- *EFA* — *supplementation—corn/safflower oil*
- *Proteins* — *2–3 g/kg/d. BCC enriched diet-Albumin infusions*
- *Vitamin A* — *3000–10,000 IU/d orally.*
- *Vitamin D* — *400–4000 IU/d orally.*
- *Vitamin E* — *50–400 IU/d orally.*
- *Vitamin K* — *5 mg every 1–2 weeks IM.*
- *Calcium* — *supplements as required.*
- *Phosphorous* — *supplements as required*
- *Magnesium* — *supplements as required.*
- *Zinc* — *1 mg/kg/d.*
- *Iron* — *3–5 mg/kg/d.*
- *Selenium* — *1–2 µ/kg/d.*

INDIAN CHILDHOOD CIRRHOSIS

Indian childhood cirrhosis as the name suggests, is one of the types of cirrhosis identified among Indian children where large amounts of copper deposition was reported. However, currently a very small proportion of children are encountered, probably due to the preventive measures adopted by households regarding use of copper/brass vessels for boiling milk for infants.

The disease was identified by Bernard Portman in 1978, in a series of children form Pune, who had liver disorders and was seeking evidence for hepatitis B infection. The confirmatory diagnosis was made by orcein staining which detects copper loading.[7]

Liver copper concentrations of 787-6654 μ/g dry weight were found in a series of children with ICC from Pune.[8]

It was postulated that hepatic copper retention may occur secondary to holestasis, but this was rejected since cholestasis was not a marked clinical feature and jaundice was a late clinical feature.

Etiology/Source

Studies from Pune group of workers discovered on reviewing the background of all the patients suffering from ICC, that all of them belonged to rural communities and their source of water was either from the wells or taps, but stored in copper or brass vessels and so was the milk stored and boiled in them. It was observed that in this group of patients none were exclusively breast fed and all received animal milk at an earlier age as compared to other diseases.[9]

Subsequent comparisons between the feeding history of 10 children with ICC and 100 age, sex and caste matched controls from the same village, led to the hypothesis that ICC was a consequence of early introduction of animal milk feeds contaminated with copper from brass vessels.[10]

Usually the brass vessels used for cooking are tinned from time to time, which can have a preventive role, but many households may not get the process done regularly due to the high expenses involved and continue to use them untinned. But gradually over a period of time, the use of these vessels has declined and very few rural households may still be found to use them.

Management

Management of ICC involves use of chelating agents like D pencilamine which unbinds copper from the cells. But it has been demonstrated that this may be beneficial only if it is given in the early stage of the disease when the child has not progressed to ascites or developed jaundice. Pencilamine is given in a dose of 20 mg/kg/d, with or without prednisolone. The mortality rate was known to decline considerably after treatment to 53% as compared to 92% in a placebo group.[11]

With treatment, liver copper levels fall to near normal concentrations in contrast with persistently high liver copper concentrations in patients with Wilson's disease receiving pencilamine. This led to the hypotheses that although pencilamine was used to chelate copper from the bound form, its benefit was not necessarily a result of its removing excess copper or even detoxifying copper,[12] but could be due to an anti-inflammatory effect by inducing metallothionein, replacing glutathione or inhibiting collagen cross linking.[13]

Prevention

In view of the above mentioned evidence of copper deposition in the liver through copper/brass vessels, which are used for storing and boiling milk for infants, it seems but pertinent that prevention is the best cure for ICC, i.e. avoiding use of copper/brass vessels for heating or storing milk or water. This fact can be corroborated by a large intervention study in the Pune District of Maharashtra.[14] In this study, one group of population received an intensive program of health education, advising them against the use of brass utensils for preparation of infant feeds. It was observed that in this group of 4.1 million population, the use of brass vessels fell from 13% to 4% and the incidence of ICC declined to zero, where as in the control population of Ahmednagar of 2.7 million, the use of brass utensils and incidence of ICC also declined, probably due to the advice to the study group being percolated into this population too. But in Chandigarh where also this incidence had been reported, and the advice had not reached, the incidence did not change.[14]

Over a gradual period of time, due to change in life style, brass vessels replaced stainless steel or hindalium vessels, which were increasingly getting popular. So, this change perhaps occurred spontaneously but gradually. Moreover, since brass vessels require more maintenance due to the tinning process (kallai), the availability of 'kallai vendors' also declined, who used to visit door to door to do the tinning of all brass vessels. Therefore, before brass vessels could completely be replaced by steel or other vessels, the availability of tinning became more expensive and less available. This led to an increase in the incidence of ICC before its decline, as it was phased out especially in the urban classes. Tinning is a process in which the uptake of copper is completely prevented from the by milk.[15]

A small percentage of the population however continue to use brass vessels even for boiling and storing milk, especially in the rural areas, which could be one reason why the incidence of ICC is still seen sporadically, especially in the referral hospitals.

REFERENCES

1. Robinson CH. Diet in disturbances of the liver, gallbladder and pancreas. In: Normal and Therapeutic Nutrition, 14th ed. Mac Millan Publishing Co. Inc. Oxford and IBH Publishing Co. 1972.pp.483-93.
2. Silva IS, Perez RM, Oliveria PV, et al. Iron overlaod and histolopathological studies. J Gastroenterol Heptal. Feb 2005;20(2):243-8.
3. Sherlock S, Dolley J. Nutrition and metabolic liver disease. In: Diseases of the Liver and Biliary System 8th ed, Oxford Medical Publication. 1991.pp.408-38.
4. Bianchi GP, Marchesini G, Fabbri A, et al. Vegetable vs. animal protein diet in cirrhotic patients with chronic encephalopathy. A randomized cross over comparison. J Intern Med. 1993;233:385-92.
5. Charton CP, Buchanan E, Holder CE, et al. Intensive eneteral feeding in advanced cirrhosis: reversal of malnutrition without precipitation of hepatic encephalopathy. Srch Dis Chil. 1992;67:603-07.
6. Bavdekar A, Bhave S and Pandit A. Nutritional management in chronic liver disease. In J Ped. May 2002;V0l. 69 .
7. Portman B, Tanner MS, Mowet MP, et al. Orcein positive liver deposits in Indian Childhood Cirrhosis. Lancet. 1978;1:1338-40.
8. Bhave S, Siddhaye D, Pradhan A etal. Pediatric liver disease in India. Arch Dis Child. 1982;57:922-8.
9. Tanner MS, Kantajian AH, Bhave SA, et al. Early introduction of copper contaminated animal milk feeds as a possible cause of Indian childhood cirrhosis, Lancet. 1983;2:992-5.
10. Bhave SA, Pandit AN, Tanner MS. Comparison of feeding history of children with Indian childhood cirrhosis and paired controls. J Ped gastroenterol Nutr. 1987;6:562-7.
11. Tanner MS, Bhave SA, Pradhan AM, et al. Clinical trials of pencilamine in Indian childhood cirrhosis. Arch Dis Child. 1987;62:118-24.
12. Scheinberg IH, Sternleib I, Scholisky M, et al. Pencilamine may detoxify copper in Wilson's disease. Lancet. 1987;2-95.
13. Mc Quaid A, Lamand M, Mason J. The interactions of pencilamine with copper in vivo and the effect on hepatic metallothionein levels and copper /zinc distribution: the implications for Wilson's disease and arthiritis therapy. J Lab Clin Med. 1992;119:744-50.
14. Bhave SA, Pandit AN, Singh S, et al. Tanner MS. The prevention of Indian childhood cirrhosis. Ann Trop Pediatr. 1992;12:23-30.
15. O'Neill NC, Tanner MS. Uptake of copper from brass utensils by bovine milk and its relevance to Indian childhood cirrhosis. J Pediatr Gastroenterol Nutr. 1989;9:167-72.

33 Diet in Kidney Diseases

NEPHROTIC SYNDROME

Nephrotic syndrome (NS) is a disease primarily confined to the glomeruli. It is most commonly seen in children but can occur in adults too. In children it is characterized by alterations of permselectivity at the glomerular capillary wall, resulting in its ability to select the urinary loss of protein.

It is estimated that the annual incidence of nephrotic syndrome ranges from 2–7 per 100,000 children and prevalence from 12–16 per 100,000.[1] There is epidemiological evidence of higher incidence of nephrotic syndrome in children from South Asia. In 95% of the cases the condition is idiopathic. In less than 5% cases the underlying causes could be systemic lupus erythematous, amylodosis and infection with HIV and hepatitis B and C virus.[2]

Nephrotic syndrome usually presenting in the first 3 months of life (congenital NS) could be secondary to intrauterine infections, e.g. congenital syphilis, toxoplasmosis and cytomegalovirus (CMV).

The classic definition of NS has been described as a clinical entity characterized by proteinuria, hypoalbuminemia and edema. The underlying physiological disturbance is an abnormal permeability of the glomerulus to macromolecules, resulting in increased filtered load of plasma proteins, part of which is reabsorbed and catabolised in the tubules, with the remainder appearing in the urine.[3]

Proteinuria in children is taken as 4mg/hr/m^2 (166 mg/24 hrs/1.73m^2).[4] In NS, it is generally associated with rates of protein >3.5g/hr, but the International Study of Kidney Disease in Children (ISKDC), has defined proteinuria as excess of 40 mg/hr/m^2, equal to 1.66 g/24 hr/1.73 m^2, accompanied by hypoalbuminemia.[5] Protein losses in the urine are commonly 5–10 g/d and may exceed 30 g/d also.

Manifestation

Nephrotic syndrome is manifested by edema which may be generalized puffiness around the eyes, extremities, especially feet and ankles, swelling of the abdomen, facial swelling, foamy appearance of urine, weight gain due to fluid retention, anorexia and hypertension. In extreme cases, complications like hypertensive encephalopathy, congestive cardiac failure, electrolyte imbalance and acute renal failure may also occur.

Dietary Modifications in Nephrotic Syndrome

The objectives of dietary management are aimed at:

1. To maintain a state of good nutrition
2. To control, or correct protein deficiency
3. To prevent edema
4. To provide palatable, easily digested meals as per individual needs.

A child with NS may require certain dietary modifications (including fluids) to be adhered to.

Fluids

Children with NS generally have problem regulating their water balance, which can cause edema. Therefore a restriction in fluids and sodium needs to be imposed. Fluids include any food which is liquid at room temperature. The fluid restriction includes insensible loss plus the previous day's output in conditions of oliguria, which is defined as urine output <1 ml/kg/hr or 25 ml/kg/d. Insensible loss of water is 400 ml/m²/d.

It may be difficult for children to restrict fluid or water especially in hot temperate climates. Some useful tips with which the child can be helped to overcome thirst or the need to consume fluids are:

- Use of small glass/cups (standardized) to keep count of the intake.
- Avoid salty foods as they increase thirst.
- Iced tea and lemonade quench thirst better than fizzy drinks.
- Frozen pieces of fruit (melon, grapes, and berries) can help quench thirst.
- Chewing gum or hand candy can help quench thirst.
- Rinsing of mouth.
- Sucking a lemon wedge can stimulate saliva and moisten the mouth.
- Staying away from sun can help avoid thirst in a child.

Proteins

Although there is excessive loss of protein in the urine, a high protein diet is contraindicated. The aim should be to replace the lost protein. Care should be taken to avoid high protein diets to prevent any tubular damage to the kidneys. A protein intake equivalent to the RDA for age is advisable which normally amounts to 1 g/kg body weight, to compensate for protein loss in the urine.

Sodium

The sodium content should be minimum to prevent fluid accumulation and edema. Foods generally high in sodium need to be restricted are:

- Salted wafers, popcorns, bakery products, snacks, chips, etc.
- Papads and pickles—all varieties.
- Salted chutneys, sauces, commercial preparations, e.g. soup cubes or powders.
- Salted cashews, peanuts, savory and other dry fruits.
- Commercial cheese, preservatives containing foods, noodle mixes and pasta.
- Foods containing baking soda and ajino motto.
- Salt to be avoided in cooking
- Generally 3–4g salt/d per day is recommended, equivalent to about 2g sodium/d.

Since a day's normal diet contains about 1 g salt without adding during cooking, an added amount of 1 g for the whole day would make it 2 g of salt for the day's diet. To explain it simply, it would mean about 1/4th level tsp (5 g) to be distributed evenly for the whole day's diet which does not contain any salt while cooking.

Calories

Calories are recommended as for RDA, plus 10% extra for infections/illness.[5]

Potassium

Potassium is generally avoided during the phase of oliguria, which means restriction of fruits and fruit juices. All high protein feeds are also rich in potassium; therefore a balance has to be maintained, while selecting low potassium diets, at the same time adequate in proteins. Pulses are also rich in potassium, therefore need to be restricted. In case complications continue to persist, the sodium and potassium levels can be stabilized by peritoneal dialysis. A list of potassium rich foods to be avoided is listed in Table 33.1.[6]

TABLE 33.1: Potassium content of various Indian foods

Low (<100 mg)	Moderate (100–200 mg)	High (>200 mg)
Rice, suji, arrowroot flour peas, cucumber, radish pink, beet root, broad beans, ridge gourd, snake gourd, tinda, fenugreek leaves tomato green, apple, banana ripe, guava, orange, papaya ripe, pine apple, pears, milk (buffalo).	Rice flakes, maize tender, wheat flour(refined), vermicelli, radish white, carrot, cauliflower, French beans, spinach, lichi, mango ripe, water melon, tomato ripe, pomegranate, cow's milk, liver (goat).	Wheat flour, maize dry, all pulses, colocasia, potato, sweet potato, tapioca, yam, brinjal, coconut, apricots, cherries, dates, lemon, sweet lime, mango, musk melon, plums, phalsa, chikoo, mutton (muscle), fish, prawn.

Refer. 6 (ICMR)

ACUTE RENAL FAILURE

Chronic glomerulonephritis, nephrosclerosis and pyelonephritis are some of the conditions which can lead to acute renal failure. Systemic lupus erythematous (SLE) an autoimmune disorder involving the kidneys, acute tubular necrosis or dysplastic/contracted kidneys can also be precipitating factors in ARF. Other common causes in children could be dehydration, burns and snake bite.

In this condition, the kidneys fail to maintain the normal composition of the blood. Some common terminologies referred to in this disease are:

Uremia: a condition arising from failure of kidney functions-literally meaning 'urine in the blood'.

Azotemia: refers to accumulation of nitrogenous constituents in the blood.

Oliguria: denotes scanty urine output (<0.5 ml/kg/hr or <1 ml/kg/hr in a neonate).

Anuria: denotes urine production <100 ml/d.

In ARF, oliguria is usually present resulting in salt and water retention, catabolism and metabolic disturbances (low bicarbonate and calcium, high phosphate, potassium and urea).

The goal of dietary management in ARF should be:

- Prevent catabolism.
- Maintain fluid and electrolyte balance.
- Control metabolic abnormalities.
- Aid recovery.

Nutritional Management

Children with ARF generally being in a state of catabolism are very anorexic and it is quite a challenge to get them to consume adequate diet. Moreover, there are quite a few restrictions imposed due to the limited amount of fluids to be given besides other protein and potassium rich foods.

Fluids

In short-term renal failure the fluid load is restricted depending upon the urine output. In case oliguria continues to persist, peritoneal dialysis is initiated. By doing so, the diet restrictions, including fluids can be relaxed, considering the urine output plus the dialysate losses.

Proteins

Protein intake is restricted to 0.5 g/kg/d, but with peritoneal dialysis (PD), it can be liberalized till 1.25 g/kg/d. It would be advisable to provide high biological value proteins for optimum utilization.[7]

Calories

A high energy diet based on the RDA for age is recommended to make up for the catabolic state of the body.

Sodium

In condition of oliguria, no added salt is used in the diet, although it becomes a little difficult to make the child accept the diet. More varieties of sweet based foods can be offered spread over the day in smaller amounts.

The presence of hypertension in most of the children necessitates limiting sodium to <2 g/d. But in case, when PD has been started, sodium restriction may be relaxed to not more than 4 g/d. Though they are in a diuretic phase, caution still needs to be maintained and if required can be relaxed a little further, once the kidneys open up.

Potassium

During the oliguric phase, potassium is strictly restricted to control hyperphosphatemia, which implies restriction of all fruits and fruit juices. Once PD is on, this restriction may be relaxed. Table 33.2 highlights the plan for management of children with ARF.[7]

TABLE 33.2: Dietary recommendations in acute renal failure

Volume	Depends on daily fluid removal (urine ± dialysate losses)
Energy	High to prevent catabolism
Protein	Low to prevent a high plasma urea, unless on prolonged peritoneal dialysis when a higher protein intake may be required
Salt	Low, except in the unusual circumstance of polyuric phase
Phosphate	Low to prevent hyperphosphatemia

Refer. 7

TABLE 33.3: List of 3 g protein exchange of common foods

Foods	Amount (g)	Serving size
Rice	50	2 small
Chappati	25	1 small
Dal	12.5	1/2 small serving
Milk	100	3/4th tea cup
Bread	30	2 slices
Coconut, fresh	50	1 big cube
Potatoes	200	3–4 medium size
Beans	100	1 small serving
Peas, fresh	50	1 small serving

Refer. 6

The choice of foods may be modified as per local availability, acceptance by the child and convenience of feeding, based on the exchange list of 3 g portion size of various foods, as given in Table 33.3.

A policy plan for nutritional management or ARF has been highlighted in Figure 33.1.[7]

CHRONIC RENAL FAILURE

Chronic renal failure (CRF) refers to a long standing progressive deterioration of renal functions. Symptoms develop slowly and include anorexia, nausea, vomiting, dysphagia, nocturia, lassitude, fatigue, decreased mental alertness, muscle twitching and cramps, water retention and under nutrition. Peripheral neuropathy and seizures may or may not be associated.

The National Kidney Foundation (NKF) has last updated the guidelines of the 2000 Kidney disease outcome quality initiative (KDOQI) in 2008, regarding the recommendations for dietary requirements of different nutrients.[8] They have graded the stages of chronic kidney disease (CKD) depending upon the rate of GFR (Table 33.4). The degree of GFR is standardized to the surface area (1.73 m^2) of a 70 kg adult and is expressed as ml/min/1.73 m^2.

TABLE 33.4: NKF/KDOQI classification for stages of CKD

Stage	Description	GFR (ml/min/1.73m²)	Treatment
One	Kidney damage with normal or increased GFR	≥ 90	1—5 T if kidney transplant recipient
Two	Kidney damage with mild or decreased GFR	60–90	
Three	Moderate with decreased GFR	30–59	
Four	Severe decreased GFR	15–29	
Five	Kidney failure	<15 (on dialysis)	5D if dialysis (HD or PD)

Refer.[6] NKF K/DOQI Guidelines 2008

Nutritional Management

Management of children with in the chronic renal failure should aim at

- Reducing N intake
- Maintain N balance
- Cover essential amino acid requirement
- Provide adequate calories.

Energy

Oral intake of children with CRF is already compromised due to various associated factors like various factors like vomiting and anorexia, therefore spontaneous intake might be very inadequate. The recommended intake for in infants range from 100–120 kcals/kg/d, while for children, it would be 80–100 kcals/kg/d.

Protein

Protein requirement of a child in CRF is mainly based on the degree of glomerular filtration rate (GRF). A high protein intake poses a risk of aggravating acidosis, hyperkalemia and hyperphosphatemia, while on the other hand a restricted protein intake can help in reducing blood urea N (BUN), improve renal function and reduce symptoms of nausea, vomiting, muscle cramps and convulsions. Certain authors have based the protein requirements of children with CRF by broadly classifying them into mild, moderate and severe CRF as shown in Table 33.5.[5]

Day 1

High energy protein-free carbohydrate containing fluids, e.g. solution of dextrin maltose (glucose polymer)

Concentation depends on degree of nausea, vomiting, diarrhea :
- Infant 15% dextrin maltose
- 1–2 years 20% dextrin maltose
- > 2 years 25% dextrin maltose

Day 2

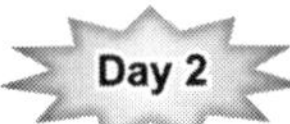

Consider introduction of protein depending on degree of uremia

Urea 30–40 mmol/l
Start 0.5 g protein/kg dry weight per day
infants - diluted baby milk + dextrin maltose
children - diluted whole protein feed
+ dextrin maltose

Urea 40 mmol/l
Protein - free high-energy
fluids for further 24 h

Day 3

Increase/introduce protein depending on degree of uremia
Maximize energy intake using carbohydrate and fats supplements as tolerated

Urea 20–30 mmol/l
Increase protein to 1 g/kg
dry weight per day

Urea 30–40 mmol/kg
As for day 2

Day 4 onwards

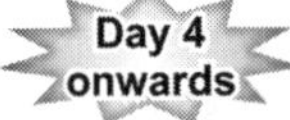

Normalized eating and drinking patterns as renal function improves

Urea 20–30 mmol/kg
As for day 3

Urea <20 mmol/kg
At least the RNI protein for height age in
infants or chronological age in children

FIGURE 33.1: Nutritional management of acute renal failure
RNI = Reference nutrient intake

Refer. 7

TABLE 33.5: Protein requirements of children with CRF based on GFR

Type of GFR	Proteins g/kg		
	0–1 year	1–5 years	5–10 years
Mild (GFR 20–40)	1.8	1.4	1
Moderate (GFR 5–20)	1.4	1.0	0.8
Severe (GFR <5)	1	0.8	0.5

Refer.[5] (International study of kidney disease in children, 1998)

In case of young children, as they begin to take more proteins from solids, milk products may need to be restricted. About 70% of proteins should be from high biological value sources, e.g. milk and milk products, fish or cheese. But, due to the high phosphate content of these, even such products may need to be given with caution. The balance of proteins can be given in the form of lower biological value protein sources, e.g. rice, pasta, bread and potatoes, which can be used liberally.

Fluids

The amount of fluids allowed will depend upon the extent of water retention. Mostly, that is taken care of by giving diuretics and restricting sodium. In case of failure to still achieve this, dialysis may be considered.

Sodium

The amount of sodium is equally restricted to take care of hypertension (if existing), and fluid retention. Salt intake can be maintained at 300–600 mg/d in infants and 1–2 g/d in older children.[5]

Potassium

Potassium levels are generally restricted in case of hyperkalemia (>6.5 mmol/l), which may involve restricting of fruits and green vegetables like potatoes, though low in proteins, are a fairly good source of potassium, therefore, these may be incorporated in the diet by soaking and discarding the water. This process allows a considerable amount of potassium to be leeched out. In fact even other green vegetables should be prepared by leeching out the water after soaking them in water for a few hours. In case if potassium levels drop, as hypokalemia may also occur in between, liberal amounts of fruit juice may be offered besides giving potassium supplement (potchlor) if required. A sample diet for a child with renal failure may be based on the pattern as shown in Table 33.6.

TABLE 33.6 Diet for a child with renal failure (Calories –100-1100; Prot. 8-10g; Sodium–< 100 mg Pot.–<250 mEq)

Sample MENU (Base diet)		
Breakfast	Sweet sago porridge (sago—25-30 g + sugar—10-15 g)	1 serve
Mid Morning	Baked potatoes (with butter optional)	50–75 g
Lunch	Rice Chappati/Parantha Curd*	1 serve (25–30 g) 1 medium (25 g) 100 g
Evening	Sago vada, sweet (sago 50 g, sugar-10–15g)**	1–2 pcs.
Dinner	Rice, plain/fried	1 serving (25 g)
	Vegetables + potato mix	1–2 serving (100–200 g)
	Sago, sweet	1 serving (25 g)

Note: * Milk may be used instead of curd.
** Potatoes may be used with sago to make the vada.
Fruit may be added in the menu if potassium not restricted.

If proteins are to be increased, equivalent exchange of protein 3 g may be suitably added (Table 33.3)

To increase calories, 1–2 exchanges of oil/sugar may be added as required.

DIALYSIS

Patients with chronic renal disease who fail to respond to conventional management may require dialysis to maintain renal functions to near normal levels.

Energy Requirements

Children with chronic kidney disease (CKD) generally have poor intake, especially those in stages 2-5 D due to reduced appetite and vomiting. Supplemental nutritional support is recommended where the usual intake of a child with CKD stages

2–5 D (Table 33.5) fails to meet the recommended dietary intake.

Early intervention is essential with introduction of tube feeds, if energy requirement cannot be met orally. A small percentage of children may have excessive energy intake, therefore dietary intervention and lifestyle changes are needed to tackle the long-term complications of obesity. The recommended energy intake as per the NKF K/DOQI pediatric guidelines (last updated in 2008), for stages 2–5 and 5D have recommended 100% of the estimated requirement for dialytic protein and amino acid losses. Based on the response in rate of weight gain or loss, suitable adjustments can be made. However, it has been recommended that tube fed children and infants be encouraged to continue some oral intake or have continued oral stimulation, e.g. sucking or a pacifier and/or positive non-threatening contact with food.[8] Advanced CKD stages are often associated with anorexia and gastrointestinal disorders, which may inhibit the ability to maintain adequate nutritional status through oral and/or enteral nutrition.

Fats, carbohydrates and proteins may be substituted for one another to meet the energy needs. Uneven distribution of calories from each of the macronutrients may be associated with an increased risk of some chronic diseases like coronary heart disease, obesity and diabetes mellitus, which are commonly seen in children with CKD over a certain length of time. Therefore, the acceptable macronutrient distribution (AMDR) in children with CKD should be as given as in Table 33.7.[8]

The use of protein supplements are recommended to augment the inadequate oral and/or enteral protein intake in children in stages 2–5 and 5D of CKD, as these children are unable to meet their requirements orally.

TABLE 33.7: Acceptable macronutrient distribution range (AMDR) in children with CKD

Macronutrients	1–3 years	4–10 years
Carbohydrates	45%–65%	45%–65%
Fats	30%–40%	25%–30%
Proteins	5%–20%	10%–30%

Refer. 6

Poor appetite and vomiting are the frequent problems seen in children with CKD and this is the main reason for their poor intake. Vomiting and irritability are along with discomfort are suggestive of gastroesophageal reflux (GER) initially can be managed by concentrated feeds to reduce the volume and increase the density, and maintaining elevated position after feeds.[9] Tube feeding is a suitable alternative under such conditions, which may be initiated by small frequent feeding. This can help achieve significant weight gain and catch up growth.[10]

The AMDR ranges for a healthy distribution of calories from carbohydrates, fats and proteins are based upon the evidence that consumption of greater or lesser than these ranges may be associated with nutrient inadequacy and increased risk of developing such chronic diseases as coronary heart disease, obesity, diabetes and/or cancer.

Generally calorie dense formulae are prescribed for infants, but since there are no AMDR guidelines for children under 1 year, care should be taken that when increasing the caloric density of the formula, the distribution of proteins, fats and carbohydrates should be kept consistent with the base formula,[11] which must adhere to strict standards (7%–12% proteins, 40%–54% fats and 36%–56% carbohydrates).

Protein Requirements

Although there is no evidence for dietary protein restriction to maintain a nephroprotective effect, it can be restricted safely to 0.8–1.1 g/kg/d in children with CKD. This will help reduce the accumulation of nitrogenous waste products and facilitate lowering of dietary phosphorous levels. It will also help delay the onset of signs and symptoms of uremia. The committee of the KDOQI, 2008 felt that implementation and maintenance of a strict low protein diet requires a major life style change and hence not very practical and acceptable by many families. Therefore moderate protein restriction aiming at 100% to 140% of the RDA in CKD stage 3 and 100%–120% of the RDA in CKD stages 4–5 as given in Table 33.8 may be a reasonable compromise in most cases.[8]

These protein recommendations refer to a stable child, assuming that energy intake will result in inefficient utilization of proteins, with increased production of urea.

TABLE 33.8 Recommended dietary protein intake in children with CKD stages 3–5 and 5D

AGE	Dietary Reference Intake (DRI)				
	DRI g/kg/d	Recommended for CKD stage 3 (g/kg/d) 100%–140% RDA	Recommended for CKD stage 4–5 (g/kg/d) 100%–120% RDA	Recommended for HD (g/kg/d)	Recommended for PD (g/kg/d)
0–6 months	1.5	1.5–2.1	1.5–1.8	1.6	1.8
7–12 months	1.2	1.2–1.7	1.2–1.5	1.3	1.5
1–3 years	1.05	1.05–1.5	1.05–1.25	1.15	1.3
4–13 years	0.95	0.9–1.35	0.95–1.15	1.05	1.1
14–18 years	0.85	0.85–1.2	0.85–1.05	0.95	1.0

Refer.[8] (NKF KDOQI Guidelines, 2008)

In case dietary protein is not achieved at 100% of the RDA, or if there is evidence of deficiency of any of the micronutrients, these should be supplemented.

Vitamins and Trace Element Requirements

Patients with CKD and those on dialysis therapy are at an increased risk of vitamin and mineral deficiency due to abnormal renal metabolism, inadequate intake and poor gastrointestinal absorption and dialysis relayed to losses.

The recommendations for various B complex vitamins (B_1), riboflavin (B_2), niacin (B_3), pantothenic acid (B_5), pyridoxine (B_6), biotin, cobalamin, ascorbic acid, retinol and tocopherol, vitamin K, folic acid, copper and zinc for children with CKD stages 2 to 5 and 5D.

In case dietary protein is not achieved at 100% of the RDA, it is suggested that supplementation of vitamins and trace elements be provided or if there is clinical evidence of a deficiency of any of these vitamins. For children with CKD 5D on dialysis, a water soluble vitamin supplement is recommended.

Calcium needs to be supplemented for children with CKD stages 2–5 and 5 D from nutritional sources and phosphate binders in the range of 100-200 of the DRI.

Fluid and Electrolyte Requirements

In children with CKD, the requirement of fluids and electrolytes varies according to the status of the kidney disease, degree of residual kidney function and type of renal replacement therapy. The sodium and potassium restriction or supplementation depends upon the volume of urine output, ability to concentrate urine hydration status and the presence or absence of hypertension or hyperkalemia. The K/DOQI recommendations for children with CKD are

1. Supplemental free water and sodium supplements should be considered for children with CKD stages 2-5 and 5D and polyurea to avoid chronic intravascular depletion and to promote optimal growth.
2. For all infants with CKD stage 5D, on peritoneal dialysis, sodium supplements should be considered.
3. Children and infants with CKD stages 2-5 and 5D, who are hypertensive, restriction of sodium should be advised.
4. For infants with CKD stage 5D on peritoneal dialysis (PD) therapy sodium supplements need to be prescribed.
5. For children with oliguria, fluid intake is advised to prevent complications of fluid overload.
6. Children with hyperkalemia, need to be advised potassium restriction, especially those with CKD stages 2–5 and 5D.

NUTRITIONAL MANAGEMENT OF TRANSPLANT PATIENTS

Children, who have undergone renal transplantation, need to be monitored and assessed for their growth and development to meet their nutritional requirements while minimizing the side effects of immuno suppressive drugs.

Management of the child with kidney transplant includes care of the graft besides care of complications of CKD stages 1–5T. They continue to require dietary modifications post-transplant. The modifications include in terms of hypertension, hyperkalemia, hypophosphatemia, hypomagnesiumia and hyperglycemia, which could be complication of immunosuppressive drugs. For children with CKD stages 2–5T, management of protein and phosphorus is done as for children with similar GFRs before transplantation.

The energy requirement of children with CKD stages 1–5T should be equal to 100% of the estimated energy requirements (EER) adjusted for BMI. Adjustments in view of loss or gain in weight can be done as per requirement.

A balance of calories from carbohydrates, proteins and unsaturated fats within the physiological ranges recommended by AMDR of the DRI is suggested for children with CKD stages 1–5T to prevent or manage obesity, dyslipidemia and corticosteroid induced diabetes.

Children with CKD stages 1–5T and hypertension or abnormal serum electrolytes concentrations which are common with immunosuppressive drugs need to be managed by suitable dietary modifications.

Calcium and vitamin D intakes need to be provided at least 100% of the DRI for children with CKD 1-5T, however, not exceeding 200% of the DRI.[6]

Fluids including water and other beverages should not be sweetened with simple sugars, to avoid excess weight gain, hyperglycemia and dental decay.

Food hygiene and safety and avoidance of foods from doubtful sources need to be ensured strictly for immunosuppressed children with CKD stages 1–5T.

REFERENCES

1. Eddy AA, Symons JM. Nephrotic syndrome in childhood. Lancet. 2003;362:629-39.
2. Mc Kinney PA, Feltbower RG, Brocklebank JT, Fitzpatric MM. Time, trends and ethnic patterns of childhood nephritic syndrome in Yorkshire, UK. Pediatr Nephrol. 2001;16:1040-4.
3. Trompeter RS, Barret TM. Treatment and management of nephritic syndrome in children. In: The nephritic syndrome ed. Cameron JS and Glassock RJ (19880).
4. Barret TH. Renal Disorders. In: Clayton BE, Round JM eds. Chemical Pathology and the Sick Child, Oxford: Blackwell Scientific Publications. 1984;120-43.
5. International Study of kidney Disease in Children. Nephrotic Syndrome in Children: prediction of histopathology from clinical and laboratory characterstics at time of diagnosis. Kidney Int. 1998;13:159-65.
6. Gopalan C, Rama Sastri BV, Balasbramanian SC. Nutritive Value of Indian Foods, National Institute of Nutrition, ICMR, Hyderabad. 2008.
7. Rees L, Webb N, Brogan p (eds): Acute Renal Failure In: Pediatric Nephrology, Oxford University Press. 2007.pp.360-84.
8. NKF/KDOQI Clinical Practice Guideline for Nutrition in Children with Chronic kidney disease: 2008 Update. Am J Kidney Dis. 2009;53(Suppl 2):S1-S124.
9. Dello Strologo L, Principato F, Sinibaldi D, et al. Feeding dysfunction in infants with severe chronic renal failure after long-term nasogastric feeding. Pediatr Nephrol. 1997;11:84-6.
10. Rudolph CD, Mazur LJ, Liptak GS, et al. Guidelines for evaluation and treatment of gastroesophageal reflux in infants and children. Recommendations of the North American Society for Pediatric Gastroenterology and Nutrition. J Ped Gastroenterol Nutr. 2001;32(Suppl 2):S1-31.
11. Spinozzi NS, Nelson PA; Nutrition support in the new born intensive care unit. J Ren Nutr. 1996:188-97.

34 Inborn Errors of Metabolism

PHENYLKETONURIA

Phenylketonuria (PKU) is a rare form of disorder, due to a recessive inherited metabolic disorder, first recognized in 1934 by Folling. In this condition, both parents are heterogeneous carriers and the risk of other children being involved is one in four.

The incidence varies from 1 in 10,000 in Caucasians to 1 in 30,000 in new borns.[1]

The disorder involves a defect in the conversion of phenylalanine (Phe) to tyrosine, due to which there is an accumulation of phenylalanine in the blood and tissues resulting in excessive production of phenylketones. This results in children having retardation of developmental progress, severe mental retardation, hyperactivity, seizures, a light complexion and eczema. The urine has a mouse like odor.

The mechanism of conversion of phenylalanine to tyrosine in a normal and affected child has been depicted in Figure 34.1.[2]

Due to low levels of hepatic phenylalanine hydroxylase, phenylalanine cannot be converted to tyrosine. As a result there is accumulation of Phenylalanine in the blood, cerebrospinal fluid and the tissues. Due to this block in the normal metabolic pathway, accessory metabolic pathways develop, which convert phenylalanine to phenylpyruvic acid and hydroxyphenyl acetic acid, which are then excreted in the urine. The subsequent accumalation of phenylalanine and other metabolites in the serum, affects the utilization of other amino acids by the cells. This results in deprivation of essential and consequent retardation in the development of the brain.

However prompt treatment of such children with diet restricted in phenylalanine results in reversal of symptoms and leads to normal intellectual development. It is recommended not to delay dietary intervention beyond 2 days for good results.

PKU is known to be of two types:

1. Classical
2. Atypical

In classical PKU, hepatic phenylalanine is low or absent and blood levels on a normal diet usually exceed 1200 μmol/l, but tyrosine levels are low or normal. The defect involves incomplete myelination of the central nervous system. A classical case of PKU will not tolerate more than 400 mg of dietary phenylalanine per day. With this level of dietary phenylalanine, blood phenylalanine level of 480 μmol/l can be safely achieved.

In atypical PKU, the enzyme block is less complete than in classical condition. The blood phenylalanine levels are usually less than 1200 μmol/l, although a high dietary protein intake or an acute catabolic episode may raise this figure. In general, these patients have a higher level of tolerance of dietary phenylalanine, managing 2–3 times the quantity of natural protein tolerated by these with the classical form, when phenylalanine levels are in safe range.[1]

DIAGNOSIS

Screening a child for PKU involves detection of raised phenylalanine levels (upper limit of normal 240 μmol/l). In the cord blood these levels are generally normal, but begin to rise steadily after

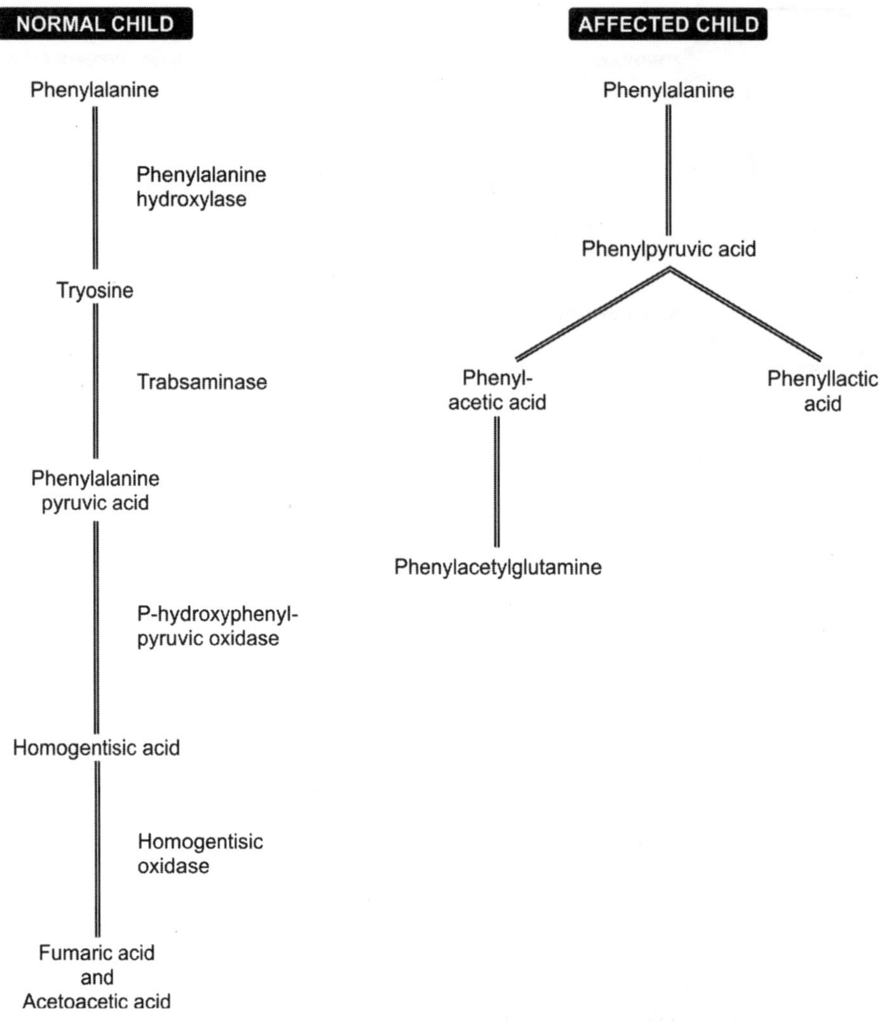

FIGURE 34.1: Mechanism of conversion of phenylalanine to tyrosine
Ref.[2], Hemalatha R

birth, following breastfeeding or even formula milk. In an unscreened child, the presenting symptoms could be seizures, albinism (excessively fair hair and skin) and a 'musty' odor to the baby's sweat, skin and urine. A tendency to hypopigmentation and eczema are also observed.

All patients with blood phenylalanine levels greater than 240 μmol/l, should be investigated further. Infants on breast feeds or otherwise should be evaluated for the protein content of their diet, as a high protein intake can artificially elevate phenylalanine levels. The tests should be repeated after 2 weeks, to confirm the diagnosis but dietary modification can however be initiated earlier. Breastfeeding should be preferred to cow's milk as it has a lower phenylalanine content.

DIETARY MANAGEMENT

Successful treatment of patients with PKU depends upon:

- Early diagnosis
- Restriction of phenylalanine intake to maintain an acceptable range of serum levels
- A nutritionally adequate diet adjusted from time to time to meet the requirements for normal growth and development

TABLE 34.1: Requirements in classical phenylketonuria per kg per day

Age (years)	Energy (Kcals)	Protein (g)	Phenylalanine from natural protein (mg)
0–1	100–130	3.4	50–60
1–2	90–100	2.5–3.5	30–40
2–4	80–100	2–3	25–40
4–6	80–100	2–3	25
6–8	70–90	2–2.5	15–20
8–14	55–75	1–1.5	As tolerated
>14	45	1	As tolerated

Source. Hemalatha R NIN, ICMR, Hyderabad, 1999[2]

- Continuing clinical and biochemical monitoring
- Education and counseling of parents.

Children diagnosed with PKU need closely monitored feeding to ensure that the protein levels of their diet does not exceed sharply, especially after weaning has been introduced. Table 34.1 gives the requirements in classical PKU patients.[2]

If breast milk is unavailable for some reason, whey based modified milk (commercially available) having the amino acid profile of human milk can be substituted. Breast fed infants have to be monitored for their phenylalanine levels in blood and weight gain at weekly intervals. If the levels are between 180–480 μmol/l, there is no need to restrict breast milk and can be continued as for normal children. However, if phenylalanine levels exceed >200 μmol/l, breast milk is withheld for 2–3 days and a low phenylalanine food supplement (LPFS), protein substitute is initiated (Table 34.2). Some of the commercially available low phenylalanine food supplements in the Western market are LPFS (low phenylalanine food supplement), PHFS (protein hydrolysate food supplement), PHFS plus minerals, under the brand names, lofenalac, aminogram, and aminogram mineral respectively. LPFS is basically a casein based hydrolysate from which 95% of phenylalanine is removed. The major constituent of these supplements are unsaturated fat, carbohydrates, vitamins and minerals.

After around 5–6 months when weaning is initiated to begin with approximately 10 g of a rice based weaning food mixed with boiled water can be offered, followed by fruits, vegetables in small amounts. Gradually an exchange of 50 mg phenylalanine food (Table 34.3), is introduced in combination with 3–4 feeds of LPFS per day, based on the blood phenylalanine levels. The aim should be to maintain a ratio of 40–50 Kcals: 1 g protein.[2] The calories can be increased by use of oil, butter, etc. By 6 months the protein requirement is increased, therefore protein hydrolysate food supplement (PHFS) is fed, gradually increasing the quantity from 1 tsp/d to 1 tsp 3 times a day, then eventually full dose of 3 g PHFS per kg/d along with 8 g PHFS mineral supplements as given in Table 34.4. Breast feeds and LPHS are proportionately reduced and finally omitted. Gradually solids are increased as per the requirement for age and blood levels of phenylalanine. The daily intake of cow's milk or pasteurized fresh milk is divided and exchanged with

TABLE 34.2: Breastfeeding regime for infants with phenylketonuria

Blood phenylalanine	LPFS	Breast feeds μmols/l 15% Sol
>2000	150–200 ml/kg/d	Nil for 3 days
1200–2000	150–200 ml/kg/d	Nil for 2 days
After 2 days, 45 ml–5 feeds	30 ml–5 feeds	On demand
<1200		
480–900	15 ml–5 feeds	On demand

Source. Hemalatha R NIN, ICMR, Hyderabad, 1999[2]

TABLE 34.3: Amount of natural foods providing 50 mg of phenylalanine (weighed after cooking)

Food item	Quantity
Milk	50 ml
Potatoes (boiled)	75 g
Potatoes (chips)	30 mg
Pear (fresh)	20 mg
Cornflakes	15 mg
Wheat flakes	10 mg
Rice (boiled)	54 mg
Porridge (with water)	65 mg
Tomato sauce	50 mg
Wheat (roasted)	25 mg

Source. Hemalatha R NIN, ICMR, Hyderabad, 1999[2]

TABLE 34.4: Low phenylalanine diets for children (1–4 years)

Age	1 month	8 months	2 years	4 years
Weight (kg)	3.63	8.2	11.8	16.3
Diet advised				
Phenylalanine (mg)	160–176	324–360	416–468	360–576
Protein (g)	14–16	27	32	40
Calories (Kcals)	440	810	1300	1700
LPFS measures (15 g)	10	18	19	23
Water (to make up volume to)	24 oz	32 oz	24 oz	24 oz
Milk	1–1/2 oz	1oz	–	–
Vegetables	–	2	4	4
Fruits	–	1	4	4
Rice/wheat exchange	–	3	5	5
Fat exchange	–	–	As desired	As desired
Free foods, US Dept				
Nutritive Value				
Phenylalanine (mg)	172	325	417	447
Protein (g)	16.8	30.4	33.1	40.4
Calories	540	944	1302	1724

Refer. Acosta PB: Nutritional aspects of Phenylketonuria. In: The Clinical Team Looks at Phenylketonuria. Children's Bureau, US Dep't of Health, Education and Welfare, Washington DC, p52.

LPFS. The total volume of feeds should not exceed 150–200 ml/kg/d.[2]

It has also been stressed that a balance must be maintained between the amount of low phenylalanine formula and the amount of natural foods that are fed. An inadequate amount of phenylalanine can lead to signs of deficiency which include anorexia, vomiting, listlessness, inconsistent growth or failure to gain weight, pallor and skin rash.[3] The low phenylalanine formula like Lofenac supplies most of the energy, proteins and other nutrients and if inadequate amounts are fed, the amino acids and other nutrient requirements of the child will not be met. On the other hand, if inadequate amounts of natural foods are given, the phenylalanine intake will be too low to meet the requirements. Although phenylalanine intake is restricted, it must be remembered that this is one of the essential amino acids.

Low Phenylalanine Diet for 1–4 year old Children

By 1 year of age the child should be consuming 5–6 times per day comprising 3 main meals and 2–3 snacks per day as shown in Table 34.4. Unfortunately, the low phenylalanine supplements are yet not available in India; therefore in the absence of these, most children show deterioration of symptoms, in spite of early diagnosis.

ATYPICAL PHENYLKETONURIA

Children diagnosed with atypical phenylketonuria, if at all require treatment, need to follow more or less the same principles as for 'classical phenylketonuria, but the protein can be more liberal with a wider selection of foods and less of low phenylalanine protein substitutes prescribed. However, these children need to be reassessed up to 1 year of age to consider the feasibility of allowing them a near normal diet.

According to observations, children with atypical symptoms, phenylketonuria treated for varying periods of time, with blood levels, 600 µmol/l generally continue to be normal even after withdrawal of low phenylalanine diets.[1] Nevertheless, parents should be apprised of the risks of maternal phenylketonuria, in case of female patients.

The National Society for phenylketonuria (UK) has formulated a list of foods allowed and restricted for patients with phenylketonuria which include detailed dietary information for treatment of phenylketonuria.[4] They have formulated a traffic light system based on the colors of various foods to be included or excluded. These are:

Red — **Stop!** - Do not eat at all

Amber — **Go cautiously**—Foods to be eaten in moderate amounts.

Green — **Go!** - These foods may be eaten in normal amounts.

The foods included under the various lights are:

Red list: *Foods high in phenylalanine to avoid—meats, fish, eggs, cheese, nuts, bread flour, cakes, biscuits, soya based foods, aspartame (artificial sweetener found in most fizz drinks, cokes, squashes, chewing gums and some drugs).*

Amber list: *Foods containing some phenylalanine to be taken with caution. Basic list of some exchanges of food to be followed should be measured accurately (Table 34.4).*

Green List

Fruits: Apple, banana (1 small), dates, apricots, fresh and dried, blackberries, cherries, currants, figs, grapes, guavas, lemon, kiwi, mangoes, melon (water, musk), oranges, peaches, pineapple, plums, raisins, raspberries, strawberries.

Vegetables: Beans, beetroot, cabbage, cauliflower, carrots, celery, cucumber, ladyfingers, lettuce, mushrooms, mustard, onions, peppers (red, yellow, green), pumpkin, radish, sweet potato, tomato, turnip

Cereals: Corn flour, arrowroot, custard powder, sago, tapioca.

Fats: Butter, vegetable oils, margarine (but not the one containing buttermilk).

Miscellaneous: Sugar-white, brown, castor, jam, honey, marmalade, baking powder, soda bicarbonate, cream of tartar, vegetarian jellies without gelatin.

Beverages: Soda water, mineral water, lemonade, squashes, tea, coffee, pine fruit, juices, coke (without aspartame).

GALACTOSEMIA

Galactosemia is another inborn error of metabolism and as the name suggests involves accumulation of galactose in the blood, which otherwise in the normal state gets converted to glucose in the liver. The defect involves.

a. Absence of an enzyme, galactose-1-phosphate uridyl transferase, which is needed in the liver for the conversion.
b. Deficiency of galactokinase which catalyses the formation of galactose-1-phosphate from galactose.

Galactose is a derivative of glucose and lactose and is derived from the hydrolysis of lactose in the intestine. Most dietary galactose is derived from lactose, the disaccharide of milk that is hydrolysed to galactose and glucose by the action of intestinal lactase, which is usually normal in these patients. Analysis of the RBC shows little or no transferase in those who have this disorder and half the normal levels in those who are carriers. This enzyme defect is inherited as an autosomal recessive trait and mothers of galactosemic infants have a diminished ability to metabolise galactose. If such mothers consume excess amounts of milk during pregnancy, the possibilities of damage to the fetus exist, as galactose may pass the placenta.[5]

Clinical Presentation

Children are normal at birth, but after a few days of birth with introduction of milk (breast or formula) symptoms like vomiting, anorexia, occasional diarrhea, drowsiness, jaundice, puffiness of face, edema of the lower extremities and weight loss begin to appear. Poor sucking is observed within 48 hours of birth. Without treatment the outcome is generally fatal, but if the child does survive, chances of developing mental retardation, cirrhosis of liver and cataract are quite high. However early diagnosis and prompt dietary intervention can lead to excellent immediate results and a favorable long-term prognosis. Diagnosis is confirmed by elevated levels of galactose-1-phosphatase in erythrocytes, which is thought to be a toxic metabolite, proteinuria, aminoaciduria and raised serum galactose and urinary galactose with depressed blood glucose levels. Cataracts may be present at birth or develop subsequently and may remain irreversible despite treatment.

Dietary Management

Dietary exclusion of galactose and lactose sources is the only intervention to prevent clinical symptoms and ensure normal growth and development. Milk especially human milk is very high in galactose and therefore breast fed infants manifest symptoms very early. A nutritionally adequate diet free of all milk sources needs to be incorporated. Substitution of non milk formula leads to rapid improvement. All symptoms except mental retardation disappear. There

TABLE 34.5: Galactose free diet for toddlers and young children

Sample menu	
Breakfast	Cereal (suji halwa/choori, parantha/idli/ dosa Egg–optional
Mid morning	Fruit/Poha/besan pura/cheela
Lunch	Rice/Chapati Dal Vegetable Tofu (soya based) Salad
Evening	Juice Idli/dosa/upma/suji halwa/veg. cutlet
Dinner	Khichdi/Rice/chapatti Dal/Chicken/Fish Potato fingers Dessert (milk free)

Note: Use only refined vegetable oil/coconut oil

are controversial opinions regarding use of soya milk as a substitute. Some authors have used it successfully while others opine that stachyose, a terasaccharide in soyabeans, is hydrolysed to galactose. Rice based formulae or other commercially available milk free baby foods need to be fed till such time the child is old enough to accept other cereal-pulse based diets. These formulae need to be supplemented with calcium, iron and vitamins. Care should be taken to avoid all milk based foods like, ice cream, bread, biscuits, puddings, chocolates, butter, margarine, toffees, etc.

By the time the child is 6–8 months old, a greater variety of foods can be available, e.g. rice, dal, khichdi, suji halwa or upma, dalia, etc. Introduction of eggs can be delayed till about 10–12 months and then given 2–4 times per week. A sample menu of a day's diet for toddlers and young children is presented in Table 34.5. Older children can gradually be permitted foods containing traces of lactose, but visible milk in the form of ice cream, custard, porridge, etc. should still be best avoided. Care should be taken to scrutinize all labels of all commercial products used or, when outdoor on social gatherings, the contents of the dishes included should always be verified.

Duration of Dietary Treatment

In the initial years, dietary treatment is very strict, but as the child grows older, the diet may be relaxed to an extent to allow minimal lactose in their diets. The enzyme defect persists for life and hence children with galactosemia growing to adolescence and adulthood should always be wary of the selection of foods in their diet. In females, especially during pregnancy, restriction of lactose containing foods is advisable to avoid consequences in the new born.

It is not very difficult to adhere to a lactose free diet for adolescents and adults as by then they have a greater variety of foods to choose from and milk and milk products is one small portion of any adult diet. With the exception of milk and milk products as a direct source, rest all other food groups can be incorporated in the menu of such patients as listed in Table 34. 6

As with phenylketonuria, dietary counseling is of great importance. Close rapport with parents and the children along with regular follow-up visits, helps in successful implementation of dietary compliance. Regular blood galactose estimates help to establish that normal limits are not exceeded.

TABLE 34.6: List of foods to be included and excluded in galactosemia

Foods	Included	Excluded
Milk group	Soya milk/curd	All milk and milk products including breast milk, curd
Cereals/ pulses	All cereals/pulses tofu (soya paneer)	
Fats/Oils	Vegetable oils, butter, cream, ghee margarine without milk margarine with milk	
Fruits/ Vegetables	Fresh fruits/ vegetables, peas, canned vegetables	
Meat group	Muscle meat, egg, fish, poultry, liver	
Miscellaneous	All cold drinks, juices, dry fruits, all sweets from khoya, milk, sweets without, milk, khoya paneer, cheese, ice cream, besan products, sugar, Custard, baby food supplements with whey/casein, Jaggery	

FRUCTOSEMIA

Fructosemia is an inborn error manifesting somewhat like galactosemia. In this disorder, introduction of fructose in the diet of the infant before 6 months of age, results in anorexia, vomiting, failure to thrive, hypoglycemia, seizures and dysfunction of liver and kidneys.[6] Older children generally remain asymptomatic or may manifest with spontaneous hypoglycemia, which is believed to be caused by reduced glycogenolysis and gluconeogenesis.

The disorder involves four enzymes in fructose metabolism-hexokinase, fructokinase, fructaldolase and fructose1, 6 diphosphatase. Deficiency of the latter three has been described, but fructokinase deficiency is a benign error of metabolism and does not warrant any dietary restriction.

Hereditary Fructose Intolerance

This is due to the deficiency of primary fructaldolase deficiency in which fructose-1-phosphate accumulates. Clinical symptoms appear on first exposure to fructose (or sucrose) generally after weaning has been initiated with foods like fruit or sweetened cereals. Mostly such patients develop a strong aversion to sweet taste, therefore unintentional fructose intake is rare.

The striking feature of HFI, are fructosemia, fructosuria and hypoglycemia with symptoms of shock on ingestion of fructose. Once diagnosed, treatment should be initiated immediately continued for life by excluding fructose, sucrose and sorbitol from the diet. Elimination of fructose from the diet brings about immediate remission of symptoms except for hepatomegaly which may take greater time to resolve[7] Minimal inclusion of fructose in the diet can cause chronic symptoms of failure to thrive, hypoglycemia and liver diseases. A list of foods to be included and excluded in HFI is listed in Table 34.7.

Fructose-1-Diphosphatase Deficiency

In this deficiency symptoms include hypoglycemia, hyperventilation, hepatomegaly, failure to thrive, vomiting and seizures. Presence of lactic acidosis puts the infants at great risk. Unlike in HFI, these patients do not have aversion to sweet foods. In these children, glycogen is not metabolized normally and cannot be used to maintain glucose homeostasis. Unlike in HFI, where fasting improves symptoms, in patients with fructose 1-diphosphatase deficiency, fasting can cause hypoglycemia, therefore care needs to be taken avoid prolonged fasting in such patients. Frequent carbohydrate intake is very essential to maintain normoglycemia even when the child is well. A late night snack of starch based carbohydrate (sucrose and fructose free) is advisable. The total dietary carbohydrate should be high, approximately ≥ 65% of dietary energy and fat intake slightly restricted. Early diagnosis and prompt treatment can prevent irreversible damage.

TABLE 34.7: List of foods included and excluded in HFI

Foods included	Foods restricted
Milk, cheese, cream, butter, curd	Sweetened condensed milk, infant feed eggs, fish chicken containing sucrose, commercial ice cream
Rice , wheat flour, barley, oats, suji, dalia, cream,	sweetened milk shakes
Tapioca, bread only 2-3 slices/day	Flavoured milk
Cakes, biscuits made from glucose, Soya and soya flour	Flavoured and fruit yogurt
Glucose and glucose drinks, starch, maltose	Baby cereals, breakfast cereals, dextrins sweetened custard, pudding mixes
Saccharine, aspartame	Cakes, biscuits, pastries,
Tea, coffee, cocoa (unsweetened)	All fruits/juices, tomato, jam
fruit sugar, invert sugar, honey syrup	Caramel, marmalades
Vegetables-all except root vegetables, beans, peas, sweet corn, carrots, sorbitol/fructose, butter, ghee sucrose salt, pepper, spices, vinegar nuts, permitted ingredients	Sorbitol, sweetening agents containing
paste/puree	Jelly, tooth paste with sucrose or foods of doubtful content

FRUCTOSE FREE DIET

Fruits are the main source of fructose as also invert sugars which are a component of sucrose; therefore these must be excluded (including cane, beet or brown sugar, icing sugar and syrup, honey, all fruits, root vegetables, pulses and tomatoes). Some of the tooth pastes also contain some fructose and sucrose from natural fruits and need to be avoided. Other fructose or sucrose containing foods include diabetic sweets which use sorbitol, chocolates and squashes. All medicines in liquid form may contain sucrose or sorbitol and must be replaced by alternatives. A list of foods allowed and restricted is presented in Table 14.7.

MAPLE SYRUP DISEASE

This disease also termed as branched chain ketoaciduria relates to biochemical defect and is an autosomal recessive disease. The missing factor is the enzyme oxidative decarboxylase in white blood corpuscles (WBC). As such the carboxyl group cannot be removed resulting in accumulation of amino acids and ketoacids in the urine. This gives the typical odor of maple syrup to the urine and hence the name. At birth the child appears normal but becomes symptomatic within first few days of life. They experience sucking problems; respiration is irregular with intermittent periods of rigidity and flaccidity. Seizures of the grand mal type are present, and if the child survives, may manifest with mental disorders. Hyperglycemia is frequently encountered in these children and due to increased tissue catabolism following infection, there is further rise in the accumalation of the offending metabolites in the circulation.

Dietary Management

Management comprises a diet restricted in the branch chain amino acids, which is only in commercial formulation. However, a formula suited specifically for such needs is not yet available in India. Small amounts of milk may be continued in view of the requirements for growth and development. The guidelines for management of PKU can be adapted for this disorder. Most fruits and vegetables are permitted having more or less 50 mg leucine per 100 g. These are apples, pineapple, raisins, banana (in limited amount), carrots, beans, cabbage, onion, pumpkin, tomato, beetroot and turnips.

HOMOCYSTINURIA

This also is an autosomal recessive disorder and in which the enzyme cystathionine synthetase is lacking. The enzyme is present in the liver and brain and is necessary for conversion of homocysteine to cystathionine, an intermediate product formed in the metabolism of methionine. The manifestations are mental disorder along with cataract and dissolution of muscles of the pelvic girdle, thrombosis and pulmonary embolism are commonly seen in these patients.

Dietary Modifications

The diet should be modified for low methionine, high cystine content. Gelatin is a good source of protein being low in methionine. It is supplemented with synthetic amino acids like leucine, iso leucine, tryptophan and valine.

WILSON'S DISEASE

Wilson's disease is a hereditary autosomal recessive disorder which involves degeneration of the hepatic cells. The defect involves very low serum levels of ceruloplasmin, a copper containing protein of the blood. This is due to the increased absorption of copper from the GI tract and an increased deposit of copper in the brain, liver and kidney.

Age of presentation is generally between 4–5 years or in some can be as late as the first decade of life also. The clinical manifestations in these patients are ascites, jaundice, live enlargement and neurological involvement. The child might show a blank dazed look with the presence of tremors, seizures and dementia. A typical diagnostic feature is the presence of Kayser-Fleischer (KF) ring in the eye (a greenish brown discoloration).

Dietary Modifications

Management in such children involves dietary modifications which involves avoiding high copper food sources. Chelating agents are used to chelate or break away the copper of the diet, thus minimizing the absorption from the GIT. The aim should be to maintain a level of 1 mg copper or less in the diet. The normal range generally is about 2–3 mg.

Most foods have some amounts of copper present, but high sources are organ meats, shellfish, mushrooms, legumes, whole grain cereals, nuts, chocolates and colas. A list of foods containing high levels of copper is listed in Table 34.8. All commercial and tinned foods should be restricted. A significant source of copper can be leached out from copper vessels used for boiling milk in a majority of Indian households, especially if they are not adequately tinned. Therefore mothers should be warned against using copper vessels for cooking or storing milk or any other food item to be consumed by the child.

Treatment depends upon low copper diet (1.0–1.8 mg/24 hours), preventing copper absorption, mobilizing these deposits and promoting their excretion. Potassium sulfide, 20 mg, three times a day with meals, prevents copper absorption.[8] Patients with Wilson's disease[10] may develop anemia, therefore iron supplements need to be given also. Zinc given orally increases fecal copper excretion.[9] Table 34.8 presents a picture of the foods to be avoided and allowed in patients with Wilson's disease.

TABLE 34.8: Foods restricted and allowed in Wilsons disease

Foods restricted	Foods allowed
(High copper-0.8-1mg %)	(Low copper-0.01-0.6mg %)
All dry fruits, nuts (coconut, peanuts)	All cereals-rice, wheat, maize
All seeds-til, mustard, saffola oil	All leafy vegetables, green peas
All organ meats-liver, kidney	All fruits
Chocolates, toffees, colas	All roots, tubers and other vegetables
Black pepper, gram whole, Bengal gram	Pulses-whole moong dal, arhar
White and kabuli gram, lentil, dry peas	Fish
Rajma, moth dal	Milk and milk products
Mushrooms	Fats and sugars

Refer.[10] ICMR

REFERENCES

1. Dorothy E M Francis. Phenylketonuria In: Diets for Sick Children, 4th ed. Blackwell Scientific Publications. 1987.pp.224-62.
2. R Hemalatha. Diet Therpay in classical Phenylketonuria, Nutrition, National Institute of Nutrition, ICMR, Hyderabad. April 1999.
3. Sutherland BS, et al. Growth and nutrition in treated phenylketonuric patients. JAMA. 1970;211:270-76.
4. National Society for Phenylketonuria (UK), London N14 4ZF, Compant No: 1256124, Charity No: 273670
5. Hansen RG. Hereditary Galactosemia. JAMA. 1969;208:2077-82.
6. Levin B, et al: Fructosemia. Observations on seven cases. Am J Med. 1968;45:826-38.
7. Baerlocher K, Gitzelmann R and Steinmann B. In: Inherited Disorders of carbohydrate metabolism. Eds. Burman D, Holten JB and Pennock CA. Lancaster. MTP press Ltd. 1980.pp.163-90.
8. FP Antia Copper In: Clinical Dietetics and Nutrition, 3rd ed, Oxford University Press Bombay. 1993.pp.125-7.
9. Brewer GJ, Hills GM, Prasad AS, Cossack ZT, et al. Oral zinc therapy for Wilsons disease, Ann Intern Med. 1983;99:314-20.
10. Gopalan C, Rama Sastri BV, Balasbramanian SC. Nutritive Value of Indian Foods, national Institute if Nutrition, ICMR, Hyderabad. 2002.

35 Nutritional Support in Juvenile Diabetes Mellitus

The increasing incidence of Type 1 diabetes among children in our country is posing a major challenge to the medical community. The changing life style patterns in terms of urbanization or modernization has brought along with, its own risks. Several studies have already confirmed some association between incidence of Type 1 diabetes with many nutrients and accompanying food additives.[1,2]

Some authors have also shown evidence of co-relation between incidence of Type 1 diabetes and cow's milk intake by the child in early infancy.[3,4,5,6] Reports also have confirmed that exposure to cow's milk before 3 months of age and having the high risk genotype resulted in an 11 fold increased risk of insulin dependent diabetes mellitus (IDDM) compared with subjects with no risk factors.[7] Eating pattern in childhood has also been associated with Type 1 diabetes at the population level. It was also observed that average daily intake of energy from animal origin like dairy products and meat, directly co-related with energy from vegetable food items like cereals.[8] It has been reported that over nutrition early in life may lead to hyperinsulinism thus acting as a predisposing factor for Type 1 diabetes.[9,10] Though there are studies to confirm a direct co-relation between long duration of breastfeeding and decreased risk of IDDM,[11,12] certain authors have failed to collaborate the findings.[10] One of the first observational studies from Finland showed that the age of introduction of dairy products is associated with risk of IDDM independent of total duration of breastfeeding.[13] In other words the length of exclusive breastfeeding might have some protective role against risk of Type 1 diabetes.

Children have characteristics and needs that dictate different standards of care. The management of diabetes in children involves considerations taking major differences between children of various ages and adults. For instance, insulin dose based only on body size are likely to be incorrect; the consequences of hypoglycemic events are distinctly different between adults and children; risks for diabetic complications are influenced by puberty and the targets of education need to be adjusted to the age and development stage of the patient with diabetes and must include the parents or the care giver.

The parents of a child who is first diagnosed as having a chronic disease like diabetes (including the child) are initially shocked and devastated. They may even feel a sense of guilt and repent their actions of having allowed the child eat sweets excessively. Or some of them who have had a family history might feel guilty of having passed on 'the bad genes' to the child.

An effective family based dietary education program targeted at the dietary modification of the child and their eating habits can only begin when parents are allowed to grieve and come to terms with the diagnosis of their child. It is vital to develop a rapport with the family for an effective and consistent dietary management. Young children including the school aged ones are unable to provide their own diabetes care and middle school and high school students should not be expected to independently provide all of their own diabetes care. Therefore, education regarding diabetes care must be provided to the entire family unit, emphasizing age and developmentally appropriate self-care and integrating this into the child's diabetes management.[14]

The aim should be a gradual transition toward independence in management through middle school and high school.

DIAGNOSIS/PRESENTATION

Although the diagnosis of Type 1 diabetes mellitus is quite simple and straightforward, it may be missed out, since the parents may not recognize the symptoms to be of significant concern initially (polyurea, polyphagia, polydipsia and weight loss). Only when the child is perhaps brought for some other problem or for not gaining weight despite eating well, is the problem clinched after a routine screening test. At times accidental discovery of the disease in children is made when the child is brought to the emergency for diabetic ketoacidosis (DKA), which may occur even in the absence of the above mentioned symptoms.

The American Diabetes Association (ADA) has laid down the criteria for classifying and diagnosing Type 1 diabetes in their position statement (2004) as given in Table 35.1.[15]

In the absence of unequivocal hyperglycemia these criteria should be confirmed by a repeat test on a different day. The oral glucose tolerance test is not recommended in routine use, but may be required in the evaluation of patients when diabetes is still suspected despite normal fasting glucose.

TABLE 35.1: Criteria for diagnosis of type 1 diabetes

1. Symptoms of diabetes and a casual plasma glucose > 200 mg/dl. Casual is defined as any time of the day without regard to time since last meal. The classic symptoms of diabetes mellitus include-polyuria, polydipsia and unexplained weight loss
2. Fasting plasma glucose ≥ 126 mg/dl. Fasting is defined as no caloric intake for at least 8 hours
3. 2-hour plasma glucose ≥ 200 mg/dl during an oral glucose tolerance test. The test should be performed as described by the WHO, using a glucose load of 75 g anhydrous glucose dissolved in water or 1.75 g/kg body weight is ≤ 18 kg.

Source. ADA[15]

In case of symptomatic children, in whom screening is done as a routine, (FPG) 120 mg/dl or a 2-hour plasma glucose ≥ 200 mg/dl, the test should be repeated on the second day to confirm diagnosis. However, in a child symptomatic for diabetes, a random plasma glucose ≥ 200 mg/dl does 'not' require a repeat test.

Glucose tolerance test (GTT) is rarely required in children except when the symptoms are atypical or where plasma glucose values are normal and the diagnosis is uncertain. Type 1 symptoms may present as incidental glycosuria or in an extreme form as diabetic ketoacidosis (DKA). This condition is usually seen in slender prepubertal age group of children. Almost 30% of the type 1 diabetes is known to present with DKA.[16]

MEDICAL NUTRITION THERAPY IN TYPE I DIABETES MELLITUS

The nutritional needs of children with Type 1 diabetes do not differ from those of healthy children. Children with diabetes do not require special food, nor do they need different amounts of vitamins and minerals.[17]

The total caloric intake should be based on the daily requirements of all nutrients based on the individual age which are appropriate for their growth and development

Children with Type 1 diabetes, have to match their food intake to the anticipated time of eating, as they are on injectable insulin. Therefore, the timings of their meals and snack consumption should be at regulated intervals and should be consistent with respect to total number of calories and proportion of carbohydrates, proteins and fats in each meal. As these children are on insulin which is released continuously from the site of injection, care must be taken that the timings of their food and snack intake is spaced such that the child does not land into hypoglycemia between the 3 main meals. Therefore, where intermediate acting insulin is used, in between snacks and a snack at bed time is advocated to prevent hypoglycemia. Similarly, adjustments of their meal pattern should be considered with respect to the activity levels of the child, either planned or spontaneous or even in the event of unexpected illness. All these factors require a well chalked out comprehensive nutrition education and counseling program which forms an important aspect of any successful management of Type 1 diabetes in children.

GOALS OF NURITION THERAPY

The main objectives of tackling a child with type 1 diabetes are:

- *To maintain blood glucose levels as near as possible.*
- *To achieve an ideal weight for height and promote normal physical and emotional growth and development.*
- *To prevent or ameliorate the complications of diabetes which are responsible for most morbidities and mortalities in such patients.*
- *To inculcate good dietary habits for good health.*

The first objective being that of maintaining normoglycemia to prevent long-term complications, a controlled diet intake has short-term benefits in avoiding large swings of blood glucose levels allows easier stabilization and minimizes episodes of hypoglycemia and ketoacidosis. This may seem a difficult task for the parents to follow as is for the child, all the same it has to be impressed upon them that a 'free diet' has its own problems in a way that it may become over restricted in carbohydrates especially where parents might curtail to an extent more than desired by eliminating many foods, or the opposite can happen resulting in excess intake. The need is for a regulated carbohydrate intake with increased dietary fiber in order to lengthen the postprandial glucose curves, thus avoiding hyperglycemic peaks and urinary loss. There is no evidence to suggest that a low carbohydrate intake is beneficial, but quite a bit to suggest that it is harmful.[18]

Energy Requirement

Mostly a child diagnosed with Type 1 diabetes for the first time presents with weight loss, therefore the dietary prescription should begin with estimating calorie requirements to restore and maintain an appropriate body weight and allow for normal growth and development.[19] Of course the calorie requirement will vary with age, height, weight and sex as well as physical activity, season of the year and stage of puberty. As per the American diabetes Association (ADA) position statement,[20] the nutrient recommendations for children and adolescents are based on requirements for all healthy children and adolescents as there is no research on this aspect so far. They should adopt a healthy life style which ensures adequate intake of all vitamins and minerals along with a good fiber and moderate fat content. According to a study on dietary intake of 4–9 years old children with type 1 diabetes, in 1996, it was found that although the calories, vitamins and minerals were adequate, the fiber intake was low.[20] Moreover, most of them consumed levels of saturated fats well above the National Cholesterol Education Program (NCEP) recommendations.[21]

Carbohydrate Requirements

The recommendations for carbohydrate allowances for children has been varying from 40%–55% by different authors from time to time. Earlier 40% of the total energy was recommended from carbohydrates, but lately the British Diabetes Association in 1980,[22] and updated in 1992 (Dietary recommendations for people with diabetes: An update for the 1990s[23] recommends at least 50% of the energy to be derived from carbohydrates mainly fiber rich polysaccharides. The British Diabetes Association has specific recommendations for children and adolescents with diabetes, according to who the total carbohydrates should never be below 40%–45% of the total energy as is generally in a mixed family diet. The committee on nutrition of the ADA in 1986 has recommended that carbohydrates should comprise 50%–60% of daily allowances of calories.[24] These recommendations are based on the fact that increase in dietary carbohydrates, without increasing the calories may actually increase sensitivity to insulin and lead to improved glucose tolerance in both Type 1 and 2 diabetes.[25,26]

Studies using diets containing 60%–85% of energy from carbohydrates have shown good control over the insulin dependent diabetes and well tolerated. With adequate treatment carbohydrate handling is resorted to a state similar to that of normal subjects.[26] In addition, distribution between carbohydrates, fats and proteins will differ depending upon the age of the child. Breast fed infants will obtain approximately 55% of energy from fats, 5% from proteins and

40% from carbohydrates, whereas, a 5-year-old may derive 35% energy from fat, 15% from proteins and 50% from carbohydrates. Traditionally, the concept of a diabetic diet was based more on a restrictive approach unlike in the present era, where a more holistic family based approach is recommended. Carbohydrates can be increased but from fiber based sources and proportionate reduction in fat sources is advised. Assuming that carbohydrates provide more than 40% of the energy, the formula used is 120 g carbohydrate (10 g for every year of life), e.g. a 2-year-old boy should have 120 + 20 g (140g) carbohydrate daily. His estimated average energy is about 1200 calories; therefore a minimum of 47% energy needs to be derived from carbohydrates.[27]

CARBOHYDRATE DISTRIBUTION FOR JUVENILE DIABETICS (CARBOHYDRATE COUNTING)

Most children of the preschool age group may find the bulk of the high fiber, high carbohydrate diet difficult to comply with, therefore to begin with a slightly lower carbohydrate with a little higher fat intake regime may be advised. Gradually, the high carbohydrate, high fiber foods can be introduced once the child gets accustomed to the diabetic regime. Adolescent boys needing almost 2600–3000 calories may even require 400 g of carbohydrates per day, which may be appropriate during the rapid growth period of adolescents. The same requirements may be lesser, i.e. about 200–300 g in case of adolescent girls who mature earlier and therefore may need lesser amounts.[28]

In short, if a child takes a regulated diet with selected protein sources of milk and pulses or lean meat/chicken, a moderate fat intake and a generous helping of vegetables and fruits along with prescribed cereal amounts, an adequate energy intake can be ensured, providing a good diabetic control with insulin.

Ideally the carbohydrate distribution should be such that it is distributed between 3 main meals and 2 mid meals and one bed time snack or drink. Bed time snack is a good idea and recommended as it can prevent the child from going into hypoglycemia at midnight or early morning. It is advisable that this late night or bed time snack be of unrefined carbohydrate with high fiber content and some protein, e.g. a whole wheat bread sandwich or toast with a glass of milk. A list of Indian foods with carbohydrate exchange of different food groups are given in Table 35.4.[29]

The distribution of carbohydrates also depends upon the type of insulin, e.g. short acting, long acting, intermediate or a combination of both. Generally, children treated with one injection of intermediate or long acting insulin with or without short acting one, require approximately an equal distribution of carbohydrate between different meal timings and activity.

Current recommendations are increasingly supporting the concept of dose adjustment for normal eating (DANE) which implies that total carbohydrate content of meals and snacks is more important in determining the post prandial glucose response and this in determining the pre meal insulin dosage.[30] The concept of carbohydrate counting is being encouraged in many centers dealing with pediatric population. This allows the users greater flexibility in the timings of meals, the amount of food eaten at each meal and the selection of specific foods. The objective of using carbohydrate counting system is to coordinate the food intake (carbohydrates) by matching the peak activity of insulin with peak levels of glucose resulting from the digestion and absorption of food.[31] This allows counting of only carbohydrates of the food, thereby allowing precise adjustment of premeal short acting insulin using an insulin/carbohydrate ratio.

The insulin carbohydrate ratio is based on the assumption that carbohydrate intake is the main consideration in determining meal related insulin requirements, together with SMBG.[32]

Therefore, it is now recommended that it is better to derive an insulin regime that suits the individual child's eating schedule or life style. It should be rather tailored to the food intake and not vice versa. So to begin with the care provider has to determine the right dose for an 'average' day of the child's routine, implying that the child be allowed to eat a normal healthy diet, maintaining the eating timings daily and using the blood glucose parameters, the timing and dose of insulin injection can be adjusted.

In the case of children and adolescents consideration should be given for the child's appetite when calculating the calorie requirements and nutrition prescription. The adequacy can be evaluated by following the weight gain and growth patterns as per the standard growth charts, on a regular basis. With holding food or forcing the child to eat without appetite should be avoided. But care should be taken to adjust the energy intake such that in case the child is overweight, it may be reduced and increased if the child has had initial weight loss.

GLYCEMIC INDEX

Glycemic index (GI) is an important term often related to foods or diets prescribed for diabetics. GI is defined as the area under the blood glucose response curve for a specific food, expressed as a percentage of the area after taking the same amount of carbohydrate as glucose.[33] In simple words, it implies to what extent the blood glucose can rise after eating a particular carbohydrate diet, and these responses can differ from one carbohydrate source to the other. Foods with a low GI cause less of a spike in past meal blood glucose than those with a high GI. So much so that the response of blood glucose to the same carbohydrate food can vary if prepared in two different ways or given in two different forms. For instance, a pureed apple can cause a greater increase in GI or blood glucose rise as compared to when an apple is eaten raw as such. Similarly rice flour or ground rice can induce a higher response as compared to rice eaten as such in boiled from. This is because the effect of food is altered by the dietary fiber which might be broken down, or certain enzyme inhibitors like lecithin, phytates, tannins, fats, proteins or the structure of the food itself. Moreover, the GI of the same food has been shown to have varied response if eaten in a mixed from in a meal or when eaten in isolation.[34] Fruits and milk may cause a lower GI response as compared to most starches, while sucrose will cause a glycemic response similar to that of bread, rice and potato. But all said and done about various glycemic responses to different foods, the consensus now according to the ADA is that whatever the glycemic index of any food is, it is the total amount of carbohydrate consumed which is important, irrespective of the source of those carbohydrates.[35] It is therefore important that the dietician when counseling the parents of the diabetic child evaluate each meal as a whole, since the fiber, fat and protein content as well as the method of food preparation, influences the glycemic response to the carbohydrate content of the whole meal.

In general, cereals like wheat and rice and root vegetables like potato, carrots, etc. have a high glycemic index (65%–75%). Fruits have an intermediate glycemic index of 45%–55% whiloe legumes and lentils such as dried beans, peas, green gram and Bengal gram have a low glycemic index of 30%–40%.[36] The glycemic index of various Indian foods are presented in Table 35.2

TABLE 35.2: Glycemic index of common Indian foods

Food item	GI index	Food item	GI index
Cereal Products		***Miscellaneous***	
Bread	70	Peanuts	13
Millets	71	Potato chips	51
Rice (white)	72	Tomato soup	38
Wheat flour	70		
Vegetables			
Dairy Products			
Beans	79	Milk	33
Potato	70	Ice cream	36
Sweet potato	48	Curd	36
Yam	51		
Fruits			
Beetroot	64	Apple	39
Dried Legumes			
Banana	69	Soyabeans	43
Orange	40	Rajma	29
Sugars			
Bengal gram	47	Glucose	100
Green gram	48	Fructose	20
Black gram	48	Maltose	105
Sucrose	59	Honey	87

Source: Jenkins, et al. 1981; Am J Clin Nutr, 34:362[33] Raghuram, et al. Diabetes Bull, 7:64;1987[36]

Fiber

The role of fiber in a healthy diet was under rated in the past century, but gradually since the past two decades or so, a great deal of focus is laid on its importance regarding the physiology of the gastrointestinal tract like digestion, absorption and metabolism of many nutrients. There are mainly 2 types of fiber present in vegetables and grains- the insoluble fiber which includes hemicelluloses, cellulose and lignin. But there are a number of foods like fruits, pulses, vegetables, etc. which have soluble fiber (i.e. water soluble) such as pectins, guar and storage polysaccharides. Ingestion of any carbohydrates with dietary fiber results in a decreased rise in blood glucose concentration as compared to a diet with little or negligible dietary fiber like in processed and refined foods.

The British Diabetic Association recommends a fiber intake of 2 g/100 kcals/d,[36] but since this amounts to a very high bulk for children, an intake of at least 1 g/100 cals/d has been accepted. This amounts to around 20–30 g dietary fiber in the whole day's diet which can be achieved by encouraging the consumption of unrefined cereals, grains and legumes, fruits and vegetables. Soluble fibers also have a beneficial effect on blood lipids, reducing LDL and VLDL cholesterol, while maintaining HDL cholesterol, while maintaining HDL cholesterol. However, very large doses of fiber too may not be always helpful as it can hinder the absorption of certain minerals like calcium, iron and zinc due to the high levels of phytates in high fiber foods. It is postulated that the attenuated rise in blood glucose concentration when a soluble guar is added to the ingested carbohydrate is due to delayed rather than incomplete absorption of carbohydrates.[36] On the other hand, cereal fibers which are mainly insoluble have long-term effects on glucose tolerance. Therefore patients with IDDM consuming a high fiber diet of at least 20 g of crude fiber, show improved postprandial glycemia but no change in fasting glycemia. The fiber contents of various Indian foods are provided in Table 35.3A and 35.3B.[37]

Proteins

The protein intake of children with diabetes actually remains the same as for any normal child. Any excess protein consumed above the normal requirement, enters the carbon pool and ultimately is converted into glucose or fat. This is about 10%–20% of the total daily energy intake which works out to be around 0.9–2.2 g/kg body wt/day. The protein can be a mix of animal and plant source. But care should be taken not to stress only on animal protein due to the risk of high fat content also of such foods like whole milk, meat, pork, etc.

Fat

Fat is essential to some extent in the diet of children and adolescents due to their ongoing growth and development besides providing adequate vitamins and essential fatty acids. Patients with IDDM and even NIDDM have also shown an increased prevalence of macrovascular disease, the main clinical consequences of which are atherosclerosis of the coronary, cerebral and large arteries of the lower extremities. Since excess dietary fat which includes saturated fat, cholesterol and total cholesterol, is also linked to an increased lipid profile, which is a major determinant of atherosclerosis, care should be taken that the percentage of fat from total calories should not exceed 30%, less than 7% from saturated fat and cholesterol not to exceed 200 mg/d. These are the recommendations laid down by the National Cholesterol Education Program step II (NCEP Step II) guidelines.[38] This can be achieved by encouraging.

- Use of skimmed or semi skimmed milk and milk products.
- Reduced consumption of fast finger foods like wafers, chips and other fried foods.
- Use of baked, steamed or grilled food preparations.
- Use of fish and poultry instead of red meat.
- Reduced total visible fat used in meal preparation.
- Avoidance of 'topping up' food dishes with cream butter, etc.

Sodium

Sodium is commonly used as common salt in all Indian foods besides being present in all bakery products and other processed foods. As high sodium foods are strongly linked to metabolic diseases like hypertension, it is prudent to maintain the levels in the day's diet to a moderate amount of 2.5–3 g/d, which is also recommended for any healthy

TABLE 35.3A: List of vegetables with their insoluble, soluble, and total fiber content

Fiber food source	Insoluble fiber (g /100 gram)	Soluble fiber (g /100 gram)	Total dietary fiber (g /100 gram)
Bitter gourd	13.5	3.1	16.6
Field beans	9.3	2.1	11.4
Broad beans	7.3	0.8	8.3
Beet root	5.4	2.4	7.8
Cluster beans	6.1	0.6	6.7
Green plantain	5.8	0.2	6.0
Carrot	4.1	1.6	5.7
Onion	0.9	1.1	5.7
Fenugreek leaves	4.2	0.7	4.9
Lady fingers	3.0	1.3	4.3
Cauliflower	3.5	0.7	4.2
Spinach	3.5	0.6	4.1
Potato	2.6	0.6	3.2
French beans	3.0	0.1	3.1

Refer.[37] (Khannum F, Swamy S)

TABLE 35.3B: List of fresh fruits, nuts and seeds with their insoluble, soluble, and total fiber content

Fiber source	Insoluble fiber content (g /100 gram)	Soluble fiber content (g /100 gram)	Total fiber content (g /100 gram)
Fruits			
Kiwi	2.61	0.80	3.39
Apple, with skin	2.00	0.70	2.70
Banana	1.80	0.60	2.40
Pear	1.10	1.30	2.40
Strawberry	1.70	0.60	2.30
Peach	1.20	0.80	2.00
Mango	1.06	0.74	1.80
Plum, fresh	0.70	0.80	1.50
Pineapple, fresh	1.10	0.10	1.20
Grapes	0.60	0.40	1.00
Pomegranate	0.49	0.11	0.60
Watermelon	0.30	0.20	0.50
Nuts, seeds			
Flax seed	10.15	12.18	22.33
Almonds	10.10	1.10	11.20
Sesame seed	5.89	1.90	7.79
Brazil nuts	4.10	1.30	5.40

Refer.[37] (Khannum F, Swamy S)

child. This implies not making the food bland or unpalatable by restricting sodium too much but by restricting processed foods available in the take away joints.

SUCROSE FOR DIABETIC CHILDREN

A normal child usually consumes about 20%–30% of his total carbohydrates in the form of simple sugar, which is incorporated in his milk, beverages and some other sweetened products like biscuits, cakes, ice creams or any other sweet. For a child newly diagnosed with Type 1 diabetes, to stop sugar completely and at the same time increase his complex carbohydrates in the form of high fiber cereals, vegetables, etc. may be quite a trauma, as would be for the parents. Besides, it may not be possible for him to accept a higher bulk in his diet, with the result there may be quite a dilemma for the parents to convince the child to eat and the child may just refuse to accept food at all. This could further destabilize his insulin regime and consequently pose a challenge for the family and the care providers to achieve his glycemic control.

In the light of this problem, many authors have now recognized that some sugar taken as a mixed meal may be safe without having any adverse affects on the glycemic levels, provided the amount of sugar is adjusted or accounted for in the total day's ration of cholesterol allowed[39, 40]. As already mentioned earlier, ADA recommendations also emphasize the significance of the total carbohydrates consumed rather than the 'source' of carbohydrates.[15] Therefore, the inclusion of a controlled amount of sugar (approximately in the diet of children with Type 1 diabetes can have some benefits like.

- Child is able to accept the diet which will not be too different from the rest of his peers.
- Dietary compliance becomes more easy and practical.
- Brings in more variety, palatability and acceptance.
- Can avoid use of sugar substitutes.

SWEETNERS

The role of sweeteners has become quite significant in the diet of most diabetics for whom 'sugar free' concept is just impossible or difficult to adhere to. This seems even more applicable in the case of children who may be consuming at least 20%–50% of their carbohydrates from sugars alone. In order to overcome this problem and to be able to achieve optimum compliance to the dietary regime, sweeteners have been well accepted and proven to be totally safe for both diabetic and normal children.[41] The sweeteners are available in two forms-nutritive and non-nutritive. The nutritive sweeteners are fructose, sorbitol and xylitol. Fructose is as sweet as sugar and is present as a constituent of many fruits and vegetables and honey in the form of free monosaccharides. However these may not be suitable for children due to its slightly adverse affects on serum lipids. Sorbitol is a sugar alcohol (polyol) half as sweet as sucrose but its use has been debatable to substitute in place of sucrose. Xylitol is also as sweet as sucrose and widely distributed in fruits and vegetables, but due to its adverse affects on the GIT, its usefulness has been debated.

Among the nonnutritive sweeteners, saccharine, aspartame and acesulfame K are commonly available and recommended by Food and Drug Administration (FDA) in the USA. Saccharine is known to leave a slightly bitter taste after consuming it, while aspartame, the most commonly used and recommended to be safe with an acceptable daily intake (ADI) being 50 mg/kg/d. As per the FDA guidelines the amount generally used ranges from 2–4 mg/kg/d, even if used consistently which falls well below the acceptable daily intake (ADI).[42] However, in routine use I would recommend against using any artificial sweeteners in case of children, especially in order to guard against any unforeseen repercussions of its prolonged use. Moreover, once a child is given to understand that these sweeteners are safe for him/her, there is a tendency of their getting dependent on them routinely. I would recommend to teach the child to get used to not taking sugar at all, or in case occasionally even if he/she might want to consume simple sugar in any form it should not make a significant difference as long as the total carbohydrates are adjusted as per the weight and age of the child.

INSULIN REGIME AND DIET PLAN

Prescription of a diet plan for a diabetic is based primarily on the type of insulin regime that is provided to any child. The commonly used regimes are:[27]

1. Single dose of isophane injection daily (no longer used).
2. Multiple injection therapy: This involves 3–5 injections per day before breakfast, lunch and evening meal and isophnae insulin before bed and or before breakfast.
3. Twice a day injection (one before breakfast and one before dinner).

This is routinely used and comprises mixed soluble and insoluble and isophane insulin or mixed insulin analogue and isophane insulin.

Isophane and isophane mixed insulin: Meals are planned such that the carbohydrates are distributed at regular intervals to avoid hypo or hyperglycemia. For optimum postprandial blood sugars the injection is given at least 30 minutes before a meal. Generally a five meal pattern of 3 main meals and 2 in between snacks and perhaps one at bed time in recommended.

Analogue and isophane mixed insulin: With this regime the meal plan is same as above except that meals can be taken directly after injecting.

Insulin analogue in multiple injection therapy: In this regime also meals can be had directly after injecting. This has a short period of action and so more appreciated by children and parents as in between snacks are not required, especially in teenage girls trying to control their weight.

Multiple injection therapy: This regime offers the advantage of more flexibility in meal and snack timings and the short acting insulin is given prior to eating.

EXERCISE AND HYPOGLYCEMIA

The role of exercise in long-term control of diabetes in children and adults is well recognized. It lowers the blood glucose levels by increasing the non-insulin dependent uptake of glucose by the cells and increasing the insulin sensitivity. In case when children are involved in strenuous outdoor activities or sports, the amount of insulin can be decreased accordingly or additional exchange of carbohydrate say, 10–20 g may be given in some form of complex carbohydrate before an event or in some cases may be given even after (Table 35.4). In events like hiking, swimming or a game of cricket, extra-carbohydrate exchange can be given in the form of some unrefined cereal, e.g. Whole wheat bread sandwich or cereal with milk as this will help to release glucose into the blood stream gradually. It is important for the parents to be aware that they should watch out for signs of post exercise hypoglycemia which can occur even several hours after the exercise, possibly extending to midnight. It would be advisable in such cases to give an exchange or two of unrefined carbohydrate with some protein base at bed time to avoid any such eventuality. A list of noncarbohydrate foods that can be allowed are given in Table 35.5. Seasonal alterations in sports activities and type of sports in which children are involved may need frequent adjustments to allow the child to participate in school team and individual sports. For this initially frequent self blood glucose monitoring (SBGM) is required to determine the dose of insulin to be adjusted along with the amount and type of food to be given. If blood glucose levels are < 100 mg/dl during the period of exercise, 15 g of carbohydrate can be given as a readily absorbable sugar. This can be in the form of electrolyte containing sports drink. These are quite helpful in preventing hypoglycemia both during and after weight exercise. The dose of insulin may be decreased rather than increasing calories as this regime can help optimum weight management for all diabetic children. Studies in pediatric population have shown that discouraging sedentary activities such as television or computer monitors are an effective method to ensure physical activity and encourage weight loss in inactive children.

To sum up the recommendations for all children with Type 1 diabetes are:[15]

- Children with Type 1 diabetes should adhere to a minimum of 30–60 minutes of moderate physical activity.

- SBGM before exercise should be done (parents can help in case of younger children). A suggested intake of 10–15 g of carbohydrate depending upon the age of the child can be given if blood glucose falls < 100 mg/dl; for vigorous activity of more than 30 minutes, additional 15 g of carbohydrate may be given.
- For prolonged vigorous exercise hourly blood glucose monitoring during the exercise as well as after the event is advisable.
- At the onset of a new sports season, frequent blood sugar monitoring during the 12 hour post exercise period should be done to adjust insulin dosage.
- Physical exercise (especially for overweight or obese) children and adolescents should be encouraged and sedentary activity discouraged.

Hypoglycemia is an important complication in most diabetic children and a cause of great concern to parents. It is generally a result of a temporary rise in insulin in the blood due to either excess dose or delayed or refusal of food intake, increased exercise or unusual exposure to cold. Delayed meals due to unscheduled assignments or emergencies can also contribute to hypoglycemia in which case it is a good idea for such children to carry a pack of some snack to be consumed to tide over such temporary crisis. The parents and children need to be explained common features of hypoglycemia to be able to tackle the situation promptly without landing into emergency situations as is commonly seen. These include sweating, pallor, and dizziness, restlessness at night or waking and altered behavior, e.g. sudden tantrums or depression.

Treatment of hypoglycemia generally involves giving an easily absorbable carbohydrate in a concentrated form, e.g. sugar or glucose. Diabetics are generally advised to keep some sugar cubes handy with them always. The dictum should be 'if in doubt, treat as hypoglycemia', especially so for a lay person who may not be sure of the hypoglycemia status. In severe cases, injectables like glucagon is required to be administered.[41] Glucagon reverses the action of insulin and is a secretion of the alpha cells of the pancreas. It is injected just like insulin and parents can be taught how and when to use it. It liberates glucose from liver glycogen, resulting in a rise in blood sugar thus reversing the affect of hypoglycemia.

However, parents need to be aware that children and adolescents may even take advantage of the existence of a state of hypoglycemia, which warrants immediate feeding. They may attempt to 'fake' hypoglycemia as an attention seeking behavior and getting sweets or any food of their own choice. In such situations a spot blood glucose monitoring can give a true picture.

CONSIDERATIONS IN DIFFERENT STAGES OF CHILDHOOD

Infants

Diabetes during infancy is generally of transient type ad very rare. Insulin may be required in minimum doses. These children should have their carbohydrate allowances based on milk feeds which should be frequent and regular. Breastfeeding should be encouraged to be continued. Their fluid requirement of 150–20 ml/kg body weight can be met by breast feeds or top feeds (150 ml breast milk will contain approximately 10 g of carbohydrate). After 5–6 months complementary feeding should be initiated with noncarbohydrate sources like pureed vegetables and fed by spoon. As the child gets acclimatized to spoon feeding, carbohydrate exchanges from cereals and pulses can be initiated. To begin with, 5 g of carbohydrate exchange can be offered, e.g. 5 g of rice or 25 g of potato. By 10–12 months, the amounts can be gradually increased to meet the energy and protein requirements during their growth and development. By one year the child should be having about 90 g of carbohydrate as solids, the remaining coming from milk. Since the first year of life is the period of most rapid growth with constantly changing eating patterns, the parents need to be inconstant follow-up with their dieticians for periodic counseling and reassurance regarding the child's feeding schedule. They need to be counseled regarding signs of hypo or hyperglycemia. In conditions of recurrent hypoglycemic spells, it may be necessary to give cereal based carbohydrates (e.g. rice) earlier than 3–4 months to prevent nocturnal hypoglycemia.

TODDLERS

Till 1 year of age whole milk can be offered but by 2 years semi skimmed milk can be started as by now the child would be on a full solid diet besides milk. This can continue till about 5 years after which skimmed milk or toned milk should be started, so as to reduce the total fat content of the diet. Gradually fiber rich carbohydrates can also be increased. There can be toddler food refusal syndromes and parents can face a tough time coping with their tantrums. In such cases slight variations in the menu or food choices can be made to avoid hypoglycemia. Too much fuss and forced feeding should be discouraged. After a long gap of food refusal with the child going into hypoglycemic levels, most often they accept food gradually. Most children on insulin feel excessively hungry- this could be due to poor control or sugar being lost in the urine. Re-evaluation of the dietary regime should be done and if required, adjust the dose of insulin as following the DANE concept.

SCHOOL CHILDREN

By the time the child stares going to school, he or she should be taught to follow a prescribed diet schedule and become as independent as possible. The carbohydrate portions can be divided into 5 meals and snacks beginning with breakfast, a mid meal packed snack and or a fruit till the child is back home for lunch.

The school teachers/authorities should be informed about the diabetic status of the child and be apprised of the importance of in between snack for such children to avoid risk and symptoms of hypoglycemia. If possible school should be able to provide suitable food or snack to deal with any crisis of hypoglycemia if at all it occurs. The child on his part also should be made aware of the importance of maintaining a regulated eating schedule and regarding the foods that he/she can take freely or need to avoid.

In case of social eating, the diabetic child should not be discouraged to participate e.g. a trip going for a picnic or some children's party. However, school authorities or the hostess if at home, should take care to include some such food/dish like a sandwich, or some peanut packing, e.g. on toast or cheese preparation which the child can take. If parents can co ordinate with the host regarding the menu offered, the child may be allowed to eat moderate helping from the party, and the carbohydrate counting can be adjusted in the latter part of the day, thus maintaining the recommended regime. Regarding consumption of sweets, children with diabetes mellitus need to be positively reinforced an explained the risks of going into hypoglycemia. They can be reassured that during exercise or some sports activity, some sweet may be offered. But still if the child is unable to cooperate or is on habitual bingeing, the services of a child psychologist need to be sought as this could suggest underlying stress.

ADOLESCENTS

Adolescent period being one of stress, exploring and rebellion, it might be quite a challenge for parents to cope with them and bring them to be convinced regarding their recommended dietary lifestyle. Snacking and eating out include use of alcohol and substance can be an added problem which needs to be tackled very patiently, yet firmly by parents and if required seek help of their psychologist or psychiatrist.

It is recommended that these children be appropriately counseled regarding the carbohydrate content of various portion sizes of various foods so that they can be aware of the choice of foods and also the importance of good control on their weight, e.g. a packet of chips may provide 10 g of carbohydrate and 150 calories, but an apple also will provide 10 g carbohydrates but only 50 calories. The carbohydrate exchange of various food groups with their portion sizes are presented in Table 35.4[35]. This table can help the parents select and interchange equivalent foods within the prescribed amounts of carbohydrates and calories.

The prescribed amount of calories for children with diabetes generally ranges from 1000 kcals to 2000 Kcals or even more depending on their weight, blood sugar levels and age. Annexure 1 gives in detail the exchanges and their portion sizes along with calories allowed at different levels and sample menus recommended.

TABLE 35.4: Portion size of carbohydrate and calorie exchange of various foods

Food Group	Foods	Carbohydrate Exchange (g)	Calories (Kcals)	Amount Raw (g)	Number/Size
Cereals	Rice, milled	20	100	30	1 serving (med)
	Rice flakes	20	100	30	1 serving
	Wheat atta	20	100	30	1 No.
	Wheat Maida	22	104	30	1 No.
	Bread brown	15	100	30	2 No.
	Bread white	15	75	30	2 No.
	Suji	20	85	25	1 serving (med)
	Dalia	20	100	30	1 serving (med)
	Maize,dry	20	100	30	1 Roti
Pulses	Beng gram	15	100	30	1 katori (med)
	Rajma	18	100	30	1 Katori (med)
	Moong dal/ whole	18	100	30	1 Katori (med)
	Soyabean	10	200	50	2 Katori (small)
	Red gram dal	17	100	30	1 Katori (med)
	Lentil	18	100	30	1 Katori
Milk, Milk Products	Milk, buffalo	10	230	200 ml	1 glass (med)
	Milk, cow's	10	134	200 ml	1 glass (med)
	Curd, cow's milk	6	120	200 ml	1 glass (med)
	Khoa, cow's milk	6	100	25 g	1 cube small
	Khoa, buffalo milk	5	100	25 g	1 cube small
	Skim milk powder, cow's milk	12	90	25 g	5 tsp
Roots and Tubers	Potato	22	100	100 g	2 medium
	Onion, big	10	50	100 g	2 medium
	Onion, small	10	60	100 g	4 medium
	Carrot	20	100	200 g	4 medium
	Radish, white	6	30	200 g	1 big
	Radish, pink	15	65	200 g	1 big

Contd...

Contd...

Food Group	Foods	Carbohydrate Exchange (g)	Calories (Kcals)	Amount Raw (g)	Number/Size
	Turnip	6	30	100 g	2–3 medium
	Colocasia	20	100	100 g	4–5 medium
	Yam, ordinary	25	100	100 g	5–6 medium
	Arrowroot flour	25	80	25 g	1 serving
	Sweet potato	30	100	100 g	2 medium
Vegetables-A	Brinjal, gourd veg/ leafy veg/pumpkin/ cauliflower/tinda	Negligible	Negligible	150 g	1 serving medium
Other Vegetables	Beans, peas, tomato	10 g	50	50–100 g	1 small serving
Fruits	Apple	10 g	50	75 g	1 small
	Banana	10	50	30 g	¼ small
	Grapes	10	50	100 g	20 No.
	Guava Papaya	10 10	50 50	100 g 120 g	1 medium 2 slices, med.
	Mango Pear Watermelon Pineapple Orange Melon, musk Plum	10 10 10 10 10 10 10	50 50 50 50 50 50 50	75 g 100 g 175 g 100 g 100 g 300 g 120 g	1 small 1 medium ¼ small 2 slices round 1 big 6–7 slices 4 medium
Animal Foods	Egg/chicken/meat/fish	Nil	100	-----	2/75g/75g/75g

Source: TC Raghuram, Swaran Pasricha, Sharma RD, Diet and Diabetes;National Institute of Nutrition, ICMR ,Hyderabad 1998[35]

COMPLICATIONS OF DIABETES MELLITUS

The common complications occurring among diabetic children are:

Hypoglycemia

Main causes of hypoglycemia and its management are already discussed earlier in this chapter.

Diabetic Ketoacidosis

This occurs as a consequence of absolute or relative insulin deficiency resulting in hyperglycemia and an accumulation of ketone bodies in the blood with subsequent metabolic acidosis. It is one of the commonest causes of emergency admissions in a Pediatric Center. Quite often DKA is the first presentation of a child being newly diagnosed with Type 1 diabetes mellitus. In a known diabetic child, the most common cause is omission of insulin dose, intercurrent illness, trauma, surgery or any other stress related factor. Children coming with recurrent episodes of DKA need special attention. These are the group who periodically default on their regular insulin injections or fail to adhere to the recommended dietary regime. The cause for this could be underlying eating disorders or depression which might warrant psychiatric intervention.

Illness and Hyperglycemia

Illness of any kind in a child with Type 1 diabetes also tends to lead to hypoglycemia and consequently DKA. Vomiting, nausea and pain abdomen may frequently be associated in most children. In such cases insulin should be continued with the dose being either increased or supplemented with short acting one. Dietary carbohydrates need to be continued or replaced with fluids of equal carbohydrate content, e.g. lemonade with sugar, milk, drinking chocolate with sugar or a biscuit or some soup with toasted bread and butter. These can be given orally in sips gradually over an hour or two and when settled, may slowly be brought back to the original schedule. If the child does not improve or vomiting persists, hospitalization should be sought.

During episodes of acute illness children avoid eating for prolonged periods. In such situations, blood levels tend to be high; therefore insulin doses should be continued. Carbohydrate should not be restricted to control hyperglycemia, but the insulin doses should be adjusted to the blood sugars. At least 70%–80% of the normal requirement should be given. This can be done by small frequent doses of rapidly absorbed carbohydrates in liquid form. Cold drinks without fizz can be given to prevent dehydration. For instance, on a diet requirement of 180 g carbohydrates, which is otherwise distributed between 3 main meals and 3 snacks. 35–45 g carbohydrates can be given as hourly drink between breakfast and lunch, 45–50 g between lunch and evening meal and 50–55 g between evening meal and night time.

TABLE 35.5: Noncarbohydrate foods allowed

Protein Foods	*Meats*–Lean meat, chicken, fish, egg (white) *Cheese*–Processed or cottage cheese (in moderation)
Fruits	Lemon, gooseberries, guava, avocado, pear, water/musk melon
Vegetables	Cabbage, broccoli, cauliflower, all green leafy vegetables, Radish, onions, mushrooms, beans, peas, tomato, salads
Beverages	Clear soups, lemonade, unsweetened tomato juice, sugar free fizzy drinks
Fats	Fried foods and cream to be used in moderation Low fat spreads, vegetable oils, butter, ghee grilling, baking steaming or pressure cooking to be preferred

Hypertension

In adults hypertension is generally associated with diabetes mellitus and may not be commonly seen among children. Nevertheless, it is advisable that blood pressure monitoring be done for them too and any sign or symptom if observed may be managed accordingly as per the guidelines of dash (dirtary appraoaches to stop hypertension) diet.[34]

SOMOGYI AND DAWN EFFECT

Somogyi effect is described as a rebound hyperglycemia name after the physician who first discovered it. The rebound is in response to undetected hypoglycemia (blood glucose <70 g/dl) which generally around or post midnight. In response to the hypoglycemia, the body releases hormones, glycogen and epinephrine which send signals to the liver to release glucose stores. Consequently, the glucose level can swing too high to cause hyperglycemia. This hyperglycemia generally is detectable towards early morning. Now on monitoring the fasting glucose, a picture of very high sugars is perceived due to which the care giver is prompted to increase the bed time or predinner insulin dose. This would further lead to mid night hypoglycemia and the situation can worsen leading to DKA. This actually was the result of too much insulin circulating in the blood. To ascertain whether it is actually hyperglycemia, or just a rebound effect, the best way to test is to set an alarm for around 2–3 am at night and monitor the blood glucose. Low levels of glucose at this point will signify the Somogyi effect. If this is so, it would mean, reducing the night time insulin and or, ensure a bed time snack preferably protein based; for instance, some cereal milk mix, cottage cheese or some nuts or even curd.

Dawn effect also has features of early morning hyperglycemia as the name suggests, but this is not due to rebound effect of hyperglycemia. Actually, this phenomenon occurs with normal subjects too when counter regulatory hormones like growth hormones, cortisol and catecholamines cause the glucose levels to rise. But, in diabetes, due to lack of sufficient insulin in the bloodstream, the glucose levels are not controlled, thus presenting with hyperglycemia in the morning. To prevent this phenomenon, it is recommended that a diabetic child

- Should exercise or indulge in some sport later in the day, so that more of glucose lowering effect occurs at night.
- Limit bed time carbohydrates and increase protein/ fat based snack (nuts, eggs, cheese).

Nutrition Counseling and Follow-Up

Counseling is an important aspect of management in children with diabetes. A positive approach to meal planning is to encourage family members and other support persons to follow the same life style recommendations as the child with diabetes. A close interaction of the parents or care giver, the child and the diabetes team (which comprises the dietician, the diabetes educator/nurse) is essential to achieve the goals of management in children with diabetes mellitus. The significance of a diabetic team has been emphasised by the landmark Diabetes Control and Complications Trial (DCCT).[43]

The focus of counseling should be based on the goal of:

- Promoting positive behavioral changes.
- Provide healthy meals and snacks.
- Focus on healthy eating habits of the entire family.

The child should be included in the counseling sessions and be reassured that he/she will not be put on a strict 'diet' and may also have some of their favorite foods. They need to be impressed upon, that they are being advised simply to establish a healthy eating plan which is not just for him/her but for the entire family.

Parents can be asked to maintain a food diary which can include all foods and snacks eaten by the child. Initially the child may feel very hungry due to glycosuria, therefore it is important to respond to their stimulated appetite. The appetite of most children stabilizes by 3–4 days of insulin therapy. The concept of exchange list of various carbohydrate foods and carbohydrate counting needs to be explained to the parents/care giver, to help them include a wider variety and liberty in choice of foods while meal planning.

The parents can be given general guidelines like consistency with timing, amount and types of foods and the relationship between food, insulin and exercise and their effect on blood glucose.

The following points need to be considered while counseling parents of a diabetic child and the child:[44]

- Parents should not promote distorted eating to maintain blood glucose control.
- Changes in food choices should be done gradually.
- Children should be include in the counseling sessions on follow-up visits, and be involved in meal planning.
- The child should not be referred to as 'diabetic'.
- Reassure children that many of the usual foods can be included in the meal plan.
- Stress healthy eating habits for the entire family rather than focusing on the child.
- Avoid negative words like 'cannot', 'do not', 'never', 'should not', because these can promote negative attitude and indicate deprivation.
- Omitting or including certain foods on the basis of one single high blood glucose reading is not advisable. It could be stress induced and in such conditions with reduction in stress, hypoglycemia may occur if food is omitted.

Continued nutrition follow-up and education are required every 6 months to 1 year as the child grows and develops. Over a period of time the family also gets trained and experienced in the nutritional management of the child, and the child too gets confident of managing his blood sugars based on his activities and eating pattern.

ANNEXURE

1000 Calories Diabetic Diet

Exchange Distribution per day

Food group	Exchange	Amount (g)	Breakfast	Mid morning	Lunch	Evening	Dinner	Bed time
Cereals	5	150	1	1	1	0.5	1	0.5
Pulses*	1	25	–	–	1	–	–	–
Milk/Curd Toned**	4	400	1.5	–		1.5		1
Fruits	1	100	–	–	–	–	–	–
Veg A&B	2.5	250	–	0.5	1	–	1	–
Fats/Oil	2	10		0.5	1	0.5	1	–

*Pulse exchange is assumed as 25 g/portion size
**Milk exchange is assumed as 100 ml/portion

Percentage Distribution of Calories

Carbohydrates	60% (148 g approx)
Proteins	17% (38 g approx)
Fats	23% (29 g approx)

Sample Menu

Breakfast

Milk/Curd	150 ml
Roti/Cereal	1/30 g

Mid morning

Roti/Parantha	1/1 small (no oil)
Vegetables	1/2 serving (Group A)

Lunch

Roti/Rice	1/30 g'
Curd	100
Vegetables	1 serving
Fruit*	1

Evening

Milk	150 ml
Biscuits	2

Dinner

Roti/Rice	1/25 g
Curd/Dal	100 g/25g
Vegetables	1 serving (Group A)
Salad/Soup	as desired

Bed time

Milk	150 ml

*Fruit may be had any other convenient time also

1200 Calorie Diabetic Diet

Exchange Distribution

Food groups	Exchange	Amount	Breakfast	Mid morning	Lunch	Evening	Dinner	Bed time
Cereals	6	180 g	1	1	2	1.5	1	1.5
Pulses*	1	25 g	–	–	0.5	–	0.5	–
Milk/Curd Toned**	4	400 ml	1.5	–	0.5	1.5	–	0.5
Fruits	2	200 g	–	1	–	1	–	–
Veg. A & B	2.5	250 g	0.5	0.5	0.5	0.5	0.5	–
Fats/Oil	3	15 ml	0.5	0.5	1.0	0.5	0.5	–

*Pulse exchange is assumed as 25 g/portion size
**Milk exchange is assumed as 100 ml/portion

Percentage Distribution of Calories

Carbohydrates 61% (180 g approx)
Proteins 17% (42 g approx)
Fats 22% (35 g approx)

Sample Menu

Breakfast

Milk/Curd 150 ml
Bread slice/Cereal/Roti 2/30 g/1
Mid Morning/Tiffin
Roti/Parantha/Idli/Poha 1/1/2/25 g + I/2 serving vegetables
Frut 1

Lunch

Roti/Rice 2/50 g
Dal/Chicken 1/2K/75 g
Vegetable 1/2 serving
Salad as deired

Evening

Milk 150 ml
Cereal/Poha/Sandwich 1 serving/1slice

Dinner

Roti/Rice 1/25 g
Dal/Chicken/Fish 1/2 Katori/50g/75g
Vegetable 1/2 serving
Salad/Soup as desired
Frut 1

Bed time

Milk/Cheese 150 ml
Biscuits (high fiber) 2

1400 Calorie Diabetic Diet

Exchange List

Food group	Exchange	Amount (g)	Breakfast	Mid morning	Lunch	Evening	Dinner	Bed time
Cereals	7	210	1.5	1.5	2	0.5	2	0.5
Pulses*	2	50	–	–	1	–	1	–
Milk/Curd Toned**	4	400	1.5	–	0.5	1.5	–	0.5
Fruits	2	200	–	1	–	1	–	–
Veg A & B	2.5	200	–	0.5	0.5	0.5	0.5	–
Fats/Oil	2	10	–	0.5	0.5	0.5	0.5	–

*Pulse exchange is assumed as 25 g/portion size
**Milk exchange is assumed as 100 ml/portion

Percent Distribution of Calories

Carbohydrates 61% (214g approx)
Proteins 17% (51.5g approx)
Fats 22% (30g approx)

Sample Menu

Breakfast

Milk 150 ml
Bread/Cereal/ Roti 3/30 g/1
Mid Morning/Tiffin
Roti/Parantha/Idli 1/1/3
*Vegetable 1/2 serving
**Fruit 1

Lunch

Rice/Roti 50 g/2
Dal/Curd/Chicken 1 K/125 g/80 g
Vegetable 1 serving
Salad/Soup as desired

Evening

Milk 150 ml
Sprout/Bread/Besan Pura/Biscuit 20 g/2 slices/20 g/2
Frut 1

Dinner

Roti/Rice 2/50 g
Dal 1 Katori
Vegetable 1/2 serving
Salad as desired

Bed time

Milk 150 ml
Biscuits-(high fiber) 2

*Vegetables from A group can be had in any amount desired
**Fruit may be selected from any low carb group

1600 Calories Diabetic Diet

Food Exchange Distribution

Food groups	Exchange	Amount (g)	Breakfast	Mid morning	Lunch	Evening	Dinner	Bed time
Cereals	8	240	2	1	2	0.5	2	0.5
Pulses*	2	50	–	–	1	–	1	–
Milk/Curd Toned**	5	500 ml	1.5	–	0.5	1.5	–	1.5 0.5
Fruit	2	200	–	1	–	1	–	–
Vegetable A and B	2.5	250	–	0.5	1	–	1	–
Fat/Oil	3	3	0.5	0.5	1	–	1	–

*Pulse exchange is assumed as 25 g/portion size
**Milk exchange is assumed as 100 ml/portion

Percentage of Calories

Carbohydrates 61% (238.6g approx)
Proteins 16% (58.5g approx)
Fats 23% (40g approx)

Sample Menu

Breakfast

Milk (toned) 150 ml
Parantha (stuffed)/Bread/Cereal 1/4/50

Mid morning

Roti/Parantha (stuffed)* 2/1
Vegetable 1/2 serving
Fruit 1

Lunch

Roti/Rice 2/50g or
Roti + Rice 1/25 g
Dal 1 k
Vegetables 1 serving
Salad as desired
Veg Soup as desired

Evening

Milk 150 ml
Biscuits/Cereal 2/10–15g

Dinner

Roti/Rice 2/50 g
Dal 1 katori
Vegetables 1 serving
Salad as desired
Veg Soup as desired
Fruit 1

Bed time

Milk 150 ml
Biscuits 2 or
Cheese Bread 25 g + 1 slice

*Parantha can be made without oil; stuffing with any vegetable of Group A.

1800 Calories Diabetic Diet

Exchange Distribution Per Day

Food groups	Exchange	Amount (g)	Breakfast	Mid morning	Lunch	Evening	Dinner	Bed time
Cereals	9	270	2	2	2	0.5	2	0.5
Pulses*	2	50		–	1	–	1	–
Milk/Curd Toned**	5	500	1.5	–	0.5	1.5	–	1.5
Fruits	2	200	–	1	–	1	–	–
Vegetables A&B	3	300	0.5	0.5	1	–	1	–
Fats/Oil	4	20	1	0.5	1	0.5	1	–

*Pulse exchange is assumed as 25 g/portion size
**Milk exchange is assumed as 100 ml/portion

Percentage Distribution of Calories

Carbohydrates	62% (260 g approx)
Proteins	16% (62 g approx)
Fats	22% (45 g approx)

Sample Menu

Breakfast

Milk/Curd	150 ml
Roti/Bread/Cereal	2/4 slices/60 g
Vegetable	1/2 serving
Oil	0.5 ml

Mid morning

Roti/parantha	2/1
Vegetables	1/2 serving
Fruits	1

Lunch

Roti/Rice	2/50 g
Dal	1 Katori
Paneer	25 g
Salad/Soup	as desired

Evening

Milk	150 ml
Biscuits-/Bread (brown)	2/1 slice
Butter	2.5 g

Dinner

Roti/Rice	2/50 g
Dal/Chicken/Fish	1K/80 g/100 g
Salad/Soup	as desired
Fruit	1

Bed time

Milk	150 ml
Biscuits	2

2000 Calories Diabetic Diet

Exchange Distribution Per Day

Food group	Exchange	Amount (g)	Breakfast	Mid morning	Lunch	Evening	Dinner	Bed time
Cereals	10	300	2	1.5	3	1	3	0.5
Pulses*	3	75	–	0.5		0.5	1 1	–
Milk/Curd Toned**	5	500	1.5	–	0.5	1.5	–	1.5
Fruits	2	200	–	1	–	1	–	–
Veg A&B	3	300	0.25	1.5	1	0.25	1	–
Fats/Oil	4	20	1.0	0.5	1	0.5	1	–

*Pulse is assumed as 25 g/portion size

**Milk is assumed as 100 ml/portion

Percentage Distribution of Calories

Carbohydrates	62% (295 g approx)
Proteins	16% (71.5 g approx)
Fats	22% (46.2 g approx)

Sample Menu

Breakfast

Milk/Curd	250 ml
Roti*/Bread/Cereal	2/4 slices/60g
Vegetables	1/2 serving(Group A)

Mid morning

Roti/Parantha*	2/1
Vegetable	1/2 serving (Group A)
Fruit	1 (low carb)

Lunch

Roti/Rice	3/75g
Dal/Chicken/Fish	1 katori/80g/100g

Evening

Milk	250 ml
Biscuits/Sandwich	3/2 slices
Fruit**	1 (low carb)

Dinner

Roti/Rice	3/75g
Dal/Chicken/Fish	1 katori/80g/100g
Vegetables	1 serving
Salad/Soup	as desired

*Roti/parantha may be made of wheat and gram flour in 2:1 ratio

**Fruit can be had at any convenient time of the day

REFERENCES

1. Davies JL, Kawaguchi Y, Bennet ST, et al. Agenome wide search for human Type 1 diabetes susceptible genes. Nature. 1994;371:130-6.
2. Dahlquist G. Environmental risk factors in human Type 1 diabetes- an epidemiological perspective. Diabetes Metab Rev. 1995;11:37-46.
3. Dahlquist GG, Blom LG, Persson lA, Sandstorm AM, Wall SGL. Dietary factors and the risk of developming insulin dependent diabetes in childhood. BMJ. 1990;300:1302-6.
4. Verge CF, Howard NJ, Irwing L, Simpson JM, Mackerras D, Silinik M. Environmental factors in childhood IDDM. Diabetes Care. 1994;17(12):1381-9.
5. Scott FW, Cow's milk intake and insulin dependent diabetes: is there a relationship? Am J Clin Nutr. 1990;51:489-91.
6. Savilhatti E, Akaerblom HK, Tainio VM, Koskimies S: Children with newly diagnosed insulin dependent diabetes mellitus have increased levels of cow's milk antibodies. Diabetes Res. 1998;47:131-35.
7. Kostraba JN, Cruickshanks KJ, Lawler-Heavner, J et al. Early exposure to cow's milk and solid foods in infancy, genetic predisposition and risk of IDDM. Diabetes. 1993;42:282-95.
8. Sandro Muntoni, Pierluigi Cucco, Gabriella Aru, Francesso Cucco and Sergio Muntoni. Nutritional factors and worldwide incidence of childhood type 1 diabetes. Am J Clin Nutr. 2000;71:1525-9.
9. Donmer G, Thoelka H, Mohnike A, Schneider H. High food supply in perinatal life appears to favor the development of insulin treated diabetes mellitus (ITM) in later life. Exp Clin Endocrinol. 1985;85:1-6.
10. Johansson C, Samvelsson U, Ludvisgson J. A high weight gain early in life is associated with an increased risk of type 1 (insulin dependent) diabetes mellitus. Diabetologia. 1994;34:91-4.
11. Borch-Johnsen K, Mandrip-Poulsen T, Zachau-Christainsen B, Joner G, Christy M, Kastrip K. Nerup J. Relation between breastfeeding and incidence of rates of insulin dependent diabetes mellitus. Lancet ii. 1984;1083-86.
12. Ayer EJ, Hamman RF, gay EC, Lezatte DC, Savitz DA, Kingensmith GJ. Reduced risk of IDDM among breast fed children: the Colorado IDDM Registry. Diabetes. 1998;37:1625-32.
13. Kyvik Ko, Green A, Svendsen A, Montensen K: Breastfeeding and the development of type 1 diabetes mellitus. Diabetes Med. 1992;223-35.
14. Ingersoll GM, Orr D, Herrold AJ, Golden MP: Cognitive maturity and self management in adolescents with insulin dependent diabetes mellitus. J Pediatr. 1986;108:620-23.
15. American Diabetes Association: Diagnosis and classification of diabetes mellitus (Position Statement). Diabetes Care. 2004;27(Suppl 1):S5-S10.
16. Scibili J, Finegold D, Dorman J, Becker D, Drash A. Why do children with diabetes die? Acta Endocrinol Suppl (Copenh). 1986;279:326-33.
17. Talbot JM, Fischer KD. The need for special foods and sugar substitutes by individuals with diabetes mellitus. Diabetes Care. 1978;1:231-40.
18. Belton NR and Farquhar JW. Diabetes mellitus. In: Chemical Pathology and the Sick Child (Eds Clayton BE and Round JM). Oxford: Blackwell Scientific Publications. 1984.pp.265-95.
19. American Diabetec Association Statement, Care of children and adolescents with Type 1 Diabetes. Janet Silverstein, Georgeanna, Klingensmith, Kenneth, Copeland, et al. Diabetes Care. Jan 2005, Vol 28, No. 1.
20. Randecker GA, Smiciklas-Wright H, Mc Kenzie JM, et al. The dietary intake of children with insulin dependent diabetes mellitus. Diabetes Care. 1996;19:1370-74.
21. American Academy of Pediatrics: National Cholesterol Education Program Report of the Expert Panel on Blood Cholesterol Levels in Children and Adolescents, Pediatrics. 1992;89:525-84.
22. Report of the Nutrition Sub-Committee of the Medical Advisory Committee of the British Diabetuic Association; Dietary Recommendations for diabetics for the 1980s. Human Nutr: Appl Nutr. 1982;36A: 378-94.
23. Nutrition Sub-Committee of the Professional Advisory Committee of the British Diab Assoc. Dietary Recommendations for children and adolescents with diabetes. Diabetic Medicine. 1989;6:537-47.
24. American Diabetic Association. Recommendations and principles for individuals with diabetes mellitus: 1986, Diabetes care. 1987;10:126-32.
25. Simpson RW, Mann JI, Eaton J, et al. High carbohydrate diets and insulin dependent diabetics. BMJ. 1979;2:523-25.

26. Simpson RW, Mann JI, Eaton J, et al. Improved glucose control in maturity onset diabetes treated with high carbohydrate modified fat diet. BMJ. 1979;1:1753-56.
27. Vanessa Shaw and Margaret Lawson. Diabetes Mellitus. In: Clinical Pediatric Nutrition 2nd ed Blackwell Publishers. p.127-35.
28. Wolfsdorf JI and Quinn M. Diabetes Mellitus In: Nutrition in Pediatrics, Basic Science and Clinical Applications. Ed Walker WA, Watkins JB. BC Decker Inc. Publishers Hamilton. London. 1997
29. Gopalan C, Rama Sastri BV and Balasubramanian SC. Nutritive Values of Indian Foods. National Institute of Nutrition, ICMR, Hyderabad. 2007.
30. Wolever TM, Hanad S, Chiasson JL, Josse RG, et al. Day to day consistency in amount and source of carbohydrate associated with improved blood glucose control in Type 1 diabetes. J Am Coll Nutr. 1999;18:242-47.
31. Diabetes Care and Education Dietetic Practice Group of the ADA. Meal Planning Approaches for Diabetes Management. 2nd ed. Alexandria, VA: American Dietetics Association. 1994;3.
32. Jenkins DJA, Wolever TMS, Taylor RH, et al. Glycemic index of foods: a physiological basis for carbohydrate exchange. Am. J Clin Nutr. 1981;34:362-66.
33. Jenkins DJA, Taylor RH, Wolever TMS. The diabetic diet, dietary carbohydrate and differences in digestibility. Diabetologia. 1982;23:477-84.
34. Position Statement, American Diabetec Association Nutrition recommendations and principles for people with diabetes mellitus. Diabetes Care. 1994;17:519-22.
35. Raghuram TC, Swaran Pasricha, Sharma RD Diet and Diabetes, National Institute of Nutrition, ICMR, Hyderabad. 1998.
36. Jenkins DJA, Wolevar TMS, Leads AR, et al. Dietary fibers, fiber analogues and glucose intolerance: importance of viscosity. BMJ. 1978;1:1392-94.
37. Farhath Khanum, Swamy S, Sudarshana Krishna KR, Sanathanam K, Viswanathan KR. Dietary fiber content of common fresh and cooked vegetables consumed in India. Plant Foods for Human Nutrition. 2000;55:207-18.
38. National Cholesterol Education Program. Report of the Expert Panel on Blood Cholesterol Levels in children and Adolescents. Pediatrics. 1992;89(Suppl). 525-84.
39. Bantle JP, Laine DC, castle GW, et al. Postprandial glucose and insulin responses to meals containing different carbohydrates in normal and diabetic subjects. N Eng J Med. 1983;309:7-12.
40. Abraira C, Derler J. Large variations of sucrose in constant carbohydrate diets in Type II diabetes. Am J Med. 1988;84:193-200.
41. Wise JE, Keim KS, Huisinga LJ, William PA. Effect of sucrose containing snacks on blood glucose control. Diabetes Care. 1989;12:423-26.
42. Council on Scientific affairs. Aspartame review of safety issues. JAMA. 1985;254:400-02.
43. Drash A. The child, the adolescent and the diabetes control and complications trial. Dibetes Cre. 1993;16:1515-16.
44. Chalmers KH. Diabetes In: Handbook of Pediatric Nutrition 2nd ed. Patricia Queen Samour, Kathy King Helm and Carol E. Lang. Jones and Bartlett Publishers, Massachusetts. 2004.pp.425-51.

36 Dietary Management in Hypoglycemia

If hyperglycemia is a problem of serious consequences, hypoglycemia too is equally significant with regards to normal growth and development of a child. Consequences of hypoglycemia are permanent damage to the central nervous system (CNS), particularly in infants under six months and hence corrective dietary measures need to be taken as soon as the problem is diagnosed.

Hypoglycemia may be asymptomatic or could be associated with features of listlessness, apathy, irritability, pallor, sweating, weakness, hunger, headache, nausea, mental confusion, convulsions and coma. It could vary considerably in their type of presentation and the mechanisms involved. In general the main types of hypoglycemia of dietary interest are:

Glycogen Storage Disease Type I (Glucose -6-phosphatase deficiency).

Glycogen Storage Disease Type III & IV (Debrancher enzyme deficiency).

Leucine Sensitive Hypoglycemia

GLYCOGEN STORAGE DISEASE TYPE I

As we know glycogen is the body's major carbohydrate reserve consisting of glucose molecules linked together into a branched chain. It is synthesized in the liver from glucose and is dependent on adequate glucose-6-phospatase activity. A regular maintenance level of glucose in the blood is required continuously and is essential for normal growth and development.

In this disorder due to the deficiency of the enzyme glucose-6-phosphatase, glucose is not released into the circulation and therefore a regular supply of it has to be ensured through dietary source, mainly carbohydrates. In the absence of continuous supply of dietary carbohydrates, serious consequences like growth retardation, hyperlipidemia and raised plasma uric acid can occur. Regular administration of carbohydrates to maintain normal blood glucose levels helps prevent secondary features of metabolic acidosis and maintain growth.[1]

Management of these children in infancy involves continuous IV glucose to maintain normoglycemia. However, such a regimen cannot be continued indefinitely over a long period. Therefore, after the initial maintenance phase, oral carbohydrate can be started to provide 0.5 g carbohydrate/kg per hour in infancy and gradually decreasing to 0.1 g carbohydrate per hour in older children. This dose can be provided in the form of glucose polymers (15–25% solution) as per requirements based on age. Overnight nasogastric feeding is advisable to maintain glucose levels during the night, while at day time 2–3 hourly glucose drinks can be given orally. However, care should be taken in overnight feeding to avoid risk of any accidental pulling or displacement of the tube or any leaks.

In older children a mixed home based diet with high source of carbohydrate is preferable at 2–3 hours intervals as absorption gets slower with oral feeds. The amount of carbohydrates calculated should be adequate to maintain normal blood glucose levels.

Another simple and established way of ensuring sustained release of glucose and thus avert any likelihood of hypoglycemia (especially during the night), is ingestion of uncooked starch which has been very beneficial in older children. When given orally, raw corn starch is slowly hydrolysed by pancreatic amylase and intestinal glucoamylase to provide a steady supply of exogenous glucose throughout the dosing interval, thereby preventing hypoglycemia. Cornstarch therapy was reported to be less effective in infants whose secretion of pancreatic amylase may be insufficient to hydrolyze the corn starch granules.[2] Compared with nocturnal intragastric feeding cornstarch therapy is less invasive, more economical and simpler to administer. These factors serve to increase patient compliance with corn starch therapy.[3] Studies have shown best results with uncooked corn starch mixed with water at room temperature. A dose of 1–2 g/kg body weight given twice daily, at night time and at lunch allows for a greater flexibility of glucose ingestion by daytime. However, this regimen is not suitable for infants, as the pancreatic amylase required to digest raw starch is absent or negligible in the new born and reaches adult levels at 2–4 years of age. For new borns and infants, it is preferable to give nocturnal infusions and frequent feeds.[4]

The dose of raw corn starch varies from one child to another and must be assessed individually. Care must be taken that children with this problem should not be allowed to remain fasting and any infections treated promptly. It has been proposed by authors that uncooked cornstarch should be postponed till pubertal growth spurt of the child has been attained.[3]

The benefit of using cornstarch as compared to continuous nocturnal glucose feeding has been reported by some workers who observed better social acceptance by patients and care givers. The only flaw reported by them is the need to take it every 6 hours which generally interrupted the sleep of the children. Moreover, they also reported that although cornstarch mixed with water did not maintain normoglycemia in infants,[5] but some other studies also showed that when it was mixed with milk or curd and given every 4 hourly could benefit young infants as young as 8 months old.[6]

Large quantities of lactose and sucrose from which galactose and fructose are most commonly derived, should be avoided in young children to avoid the risk of metabolic acidosis. Metabolic acidosis occurs due to failure of conversion of galactose and fructose to glucose, resulting in production of lactate.

Glucose Polymers

Glucose polymers are commercially available in the Western market as Polycose glucose polymers. These are easily digestible source of carbohydrate calories for use when additional carbohydrate calories are required, especially in electrolytes or fat restricted diets. These are derived from controlled hydrolysis of cornstarch. The main features of these polymers are:

- Rapid absorption (peak glucose response in 30 minutes).
- Longer glucose polymers reduce osmolality, thus reducing risk of osmotic diarrhea.
- These have a low renal solute.
- Mix easily with food and beverage.
- Minimal sweeteners to enhance acceptance.
- Lactose and gluten free.

The main criterion for preparing a diet for children with Type 1 glycogen storage disease is summarized as follows:

- 0.5 g/kg of carbohydrates per hour to be initiated as 1–2 hourly oral drinks by day and as overnight continuous nasogastric drip. To decrease to 0.01 g/kg /hr in older children.
- Milk should be minimal or avoided initially and substituted by glucose or starch or glucose polymers if available.
- Vegetable oils and polyunsaturated fatty acids are preferable to saturated fats.
- Honey should be avoided due to the high content of fructose.
- Artificial sweeteners like sorbitol or fructose based should be avoided.
- Fruits to be avoided due to their high fructose content.
- Medicines containing sorbitol, lactose or sucrose should be avoided.
- All vegetables may be permitted.
- All cereals without sugar may be allowed.
- Diet should be adequate in all other nutrients as per the RDA for individual age.

GLYCOGEN STORAGE DISEASE TYPES III AND VI

Debrancher Enzyme Deficiency

These types of glycogen storage disease also manifest features of hypoglycemia, hepatomegaly, growth failure and hyperglycemia, but in a milder form as compared to the Type I. In this condition glycogen cannot be broken down to release glucose, thereby favouring conditions of starvation as a result of hypoglycemia.[1] But plasma glucose levels can be maintained through other pathways since the metabolism of amino acids, galactose and fructose are not affected. Therefore, there is a wider choice of carbohydrates from dietary source. To avoid hypoglycemia, fasting is advised against and a high protein diet with frequent meals and or drinks should be continuously offered. A protein and starch based snack is advisable to be given at bed time to avoid feeding in the middle of the night.

A normal diet with high protein sources, low fats preferably polyunsaturated type and moderate carbohydrates is ideal for patients with these types of storage disorders. A comparison between the two types of storage disorders is summarized in Table 36.1.[1]

The use of uncooked starch has also been advocated in Type III glycogen storage disorders with beneficial results.[7,8] Experience of other workers has suggested that oral corn starch can be effective as an initial therapy as well as a maintainenance therapy for children with GSD III. Besides, the clinical response in their patients suggested that corn starch therapy may be as effective as other proposed forms of treatment for GSD III, like protein supplementation or nasogastric formula infusion. However, it was also cautioned that poor linear growth velocity should be considered as an indication of this treatment of patients with GSD III.[9]

Leucine Sensitive Hypoglycemia

This condition is a very rare disorder which involves leucine sensitivity. It manifests in the form of acute fall in blood sugars in certain infants and young children. The onset is generally observed in the first year of life and if the condition goes undetected, it may also lead to mental retardation and neurological symptoms. There is no abnormality in the metabolism of leucine but it is considered that there may be an accumulation of excess leucine in the blood. A high protein diet generally triggers the situation.

Management of the condition involves immediate administration of glucose for brain metabolism either orally or intravenously. It is speculated that this condition may disappear by age of 4–6 years.[10] Drugs like diazoxide with or without diet is considered to be effective in treating the condition. Dietary treatment involves limiting of leucine rich diets which can be done by selecting infant formulae which are modified for their protein content with reduced leucine composition. As for any other form of hypoglycemia it is advised that frequent feeding of the child may be continued and keep a watch on any signs of hypoglycemia. Some children may require as much as 1 g of carbohydrate for each 5 mg of leucine to prevent hypoglycemia, necessitating 4–6 hourly feeds daily and boosting up with carbohydrate drinks during

TABLE 36.1: Summary of diets in hepatic glycogen storage diseases

Type I	**Types III &VI**
Glucose-6-phosphatase deficiency	Debrancher enzyme deficiency
Carbohydrates: Glucose, glucose polymers starch/ slow and starch providing 50% to 70% energy Limit galactose, fructose, lactose and sucrose in diet of young children Avoid sorbitol	All carbohydrates esp. release
Protein: Normal intake for all ages	High protein intake up to twice the normal requirement for all ages
Fat: Preferably polyunsaturated	Preferably polyunsaturated
Frequency: Young children overnight glucose as continuous drip and 1-2 hourly drinks by day	Late night protein-rich carbohydrate supper or overnight drinks
Older children: uncooked starch	Frequent meals and drinks uncooked starch

Source: Francis DEM, Diets in Hypoglycemia, In: Diets for sick children pp 348-56.

the night time too. In acute illness when the child is unable to ingest adequate amounts, drinks of 15–20 g carbohydrates should be offered at frequent intervals.

Ketotic Hypoglycemia

This type of hypoglycemia occurs more frequently among the male children in the toddler age group. Symptoms include apathy, listlessness, convulsions and coma, which revert with ingestion of food. Management involves avoiding long duration of fasting and feeding frequently. Dietary carbohydrate source should be higher and spaced out during the day. However excess of fats and fried foods should be avoided. In conditions when the child is sick and refuses to eat, carbohydrate based drinks can be offered every 2–3 hourly over the day to avoid long hours of fasting. Any leftover food should be reserved after a small interval or be replaced any carbohydrate based drink, e.g. 15 or 20 g of carbohydrate increasing to 40–50 g in the older age group.[1] (See chapter 35, Table 35.5 for CHO exchange).

It is advisable to counsel parents to test for ketones in the urine and if positive, to give carbohydrate drinks as explained above along with sodium bicarbonate.

REFERENCES

1. Francis DEM. Diets in hypoglycemia In: Diets for sick Children 4th ed. Blackwell Scientific Publications. 1987.pp.348-56.
2. Chen YT, Cornblath M, Sidbury JB. Cornstarch therapy in Type I glycogen storage disease. N Engl J Med. 1984;310:171-5.
3. Borowitz SM, Greene HL. Cornstarch therapy in a patient with Type 1 glycogen storage disease. J Pediatr Gastroenterol Nutr. 1987;6:631-4.
4. Smit GPA, Berger R, Potasnick R, Moses SW and Fernandes J. The dietary treatment of Type I glycogen storage disease with slow release carbohydrate. Pediatr Res. 1984;18:9879-81.
5. Chen YT, Bazzare CH, Lee MM, Sidbury JB and Coleman RA. Type I glycogen storage disease: nine years of management with cornstarch. Eur J Pediatr. 1993;152(Suppl):556-9.
6. Wolfsderf JI, Keller RJ, LandyH, Crigler JF, et al. Glucose therapy for glycogenolysis Type I in infants: comparison of intermittent uncooked cornstarch and continuous overnight glucose feedings. J Pediatr. 1990;117:384-91.
7. Gremse CS, Bucuvalas JC, Balistrerri WF. Efficacy of cornstarch therapy in type III glycogen storage disease. Am J Clin Nutr. 1990;52:671-4.
8. Ullrich K, Schmitt H, van Teefelen Heithoff A. Glycogen storage disease type I and III and pyruvate carbohydrate deficiency: results of long-term treatment and uncooked corn starch. Acta Pediatr Scand. 1988;77:531-6.
9. Wolfsdorf JI, Rudlin CR and Crigler JF Jr. Physical growth and development of children with type I glycogen storage: comparison of the effects of long term use of dextrose and uncooked starch. Am J Clin Nutr. 1990;52:1051-7.
10. Cornblath M and Schwartz R. In: Sohaffer/AI (Ed) Disorders of Carbohydrate Metabolism in Infancy (Vol. III in the series- Major Problems of Clinic Pediatrics). 2nd ed. Phiadelphia: WB Saunders. 1976. pp.231-93.

37 Nutritional Support of the Critically Ill Child

INTRODUCTION

Adequate nutrition is an important aspect of management of a critically ill child. The outcome of a child in the critical phase is largely dependent upon the appropriate nutritional support (nor too less nor excess) and has the potential to reverse or reduce adverse long-term consequences. Patients most likely to benefit from nutritional support are those with base line malnutrition in whom a protracted period of starvation would otherwise occur. In well nourished children with short (<1 week) anticipated duration of mil by mouth feeding, improvement in nutritional status may be difficult to demonstrate.

Indications for nutritional support in the critically ill child include pre-existing malnutrition, excessive metabolic demands and the inability to ingest nutrients for prolonged periods.

Nutritional management of the critical ill child involves:

- Assessment
- Administration
- Monitoring

Nutritional Assessment

Nutritional assessment in a pediatric intensive care unit (ICU) is almost similar to that done for adults. These include anthropometry, clinical, laboratory and review of previous and current intakes. Accurate assessment in terms of nutritional and metabolic parameters can go a long way in providing optimal nutritional support with a minimal number of complications.

In a critical child the most important anthropometric data is the weight and length or height. But given the conditions the child is in, one can obtain history of recent, involuntary weight loss (exceeding 5% within 1 month or 10% over 6 months). Of course, factors like fluid overload (in case of edema) may prevent the accurate determining of dry weight in the ICU.[1]

Physical examination should focus on signs of protein energy deficiency (such as temporal wasting), signs of specific micronutrient deficiency (such as anemia, glossitis or rash), hydration state and edema. Dry weight and height are used to calculate the ideal body weight, the percentage of ideal body weight and the basal metabolic index (BMI). If the onset of the illness is indolent, preadmission weight changes become easier to interpret. Obtaining a general idea of the patient's health status and nutrient intake helps determine the nutritional goals. Body status, edema, overall muscle bulk and evidence of pre-temporal wasting should be assessed. Signs of depletion of muscle stores are indicative of pre-existing malnutrition.

Serum albumin levels also help to identify malnourished patients and their risks for morbidity. This marker is considered a strong predictor of outcome of the disease status, but may be influenced by factors like protein synthesis, catabolism, renal losses and dilutional effects.

Balance studies also are used to assess the protein and energy requirements, like nitrogen (N) balance studies, which should be in the range of 2–4 g N/day (indicating an anabolic state). This may be difficult to achieve in a critically ill child, especially when hyperventilation is present.

Formulae using Harris Benedict equation or indirect calorimetry are often used for energy requirements. This equation is modified using correction factor adjustments which are easy to use, but the limitation of this study is the tendency to overestimate the caloric needs of a child in the ICU.[2]

Loss of body weight is a definitive accompaniment of protein energy malnutrition and provides a readily accessible indicator of altered nutritional status (>10% of ideal body weight indicating malnutrition), but as mentioned already, may not reflect the true status in presence of edema. Hepatic secretory proteins like albumin, transferrin, retinol binding protein and pre albumin are markers of visceral protein stores and used as methods of nutritional assessment, but are also influenced by other factors like disorders of hepatic function, protein losing states and acute infections or inflammation. Hence these tests also may be of limited use in a child in the ICU.

Finally, in light of the above factors, consensus recommendations suggest that though there are multiple tests and combination of tests to assess nutritional status, no simple recommendation can be given regarding the 'best' test for assessing nutritional status. Use of any of these methods can be appropriate, providing the limitations are clearly understood. Although not studied in ICU patients, it is important to note that data in hospitalized patients suggest that clinical assessment of nutritional status, including weight loss (>10% of ideal body weight), is as reliable an indicator of malnutrition as more complex tests of nutritional assessment.[3]

Indications for Nutrition Support in the ICU

It has been indicted that nutrition support for any critically ill patient is required where there is evidence of malnutrition or likelihood of development of malnutrition from inadequate oral intake because of a prolonged clinical course.[4]

In patients with respiratory failure, the presence or absence of mechanical ventilation is often the first cofactor in consideration of nutritional support. Mechanically ventilated patients with respiratory failure also fall into one or two general categories-malnourished or hypermetabolic. However, if the respiratory failure is likely to be of short duration, aggressive nutritional support is not indicated.

Hypermetabolic patients, e.g. those with sepsis or acute respiratory distress syndrome (ARDS) are also fit candidates for nutritional support. The goal here is more to prevent further catabolism rather than repletion of nutritional status. The aim for nutritional support is mainly to minimize excessive protein losses, while at the same time provide maintenance substrates at levels that the body can deal with.

GENERAL GOALS AND PRINCIPLES

Goals of Nutritional Support

The general goals of nutritional support in the ICU patients are:

- To provide nutrients consistent with the patient's medical condition, nutritional status and available route of nutrient administration.
- To prevent or treat macronutrient and micronutrient deficiencies.
- To provide doses of nutrients compatible with existing metabolism.
- To avoid complications related to the technique of dietary delivery.
- To improve patient outcome such as those related to disease morbidity, e.g. body composition, tissue repair, organ function and those affecting medical mortalities and subsequent patient outcome.

Principles of Nutritional Support

Macronutrients (Calories and Protein Requirement)

In the critically ill patient the goal of nutritional support is primarily maintenance rather than repletion. Aggressive nutrition support in order to bring the patient to a metabolic state from that of catabolic phase is not advisable, because by attempting to do so, complications, like increased carbon dioxide production, deposition of fat and glycogen in the liver and hyperglycemia may be encountered. Once the hypermetabolic phase is corrected, anabolism is favored and repletion occurs. During starvation, the body adapts to the decreased supply by decreasing its metabolic rate. Glycogen stores are first utilized within 24 hours and fat conserved till quite late in the process.

Carbohydrates and lipids should be so administered, so as to minimize lypolysis and protein degradation. Underfeeding and overfeeding both can be detrimental.[5] The hazards of overfeeding are well established:

1. Increased metabolic rate.
2. Increased oxygen consumption.
3. Hyperglycemia.
4. Dehydration secondary to osmotic dieresis.
5. Fatty liver.
6. Increased carbon dioxide production.
7. Ventilator dependency.
8. Immunosuppression.
9. Fluid overload.
10. Electrolyte imbalance.

For most patients administering 25 cals/kg/d appears to be adequate. These should be provided in a volume consistent with the total fluid needs of the patient which is generally 1 ml water/calorie. About 30–70% of the total calories administered can be given as glucose, i.e. up to 2–5 g glucose/kg/d. The dose should be so adjusted as to maintain a blood glucose level >225 mg/dl, including regular insulin if required.[6]

Fats should comprise about 15–30% of the total calories administered per day. These should include omega 6 polyunstaurated fatty acids (PUFA), triglycerides in adequate dose, so as to prevent deficiency of essential fatty (EFA), i.e. about 5%–7% of the total calories. Medium chain triglycerides (MCT) can also be used to provide calories.

Proteins should comprise about 1.5–2 g/kg body weight/d. This works up to about 15%–20% of the total calories. Patients are known to lose up to 1% of their body proteins per day. In hypermetabolic critically ill patients, protein degradation and synthesis typically increases but with a net protein decrease or catabolic effect.[7] However it is recommended that the protein intake in any case should not exceed 1.8 g/kg/d, except in severe losses and even then it can vary between 1.5–2.0 g/kg/d.[8] Prolonged lack of protein support can cause nutritional deficiency.

The recommendations for an appropriate mix of carbohydrates and fats vary, but generally 60%–70% carbohydrates are given with 20%–30% fats.[9] The proportion is as follows:

	Substrate Mix
Protein	20% of the total calories (1–2 g/d)
Carbohydrates	60%–70%
Fats	20%–30%

The role of certain amino acids like glutamine also has been stressed, as a semi essential amino acid. It serves as a major source of energy, being absorbed from the bowel lumen and is required for the rapidly dividing cells of the immune system.

The role of other essential semi essential amino acids contributing to multiple metabolic processes, like arginine and branched chain amino acids has been described but the benefit of their roles in the critically ill patient has failed to document any positive effects.[10]

Administering Nutrition

Having assessed the base line nutritional status and requirements of a child in the ICU, the next step is to actually deliver the nutrients-when, how and what.

The optimal time to administer nutrition to an infant or child in an ICU may differ from one center to another. Assuming that the nutritional stores are already depleted, some authors have suggested initiating feeding in these children within a few days in infants, within 5 days in older children and within 7 days in adolescents.[11,12] Current data supports the initiation of enteral nutrition (EN) at the earliest possible after resuscitation. Small bowel feedings can usually be performed, even in the presence of gastric atony and colonic ileus. The role of agents formulated to improve gastric and intestinal motility is still controversial.

The presence of bowel sounds and the passage of flatus or stool are not necessary to initiate enteral feeds, especially when feedings are administered distal to the pylorus. However any indication of abdominal distension might call for withholding of feeding and reevaluation.

Nutrition support may be provided using either the enteral route (EN) or through the pareneteral route (PN).

Enteral Nutrition

Oral feeding when ever feasible is the route of choice in any set up as it is the least invasive way of administering nutritional support in a functioning gut. Through this route the gastrointestinal tract (GIT) is used and this helps to maintain the gut integrity and preserves the gut barrier function. The benefits of EN far outweigh those of PN:

1. It corrects the pH balance of the gut and helps reduce bacterial overgrowth. It is also known to reduce bacterial overgrowth.
2. It is known to reduce risk of gastrointestinal bleeding.
3. The gut motility also minimizes the delay in gastric emptying.

In short the accepted dictum is, 'where the gut works, use it'. It has also been demonstrated that early EN (within 3 days of onset of illness on admission to ICU) is safe, efficient, cost effective and associated with improved outcome.[13,14]

However, when there is risk of high aspiration, the decision of oral feeding should be deferred. Small frequent feedings, as opposed to large bolus feeding should be the standard norm to be followed. In conditions when large volumes of feeds are not possible, the feeds may be concentrated to increase the caloric and protein density.

Secretory diarrhea may sometimes be encountered but this does not warrant cessation of enteral feeding, unless it exceeds 1000 ml/d. Generally, in the absence of any specific medical or surgical cause for the diarrhea, e.g. enterocolitis, anti-diarrheal agents can help tide over the problem.

In conditions where the enteral route is not available in patients with respiratory failure who may not have a functioning GI tract, total parenteral nutrition (TPN) needs to be resorted to. The use of minimal EN feeding as 'trophic feeds' is also practiced by some experts along with TPN where possible.

Some of the conditions where oral route is inaccessible, and naso gastric (NG) feeding has to be resorted to are neurological disorders, in born errors of metabolism like glycogen storage disease, cystic fibrosis, bronchopulmonary dysplasia, cerebral palsy and congenital heart diseases.

Certain complications are also known to be associated with enteral feedings like vomiting, diarrhea, abdominal distension and aspiration.

Enteral feedings are generally initiated as a continuous infusion pump with initial rate of 1-2 ml/ kg. body weight per hour. As the tolerance is built up, infusion rate is gradually increased every 6-8 hours. In case of NG feeding the general rule is to check the gastric residue. If found in excess of the previous hour's feeding, it is considered significant and hence the subsequent feed is withheld for an hour or two. If there is recurrent high gastric residue, use of prokinetics are indicated. In children who have been nil by mouth for longer periods, enteral feedings should be initiated very gradually.

Regular monitoring of the feeds for their electrolyte content as well as daily intake of calories, proteins and fluids should be monitored.

Parenteral Nutrition

When the nutritional route is inaccessible for any reason, over a fairly prolonged period parenteral nutrition is the alternative means of providing adequate nutrition. However, it may be kept in mind that PN is only the second line of choice and hence not without its own limitations. The debate over EN vs PN has been since the time PN was introduced, with no clear cut decisions yet as to which outweighs the other. It is observed that the choice of administering nutrition still largely depends upon case to case basis. Contraindications to enteral feeding include diffuse peritonitis, intestinal obstruction, intractable vomiting, paralytic ileus and severe prolonged diarrhea, hypotension and hemodynamic instability. Tables 37.1 and 37.2 give a comparative picture of the advantages and disadvantages of both EN and PN respectively. In such cases total parenteral nutrition (TPN) plays an important role. Administration of 25 kcals/kg of expected body weight is adequate for most patients with normal BMI. In patients with lower BMI (<19), overfeeding is unlikely to result in refeeding syndrome which is manifested by electrolyte abnormalities, volume overload and congestive heart failure.[15] Therefore gradually introducing TPN can ameliorate the risk of refeeding syndrome. To begin with 100–150 g dextrose and low concentration of

TABLE 37.1: Advantages and disadvantages of enteral nutrition

Advantages	Disadvantages
Physiologic Preserves immune functions Preserves gut barrier function Less costly than TPN May blunt hypermetabolic response	More time needed to reach full support Depends on functional status of GIT Depends on functional status of GIT Multiple contraindications; intestinal obstruction Hemodynamic instability: high output enterocutanous fistula, severe diarrhea

TABLE 37.2: Advantages and disadvantages of parenteral nutrition

Advantages	Disadvantages
Available when enteral route contraindicated can augment inadequate oral intake Full support in less than 24 hours Contraindications are few	Intestinal atropy Higher septic morbidity

sodium chloride can be administered with regular monitoring of electrolytes and blood sugars to achieve a state of euglycemia.

Overfeeding of carbohydrates results in respiratory quotient (RQ) close to 1.0, while fat based energy can yield an RQ close to 0.7 (mixed fuels, 0.8–0.9).[16]

The TPN composition has to be modified as per individual case to prevent refeeding in general especially carbohydrates. The protein requirement in TPN ranges from 1.2–1.5 g/kg/d, which needs to be adjusted with periodic monitoring, to promote nitrogen (N) retention, and also support protein synthesis.[17]

Generally, observations in a critical care set up show that a positive nitrogen balance is rarely achieved due to the cytokine and catabolic hormone cascade preventing anabolism. There is not much risk of providing protein in higher amounts. In conditions where blood urea nitrogen (BUN) values exceed 100 mg/l, N intake might need to be decreased due to manifestation of symptoms of azotemia. In conditions of acute renal failure due to restriction of volume, the quality of feeding is limited in any case, but with chronic renal insufficiency, 0.8 g/kg /d of protein is adequate. Similarly in conditions of hepatic encephalopathy, the protein content in the TPN might need to be reduced, but still the use of branched amino acids (BCCA) have shown good results.[18]

The lipid component of TPN comprises omega 6 polyunsaturated fatty acids which are administered separately or as part of a 3-in 1 solution. The calories provided by fats up to 30% of total calories is considered safe especially when it is infused slowly as in the 3-in-1 solution. The main contraindication to lipids in TPN could be triglyceride levels > 400 mg/l.

The remainder of the total calories can be provided as carbohydrates-between 3–5 g/kg/d. The aim should be to maintain a blood glucose level <200 mg/l and the dose can be adjusted accordingly. Mostly coinfusion of insulin is required on a sliding scale if indicated. Hyperglycemia >200 mg/l has been shown to be associated with nosocomial infections which can in fact nullify the benefit of nutritional support itself. TPN induced hyperglycemia may also be associated with severe stress (e.g. in post operative patients) accompanied by rising plasma levels of counter regulatory hormones glucagon, epinephrine and cortisol.[17]

The fluid volume of TPN can be maintained at 1 l/day for patients of cardiac, pulmonary, post-operative and renal conditions in the ICU. This can provide approximately 1000 calories and 70 g of proteins which is usually adequate for the required feeding goal.

Vitamins and minerals are generally administered along with the TPN at the desired levels, along with any medications, e.g. histamine-2-receptor antagonists and metaclopramide.

In the pediatric ICU, PN is usually given as a continuous infusion, which makes it easier to manage the electrolytes, acid base and fluid disturbances which may be generally encountered in this patient population.

MONITORING

There are no standard monitoring techniques for children on TPN, but electrolytes and glucose levels are usually done on a daily basis. Liver function tests may be monitored from time to time, due to the risk of vulnerability of this population to cholestatic liver disease.[19] Transition to EN is done as soon as the patient is able to tolerate it either orally or through the nasogastric route.

However, certain parameters may be checked to minimize complications and maximize the benefits of nutrition support, which may be summarized as follows:

1. Avoid overfeeding a respiratory quotient of over 1 is indicative of overfeeding and may call for reduction of total calories (glucose and fat) to decrease carbon dioxide production.
2. Promote N retention and avoid protein overload.
3. Monitoring triglyceride clearance is recommended.
4. Adequate monitoring of fluid and electrolyte status is essential especially for potassium, phosphate, magnesium, calcium and zinc.
5. Periodic assessment of liver function tests.

Specialized Dietary Foods in the ICU

Besides the role of macro and micronutrients in the overall nutritional support of the ICU patient, a number of specific nutrients have evolved and their individual effects on specific metabolic functions are increasingly being recognized but the definitive role of each of them still remains to be defined clearly.[17]

Glutamine: Is an amino acid involved in a host of metabolic processes like during catabolic states, it is mobilized in increased amounts from peripheral tissues such as skeletal muscle. The outcome of administering glutamine in patients with catabolic states is still not clearly defined.

Branched chain amino acids (BCAA): These are the essential amino acids (leucine, isoleucine and valine), crucial for protein synthesis. Given in dose of 0.5–1.2 g/kg/d has demonstrated improved N retention with reduced urea genesis and increased protein synthetic functions.

Peptides in enteral formulations: These are proteins in their hydrolysed forms and if added in enteral formulae may enhance enteral protein absorption.

Growth hormones: These are known to have a variety of metabolic effects like increased fat oxidation, increased rate of protein synthesis and improved immune responsiveness. Again their role in patient outcome is not defined.

Arginine: This is an amino acid having a role in a number of metabolic functions but its role in improving outcome in a patient in the ICU is yet unclear.

REFERENCES

1. Blackburn GL, Bristrain BR, Maini BS, et al. Nutritional and metabolic assessment of the hospitalized patient. JPEN. 1991;1:11-12.
2. Daly JM, Heymsfield SB, Head CA, et al. Human energy requirements. Overestimate by widely used prediction equation. Am J Clin Nutr. 1985;42:11170-74 (Abstarct).
3. Thonnart N, Cuvelier B, Bracamonte M, et al. Metabolic utilization of LCT vs mixed MCT/LCT emulsion during IV infusion in man. Clin Nutr. 1984; 4suppl):50-7.
4. Heyland DK: Nutritional support in the critically ill patient. Crit Care Clin. 1998;14:423-40.
5. Dabrowski GP and Rombeau John l. Practical Critical Nutritional Management in the Trauma ICU. Surgical Clinics of North America. 2000;80:3.
6. Cerra FB, Benitez MR, Blackburn GL, Irwin RS, et al. Applied Nutrition in ICU Patients, ACCP Consensus Statement. Chest. 1997;111:769-78.
7. Streat SJ, Hill GL. Nutrition in the management of critically ill surgical intensive care patients. World J Surg. 1987;11:194-201.
8. Jolliet P, Pichard C, Biolo G, et al. ESCIM statement: Enteral nutrition in intensive care patients: A practical approach. Intensive Care Med. 1998;24:848-59.
9. Pingleton SK. Nutrition in chronic critical illness. Clinics in Chest Medicine. March 2001, Vol 22, No.6.
10. Alexendar JW. Immunoenhancement via enteral nutrition. Arch Surg. 1995;128:1242-45.
11. Norris KKG, Steinhorn DM. Nutritional management during critical illness in infants and children. Crit Care Med. 1981;9:580-3.
12. Ford EG. Nutritional support of pediatric patients. Nutr Clin Prac. 1996;11:183-91.
13. Adams S, Dellinger EP, Wertz MJ, et al. Enteral vs Parenteral nutritional support following laprtomy for trauma: a randomized perspective trial. J Trauma. 1986;10:882-91.

14. Kudsk KA, Croce MA, Fabian TC, et al. Enteral vs parenteral feeding: effects on septic morbidity after blunt and penetrating abdominal trauma. Ann Surg. 1992;215:503-10.
15. Apovian CM, Mc Mohan, MM, Bistrain BP. Guidelines for refeeding the marasmic patient. Crit Care Med. 1990;18:1030-33.
16. Guenst JM, Nelson CD. Predictors of total pareneteral nutrition induced lipogenesis. Chest. 1994;105:553-59.
17. Cerra FB, Benitez MR, Blackburn GL, et al: Applied Nutrition in ICU patients: a consensus statement of the American College of chest Physicians. Chest. 1997;111:769-78.
18. Fischer JE. Branched chain amino acid solutions in patients with liver failure: an early example of nutritional pharmacology. JPEN. 14 (suppl):249S-56S.
19. Hofmann AF. Defective biliary secretion during total parenteral nutrition: possible mechanisms and possible solutions. J Pediatr Gastroenterol. 1995;20:376-90.

38 Nutritional Management of Pediatric Heart Diseases

INTRODUCTION

In the pediatric group, cardiac issues of nutrition can be discussed from mainly two aspects. First, is the congenital heart ailments and second from the perspective of dyslipidemias. The later aspect is gradually assuming more significance over the past decade or so, due to the rising incidence of this problem being encountered in the pediatric population. More so, because it is now well established that the lifestyle diseases earlier occurring in the late fourth to fifth decade of life, now are being observed in the younger age group of around the third decade and that too in the fairly well advanced stage. It is now believed that prevention at the pediatric age, in terms of dietary habits and lifestyle can alter the scenario and avoid complications of dyslipidemias later in life, thereby reducing the incidence of morbidity and mortality in the population.

CONGENITAL HEART DISEASE

The role of diet and nutrition is greatly associated with congenital heart disease (CHD). Growth retardation and malnutrition is frequently seen in most children born with CHD.[1,2]

An estimated 27% of children with CHD fall below the third percentile for height and weight. Increased metabolic demands and decreased energy intake contribute to growth failure in these children. This is due to the fact that their basal metabolic (BMR) is higher due to an increased proportion of metabolically active tissue and decreased fat stores.[3]

The fact that the severity of the effect of the cardiac defect is correlated to the degree of growth failure and malnutrition is controversial. Cardiac lesions may be found to be of two types, cyanotic and acyanotic as given in Table 38.1.[3]

Whatever the cardiac lesions be, it is crucial that nutrition of the child should be taken care of, since the optimal outcome depends on maximizing weight gain and linear growth. Different types of congenital heart diseases may alter the pattern of growth impairment in their own way. Cyanotic patients have both parameters of weight and height compromised, while acyanotic patients tend to have more problems of weight gain as compared to linear growth. With left to right shunts, the degree of linear growth impairment is proportional to the size of the shunt and severity of the pulmonary hypertension.[4] Failure to thrive is more pronounced in cyanotic patients

TABLE 38.1: Types of cardiac lesions

Acyanotic		Cyanotic
Obstuctive Malformations	Left to Right Shunt Malformations	
Pulmonary stenosis	Patent ductos arteriosus	Transportation of great arteries (TGA)
Aortic stenosis	Ventricular septum disease (VSD) Atrial septum disease (ASD)	Tetrology of Fallot (TOF)

Refer. 3

with congestive heart failure. However, growth impairment does not correlate well with degree of hypoxemia. In cyanotic patients iron deficiency has been attributed to growth failure besides stroke and behavioral problems. Patients with pressure overload lesions without intracardiac shunts grow normally.[3]

Etiology

Congenital heart disease refers to problems in the function of the heart caused by abnormal heart development before birth. According to National Library of Science, congenital heart disease is the most common type of birth defect and accounts for more deaths in the first year of life than any other birth defect. A few of these defects can be prevented during pregnancy by avoiding toxic substances. Some of the common causes of CHD are:

- *Gene mutations*: Gene changes in the ante natal period are attributed to isolated heart defects, e.g. atrial septum disease (ASD).This involves a condition where in the wall separating the upper chambers of the heart does not close completely at birth. The opening allows blood to flow between the left and the right chambers causing pressure to build in the lungs. Patent ductus arteriosus (PDA) is another example of gene mutation which involves the blood vessel failing to close since birth leading to abnormal blood flow between the heart and the pulmonary artery. As per the US National Library of Medicine,[5] the symptoms of genetic mutations may be subtle and progress as the child grows.
- *External factors*: In about 2% of the cases, environmental or maternal factors may cause CHD as per Lucile Packard Children's Hospital at Stanford, e.g. cigarette smoking, medications for treating seizures or lithium used for bipolar disorder treatment.[6]
- *Chromosomal abnormalities*: In some cases, chromosomal abnormalities can also cause CHD. Children with chromosomal abnormality causing Down's syndrome, typically have heart defects.

Factors Affecting Growth Failure in CHD

A number of factors have been attributed to growth failure in CHD (Table 38.2). Increased demands on one hand and decreased or inadequate intake on the other is the chief causative factor. These children have a higher BMR due to increased proportion of metabolically active tissue and decreased fat stores. Infants with CHD need significant higher daily calorie intakes than recommended for their healthy counter parts. This could be almost 160 kcals/kg/d. Tachypnea, diminished strength, easy fatigueability and lack of coordination between their sucking and swallowing reflexes can all contribute to decreased intake.[7,8,9]

Management of CHD

Management of infants and children with CHF is quite a challenge for reasons mentioned in Table 38.2.[7,8,9] The goals for management need to be first

TABLE 38.2: Factors affecting growth failure in CHD

Factors	Effect
Type of cardiac lesion Cyanotic Acyanotic Obstructive Left to right shunt	Reduced height and weight Linear growth more affected than weight Reduced weight more than ht. in early stages. Weight less in cyanotic children. Large shunts affect body fluid compartment
Inadequate energy Decreased energy for feeding anorexia, early satiety observed, increased metabolic rate, increased energy cost for infants/ children with CHD.	Intake varies; 80%–90% of required may attempt feeding but tires soon. Poor intake. 36% increase in BMR observed
Dysmotility and malabsorption CHD may cause compressive hepatomegaly, reduced gastric capacity. Mild abnormality in absorption of nutrients; malabsorption with increased total body water	Premature satiety, increased potential for gastroesophageal reflux (GER) Increased potential for GER/aspiration mild steatorrhea, bile salts loss sicker infants with raised body water. May have lower intake and mild malabsorption
Prenatal factors Trisomy 21 (Down's Syndrome)	Postnatal growth delay may be characterstic of syndrome

Refer. 7, 8, 9

defined to be able to plan a feeding pattern for them. These are:

- Optimum nutritional support for possible planned surgery
- Minimize catabolism
- Preserve lean body mass
- Correct abnormal parameters
- Support normal feeding skill development.

Planning a diet to meet the above goals involves considering certain factors like:

- Age of the child and nutrient requirement
- Current intake pattern and deficiencies which correction
- Various stress factors, medications
- Socioeconomic factors.

Neonatal Period

Early neonatal period being a period of rapid growth, babies are very vulnerable to growth failure especially those born with birth defects like CHD. Their requirements for macronutrients need to be addressed seriously.

Energy

The energy requirement of a neonate on the first day of life is estimated to be around 50–60 kcals/kg/d, gradually increasing to 120–150 kcals/kg/d by the end of the first week. Babies born with CHD can require up to 200 kcals/kg/d. This target can be achieved by resorting to parenteral nutrition in the early acute phase of the illness. Term neonates may gain up to 10–15 g/d, but in preterm this gain can be slower. For pre term babies, the parameters used for assessing their growth is based on the corrected age.

It is usually not possible to provide for growth at this phase, therefore parenteral nutrition (PN) is generally resorted to. In the second phase, enteral nutrition (EN) is initiated. Ideally PN and EN are used simultaneously and gradually go on to enteral feeding solely. In the third phase energy is increased to achieve optimal growth. The energy may be enhanced by making the feeds denser, especially when the total volume of fluids permitted is also restricted. Since the calorie needs of a pre term baby is greater than that for a noncardiac infant, as shown in Table 38.3,[10] supplementation of feeds is recommended from the time of diagnosis itself.[11]

TABLE 38.3: Macronutrient requirements in healthy term and preterm infants

Nutrient	Normal requirements	
	Term	Preterm
Energy (kcals/Kg/d)	100	120
Carbohydrates (g/Kg/d)	10	12–14
Fat (g/Kg/d)	3.3–6	4–7
Protein (g/Kg/d)	1.5–2.2	3–4

Refer. Premmer DM, Georgieff MK. Nutrition for ill neonates. Pediatric Review. 1999;20:56-62

It was also observed that feeding and growth of breast fed infants was better as compared to those on bottle feeds.[12]

The energy requirement of term infants is about 135–155 kcals/kg/d in the enteral nutrition. Toddlers and older children may need about 20%–30% more than normal estimated needs. Post-surgery (repair) the calories needs will decrease, but may still be about 10–15 cals/kg above the normal.[13] Energy from fats may be almost 50%–60% of the total requirements while 10%–20% of the energy may be provided by proteins. The remaining 20%–25% of the energy can be derived from carbohydrates.[14] The calorie needs for a particular infant is best derived by assessing growth parameters and making adjustments as needed until appropriate growth is achieved.

Fortification

To increase the density of the feeds, various fortifiers have been used like human milk fortifier (HMF), MCT oil, etc. to maintain a maximum energy density. Of 1 kcal/ml. One sachet of HMF (2 g) added to 50 ml of EBM will provide an additional 6.5 calories and a good amount of other nutrients too. The calorie density of a feed with added HMF to EBM (0.67 cals/ml) will provide a density of 0.8 cal/ml.[14]

If using formula feeds, the dilution prescribed on the instructions can be decreased, e.g. instead of 30 ml water per scoop, 25 ml water may be used or the amount of scoops may be increased in the same 30 ml of water.

Medium-chain triglycerides oil (7.7 cal/ml) is safe to use to increase the density without increasing the osmolality of the feed.

Beyond 6 months of age, complementary feeds can be initiated, taking care to introduce calorie dense

TABLE 38.4 Estimated daily fluid requirement in the first year of life

Birth weight	Day 1	Day 2	Day 3	Day 4	Day 5	Day 6	Day 7
<1000 g	80	100	120	130	140	150	160
1000–1500 g	80	95	110	120	130	140	150
>1500 g	60	75	90	105	120	135	150

Refer. 12

foods. Fats/sugar is added to the preparations as required. Certain calorie dense pediatric supplements may be used in chronically ill children even below 2 years.

Fluids

Preterm babies especially those with very low birth weight (VLBW), having weights <1500g need to be kept on restricted fluid intake in the first week of life, particularly in conditions requiring restricted fluid intake, like in those with respiratory distress syndrome (RDS) and PDA as given in Table 38.4.[15]

The intake is generally restricted to two third of the estimated requirement per day. The use of diuretics in the infants may lead to hypokalemia. Body stores of calcium, magnesium and phosphorous may also be deleted. Acid base state may be altered, further complicating the management.

PEDIATRIC DYSLIPIDEMIAS

Dyslipidemias are disorders of lipoprotein metabolism resulting in abnormal excesss of total cholesterol (TC), low density lipoprotein (LDL-C) or triglycerides (TG), or deficiency of high density lipoprotein cholesterol (HDL-C).[16]

In children the most common type of dyslipidemia is the idiopathic type (polygenic risk factor associated or multifactorial), while a minority will have monogenic or secondary dyslipidemia. The more common genetic dyslipidemia include familial hypercholesterolemia (FH), familial combined hyperlipidemia (FCH), familial defective appoprotein B and familial hypertriglyceridemia.

There is increasing prevalence of risk of CHD among children, including metabolic syndrome and obesity as well as continued emphasis on primary prevention of CHD.[17,18]

It is considered that childhood dyslipidemia by itself may not lead to any adverse affects at that stage, but can have serious consequences later in life. Large epidemiological studies have proven that the lipid levels of children correlate well with those of adult family members.[19]

Management of Dyslipidemia

The goal of nutritional support in pediatric hyperlipidemia is to provide nutrition for normal growth and development, to normalize lipid levels and also to decrease the risk of cardiovascular diseases.[20]

The guidelines for diet modification as advised by American Heart Association (AHA) are for children above 2 years of age. Restriction of fats below 2 years is not recommended[21] as it may interfere and hamper growth and development of the child.

Additional intervention for children includes dietary supplements (fiber, sterols, omega 3 fatty acids), exercise, weight loss for overweight children and identification and treatment of diabetes mellitus or other causes of dyslipidemia. Although children and adolescents with idiopathic dyslipidemia generally have less severe lipid abnormalities than children and adolescents with monogenic disorders, such abnormal levels would still potentially improve with intervention.

The dietary changes included are similar to Step 1 guidelines[21] (Table 38.5) and can be incorporated with low fat dairy products. The American Academy of pediatrics recommends that total fat intake should not fall below 20% of total calories for children and adolescents.[21]

TABLE 38.5 Steps 1 and 2 dietary modifications

Nutrient	Step 1 diet	Step 2 diet
Total Fat	No more than 30% on average of total calories	Same
Saturated fatty acid (SFA)	Less than 10% of total calories	Less than 7% of total calories
Polyunsaturated fatty acid (PUFA)	Up to 10% of total calories	Same
Monounsaturated fatty acid (MUFA)	Remaining fat calories	Same
Cholesterol	<300 mg/d	Same
Protein	15–20% of total calories	Same
Calories	To achieve normal weight and promote growth and development	Same

Refer. 21

REFERENCES

1. Greecha CP. Congenital heart disease. In: Nutritional Care for high risk new borns. Groh Wargo S, Thompson M, Cox J (eds). Chicago: Precept Press. 1994;266.
2. Mehrizi A, Drash A. Growth disturbances in congenital heart disease. J Pediatrics. 1962;61:418-29.
3. Wright GE, Rochini AP. Primary and General Care of the child with congenital heart disease. American College of Cardiology (ACC), Current Journal Review 2002, March/April.
4. Varan B, Tokel K, Yilmaz G. Malnutrition and growth failure in cyanotic and acyanotic heart disease with and without pulmonary hypertension, Arch Dis Child. 1999;81:49-52.
5. US National Library of Medicine: healthorg.com/...../ genemutation linked to congenital heart disease.
6. Lucile Packard Children's Hospital at Stanford: Factors contributing to congenital heart disease.
7. Umansky R, Hauck AJ. Factors in growth of children with patent ductus arteriosus. Pediatrics. 1992;146:1078-84.
8. Salzer JR, Haschke M, Wimmer M, et al. Growth and nutritional intake of infants with congenital heart disease. Pediatric Cardiol. 1989;10:17-23.
9. Stranway A, Fowler R, Cunnigham K, et al. Diet and growth in congenital heart disease. Pediatrics. 1976;57:75-86.
10. Premmer DM, Georgieff MK. Nutrition for ill neonates. Pediatric Review. 1999;20:56-62.
11. Jackson M, Poskitt EM. The effects of high energy feeding on energy balance and growth in infants with congenital heart disease and failure to thrive. Br J Nutr. 1991;65:131-43.
12. Combs VL, et al. A comparison of growth patterns in breast fed and bottle fed infants with congenital heart disease. Pediatr News. 1993;19:175-79.
13. Nydegger A, Bines JE. Energy metabolism in children with congenital heart disease. Nutrition. 2006;7(8):679-704.
14. Poonam Sadana. Nutritional management of infants with congenital heart disease, Cardiology chapter of IAP, http://cardioiap.org/drpoonam_nutrition.php.
15. Wernovsky G, Ades AM, Spray TL. Management of congenital heart disease in the low birth weight infant. In: Avery's Diseases of the Newborn 8th edition, Taeusch HW, Ballard RA, Gleason EA (Eds) (888-895) Saunders. 2005.
16. Ahmed SM, Clasen ME, Donnelly JE. Management of dyslipidemia in adults. Am Fam Physician. 1998;57 (9):2192-204.
17. Kavey R-EW, Daniels SR, Laura RM, Atkins DDL, et al. American Heart Association guidelines for primary prevention of atherosclerotic cardiovascular disease beginning in childhood. J Pediatr. 2003;142(4):368-72.
18. Williams CL, Hayman LL, Daniels SR, et al. Cardiovascular health in childhood: A statement for Health professionals from the Committee on

Atherosclerosis, Hypertension ad Obesity in the young (AHOY) of the Council on cardiovascular disease of the young, American Heart Association. Circulation. 2002;106(1):143-60.
19. Schrott HG, Bucha KA, Clarke WR, Lauer RM. The Muscatine hyperlipidemia family study program. Prog Clin Biol Res. 1979;32:619-46.
20. American Academy of Pediatrics. Committee on Nutrition, Statement on Cholesterol. Pediatrics. 1992; 90:469-73.
21. NCEP Expert panel on Blood Cholesterol Levels in Children and Adolescents. National Cholesterol Education Program (NCEP), Highlights of the report of the expert panel on blood cholesterol levels in children and adolescents. Pediatrics. 1992;89:525-27.

39 Nutrition Support in Children with HIV/AIDS

Acquired immunodeficiency syndrome (AIDS) is a serious condition comprising a deficiency of the immune system and other complex and severe diseases, leading to death. It is the final stage in progression of diseases resulting from human immunodeficient virus infection (HIV+) which can be transmitted to other persons.[1]

The disease was first identified in 1980s around Africa and identified as 'slim' disease since the affected patients looked very lean and was later named as AIDS in 1982 and in 1986, reported to be an HIV infection.[2] The number of people living with HIV increased 3-4 times from 1990-2008 and is still rising. Young people (15-24 years old) account for half of all new HIV infections worldwide and about 6,000 become infected with HIV everyday.[1]

Infants born to mothers who are HIV+ are generally of low birth weight related to low gestational age, having high viral loads.[3]

Pathophysiology

The AIDS is caused by the human immunodeficiency virus (HIV-1). HIV enters the cell and after replication, induces cell dysfunction or death. Cells of the immune system are the most commonly affected.

The lymphocytes which are part of the immune system are of two types-B cells, responsible for humoral immunity and T cells, responsible for cell mediated immunity.

The T cells are either helper (CD 4+) or suppressor (CD 8+). CD4 cells enhance the operation of the entire immune system, while the CD8 cells shut down the immune response after the foreign antigens have been destroyed. In healthy individuals, the numbers of helper cells (CD4) are twice as the CD8 cells, where as in patients with AIDS, it is vice versa, i.e. the CD 4 counts are suppressed drastically.[4]

Breastfeeding is one of the commonest and easy routes of transmission of the disease from HIV infected mothers to their infants. The rate of the infection in babies is cumulative and roughly constant throughout the breastfeeding periods.

There are a number of factors, which influence the rate of transmission from mother to child, while breast feeding. These are maternal clinical immunologic status, plasma and breast milk viral load and condition of the breast (e.g. mastitis, cracked nipples, etc.).

Effect of HIV on Nutrition

Nutrition plays an important role in HIV affected mothers and their infants. Poor nutrition is commonly seen in such mothers and malnutrition can play an important role in the progression of the disease. In children HIV infection can result in failure to thrive, stunting and wasting. There is poor feeding, malabsorption, tissue catabolism and psycho social factors. Figure 39.1 highlights the effects of HIV on the nutritional status of the children. Higher viral load can further accelerate growth failure. Infected children born to HIV + mothers have early stunting which is sustained, and are malnourished but not necessarily wasted.[5] It has been postulated that HIV does not affect the birth weight of the child, but significant postnatal growth abnormalities even

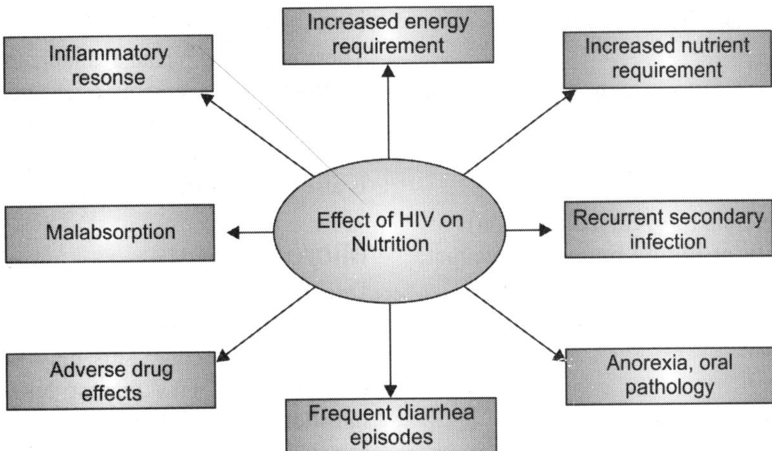

FIGURE 39.1: Effect of HIV on nutrition

in the asymptomatic child can occur rapidly.[6] The impairment of growth is generally observed by 2 years of age, while some have also reported such deficits as early as 4 months also in some infected infants.[7,8] Children with HIV, manifest preferential loss of lean body mass as compared to fat mass, which may or may not be associated with weight loss.[6]

Causes of Malnutrition in HIV Infected Children

The main obvious cause of failure to gain weight is attributed to increased expenditure. They tend to burn 10% more calories while resting, compared to those who are in infected. Besides this decreased energy intake is an added contributory factor. This could be aggravated by associated anorexia and inability to eat. Conditions like oral thrush, diarrhea, nausea and vomiting may all be linked to decreased intake by these patients. Malabsorption of the GIT of all the nutrients, especially fat from food is another significant causative factor of decreased intake.

Oxidative Stress in HIV+/AIDS Patients

Children with HIV+ infection may have decreased levels of antioxidants like vitamins, sulfhydryl (SH) potential and total glutathione (GSH). Malnutrition and diarrhea can also cause a decrease in the levels of vitamins and SH compounds.

The AIDS progression can also be caused by some toxic foods and drinks and certain toxic chemicals, herbicides, alcohol and tobacco.

Studies have demonstrated significantly decreased blood levels of vitamin A, beta carotene, vitamin E and the antioxidative status in HIV+/AIDS patients, as compared to healthy individuals. This is mainly as a result of poor nutrition with lowered dietary antioxidants.

Immunity and Other Cofactors in AIDS

Even if people are infected with HIV, they may remain asymptomatic for a long duration, but their immune system gradually becomes weak till the symptoms appear. The immune system in these patients is severely affected, thereby exposing them to increased susceptibility to opportunistic infections, which are unlikely in healthy individuals. Common symptoms are fever, chills, sweats, lymphadenopathy, weakness and weight loss. They are prone to be infected by harmful infectious microorganisms like bacteria, viruses, fungi and parasites. These opportunistic infections accentuate malnutrition and wasting syndromes.

Role of Nutrition in HIV+/AIDS Children

Nutrition interventions have a wide range of benefits for HIV related outcomes.[9] The goal of nutrition support in HIV+/AIDS patients should be

- Promote optimal growth
- Lean tissue repletion (prevent malnutrition)
- Enhance quality of life by providing adequate calories and nutrients
- Improve immunity (increase in CD4 count) by improving intake.

Nutritional Requirements for HIV Infected Child

Energy

The HIV infection affects nutrition through increases in resting energy expenditure, reductions in food intake, nutrient malabsorption and loss and complex metabolic alterations, leading to weight loss and wasting in AIDS. There is need to increase energy intake by at least 10% of the recommended dietary intake (RDA) in asymptomatic HIV infected children to maintain growth. But if there is already significant weight loss and the patient is symptomatic, an increase of 50%–100% energy above the RDA for healthy children is recommended.[10]

An oral intake of a wide variety of nutrient dense foods combined with oral supplementation and nutritional counseling should help to meet the increased needs. A high fat supplement or recipe which includes high amounts of oil, cream or butter can help meet the increased demands.

In children unable to accept orally, as per required amounts, nasogastric feeding should be considered. In children unable to accept orally, as per required amounts, nasogastric feeding should be considered. His can be done in addition to a free oral intake during the day, as a night time regimen. Commercial supplements can be helpful in supplementing the oral intake if the child is unable to consume adequately. Parenteral nutrition should be reserved for HIV infected children, who continue to lose weight on an aggressive enteral program, or for children who have persistent diarrhea with weight loss or severe recurrent or chronic pancreatic or biliary tract disease.

Protein

There is not much data available to support increase in protein requirements over and above the RDA (12%–15% of total energy intake). However, with an increase in the total energy, the intake of protein is also proportionately increased.

Micronutrients

Due to the decreased intake by children with HIV/AIDS infected children, deficiency of micronutrients are bound to occur. This may further accelerate progression of HIV disease leading to worsened nutritional status.[10] Nutritional supplement may also restore intestinal absorption and increase CD4 count in affected children. As per WHO recommendations, children younger than 5 years born to HIV infected mothers, living in resource limited settings should be supplemented periodically (4–6 months) with vitamin A in doses as per healthy children.[10] Suggested vitamin A doses are 1 lac IU for children 6–12 months and 2 lac IU for children above 1 year.

Various workers have proposed high and specific doses of vitamins (A, B_1, B_2 and folic acid, C, D and E) for children with HIV/AIDS infection.

Vitamin A and β carotene are considered to have a role in maintaining and protecting skin and epithelium and increasing immune functions.[11]

Vitamins B complex functions as co-enzymes for energy metabolism and increase in lean body mass.[12,13]

Vitamins C and E exert an antioxidant role and act in preventing oxidative stress, while minerals like iron, selenium and zinc are known to act as co factors for antioxidant enzymes.[14]

Affect of Antiretroviral Therapy

The nutritional status of individuals put on highly active antiretroviral therapy (HAART) is known to improve independent of its effects suppression and immune status, although wasting can still be seen in some patients.[15] The first beneficial effect to be noticed after beginning of HAART, are gains in arm and muscle circumference. The improvement is seen maximum in children with lowest base line BMI and who have more advanced HIV disease.

Antiretroviral therapy (ARV) is also known to cause severe nausea and vomiting which can decrease the intake of the child. Besides, there are other metabolic complications like derangement in glucose metabolism, bone metabolism and lactic academia, associated with initial treatment of ARV drugs. Like in adults, children are also affected by the metabolic effects of HAART and have a significant risk of lipodystrophy.

Feeding of the HIV Exposed Infant

Infants on breast feeds are also at risk through-breastfeeding. The risk of HIV transmission-through breastfeeding is directly related to the health, viral load and immune status of the mother. Infection occurs at an average rate of about 8.9 HIV transmissions per 100 child years of breastfeeding.[16]

The HIV positive mothers are recommended to avoid breastfeeding if replacement feeding is affordable, feasible, sustainable and safe (AFASS).[17] Very often in poor socioeconomic strata, mothers tend to initiate breastfeeding. WHO recommends exclusive breastfeeding for these mothers and also early cessation of feeding. Infants who are not breast fed or who stop breastfeeding early and do not have access to safe and nutritious replacement foods are at increased risk of malnutrition, diarrhea and other illness and death.[18]

World Health Organization/United Nations Children's Fund/United Nations AIDS/United Nations Population Fund[19] has framed certain guidelines which can help in deciding which feeding option would best suit an individual HIV infected mother depending upon various social and environmental factors.[20] These are summarized in Table 39.1.

WHO, UNICEF, UNAIDS, UNFPA[20] recommends several variations of exclusive breastfeeding and replacement milk for infants of HIV infected mothers[19] (Table 39.2).

Breastfeeding

Mothers who do breast feed due to conditions mentioned earlier need to exercise some preventive measures so as to minimize the risk of transmission

TABLE 39.1: Considerations for deciding on the most feasible option for HIV+mothers

	Most feasible option		**Replacement feeding or expressed, heat-treated breast milk**
	Breastfeeding/ wet-nursing	**Unclear**	
Drinking-water supply	River, stream, pond, or well	Public standpipe	Piped water at home or ability to purchase clean water
Latrine	None or pit latrine	VIP latrine	Waterborne latrine
Income	Less than USD 15 available for formula each month	USD 15 available for formula most months	USD 15 available for formula every month (unless using expressed breast milk)
Food storage	No refrigerator or regular electricity supply available	Access to refrigerator with regular electricity supply, but not at home	Refrigerator at home with regular electricity supply
Preparation and fuel	Inability to boil water and utensils for every feed	Ability to boil water for every feed but with effort	Ability to boil water for every feed
Ability to prepare night feeds	Preparation of replacement feeds at night difficult	Preparation of replacement feeds at night possible but with effort	Preparation of replacement feeds at night possible
Family and community support	Breastfeeding expected, and family unaware of HIV status	Replacement feeding acceptable, but family unaware of HIV status; or breastfeeding expected, but family aware of HIV status and willing to help with feeding	Family aware of HIV status and willing to help with feeding

Refer. 20

TABLE 39.2: WHO/UNAIDS/UNICEF feeding options for infants on HIV infected mothers

Breast milk	Replacement milk
Exclusive breastfeeding by the mother for 6 months and continuing till age of 2 years or as long as mothers choose. Exclusive breastfeeding by the mother with early cessation, with rapid weaning to replacement milk as early as feasible. Breast milk expression with heat treatment; expressed milk fed by cup. Wet nursing by an HIV uninfected mother	Commercial infant formula prepared as per manufacturer's directions Fresh full cream milk; with added water, sugar and micronutrients, boiled before use Evaporated full cream milk or powdered full cream milk; with added water, sugar and micronutrients

All feeding options recommend introduction of complementary foods at 6 months of age.
Refer[19]. WHO,UNAIDS,UNICEF (2000)

through breast milk which can be summed up as follows:

1. Practice exclusive breastfeeding ideally for 6 months.
2. Stop breastfeeding as soon as replacement feeding is acceptable. Feasible, affordable, sustainable and safe-preferably not later than 6 months.
3. Good lactation management (early initiation, attachment, positioning, frequent feeding, learning to express) can prevent breastfeeding problems like cracked nipples, engorgement and mastitis.
4. When cracked or bleeding nipples, mastitis or abscesses do occur, continue feeding from the unaffected side, and regularly express from the affected side and discard.
5. Oral thrush or mouth ulcers in the infant should be promptly treated.
6. Expressed milk can be heat treated in conditions during periods of increased risk of transmission, secondary to cracked nipples or during transmission from exclusive breastfeeding to replacement feeding.
7. Condoms should be used by sexually active mothers throughout the lactation period.

Replacement Feeding

Replacement feeding is given as a substitute for breastfeeding, in the form of formula milk before six months. After six months, this feeding is continued but with introduction of semi solid food. This is especially important for mothers diagnosed recently with HIV infection or progressed to AIDS (or whose CD4 count is less than 200/μl) who should offer replacement feeding to prevent high risk of transmission to the infant. Most commercial infant formulae are appropriate if prepared hygienically and as per directions on the packing. Infants who also test positive for HIV infection can be offered breastfeeding by mothers testing positive for HIV, since preventing breastfeeding for them will not make any difference. It would be advisable for such mothers to continue on exclusive breastfeeding for 6 months, but beyond that complementary feeding should be started in any case, in the form of juice, rice, potatoes, dark green vegetables, etc.

Mothers who wean from exclusive breastfeeding to replacement feeding need to consider some important factors for smooth transition:

1. Infants should be allowed a period of 2 days to 2 weeks to adjust to the new feeding pattern.
2. The infant should be acclimatized to the use of cup feeding by using expressed breast milk (EBM).
3. Breastfeeding can be eliminated for one cup feed and EBM can be replaced in the cup.
4. The EBM should be discarded if nipples are sore, cracked or engorged. Cold compresses can help mitigate inflammation due to engorgement.
5. Once cup feeding has begun and accepted by the infant, reintroduction of breast feeds should be avoided, nor should breastfeeding be used to pacify the child.
6. In case EBM has to be given, it should be heat treated and given by cup.

At six months, if it is still not conducive to 'AFASS', continuation of breastfeeding is recommended along with complementary foods. EBM of HIV+ mothers, if adequately heat treated, will not transmit HIV infection and nutritionally and immunologically safe. This can also be done in conditions when there is increased risk of transmission through cracked nipples. Wet nursing is a good option for feeding infants, in communities where it is acceptable and feasible, but care should be taken that they be tested before and after six weeks of starting.

REFERENCES

1. http://www.who.int (WHO and FAO)
2. http://www.aids.org (How many people have HIV and AIDS? AID.ORG, Inc-A-A project of Community Partners, 2007).
3. Katz A. The evolving art of caring for pregnant women with HIV infection. J Obstet Gynecol Neonatal Nurs. 2003;32:102-8.
4. Olsen LG, Cutroni R and Furuta L. Pediatric Acquired Immunodeficiency Syndrome. In: Handbook of Pedutric Nutrition 2nd ed. Samour PQ, Helm KK and Lang CE. Publishers Joes and Barlette. 2004.pp.453-63.
5. Bobat R, Coovdia H, Moodley D, Coutsoudis A, Gouws E. Ann Trop Pediatr. Sep 2001;21(3):203-10.
6. Miller TL. Nutritional aspects of pediatric HIV infection. In: Walker WA, Watkins JB eds. Nutrition in Pediatrics. 2nd ed. Hamilton, Ontario; C Decker. 1996:534-50.
7. Miller TL, Evaas S, Orav EJ, Morris V, et al. Growth and body composition in children with human immunodeficiency virus-1. Am J Clin Nutr. 1993; 57:588-92.
8. McKinney RE, Robertson JR. Effect of human immunodeficiency virus infection on the growth of young children. Duke Pediatric AIDS Clinical Trials Unit. J Pediatr. 1993;123:579-82.
9. Baruchal S, Wainberg MA. The role of oxidative stress in disease progression in individuals infected by the human immunodefiecient virus. J Leukoc Biol. 1992;52:111-4.
10. WHO: Requirements for People Living with HIV/ AIDS: Report of a Technical Consultation. Geneva, WHO. 2003.
11. Falio FN, Helio V, Alceu A, et al. Recommended dose for repair of serum vitamin A levels in patients with HIV infection/AIDS may be insufficient because of high urinary losses. Nutrition. 2006;22:483-9.
12. Davidhizae R and Dunn C. Nutrition and the client with AIDS. J Pract Nurs. 1998;48:16-25; quiz 26-8.
13. Lands L. A Comprehensive Approach to HIV: The synergism of Complementary Therapies Combined with Aggressive Medical Management, Carl Vogel Foundation, Washington DC. 1992.
14. Chandra RK. Nutrition and the immune system: an introduction. Am J Clin Nutr. 1997:19:460 S.
15. Rousseau MC, Molines C, Moreau J, Delmont J. Influence of highly active antiretroviral therapy on micro nutrients profiles of HIV infected patients. Ann Nutr Metab. 2000;44(56):212-16.
16. The breastfeeding and HIV International Transmission Study BHITS Group. Late postnatal transmission of HIV-1 in breast fed children: an individual patient data meta analysis.
17. WHO. New Data on the prevention of Mother to child transmission of HIV and their Policy Implications: Conclusions and recommendations. Geneva. Oct 2000;11-13.
18. WHO Collaborative Team on the role of breastfeeding in the prevention of Infant mortality. Effect of breastfeeding on infant and child mortality due to infectious diseases in less developed countries. A pooled analysis. Lancet. 2000;353:451-55.
19. WHO, UNAIDS, UNICEF: HIV and Infant Feeding Counseling: A Training Course, Geneva, WHO/ UNAIDS/UNICEF, 2000. WHO document WHO/FCH/ CAH/00.2-4.
20. WHO, UNICEF, UNAIDS, UNPFA: HIV and Infant Feeding: A guide for Health Care Managers and Supervisors. Geneva, WHO. 2003.

40 Nutritional Management of Cancer and Bone Marrow Transplant in Children

INTRODUCTION

Adequate nutrition for a child with cancer plays a crucial role in several clinical outcome measures, such as treatment response, quality of life and cost of care.[1] The importance of nutrition in children and adolescents with malignancies meet to be reinforced keeping in view that the nutritional status of the cancer patient is of major concern due to the fact that such patients offer a narrow safety margin for aggressive treatment.

The survival of children with cancer has increased significantly over the last few decades due to various reasons like early detection, improved multimodality treatment and enhancement of supportive care, including prevention and efficient management of infections.[2] Children with cancer are particularly vulnerable to malnutrition since they exhibit elevated substrate needs due to the disease and its treatment. On the other hand they have increased requirements of nutrients to attain optimal growth and development.[3]

Nutritional Implications of Cancer in Children

Protein Energy Malnutrition

Protein energy malnutrition is one of the major secondary diagnosis in children with cancer as a result of decreased intake, increased energy requirements and malabsorption. The incidence at diagnosis ranges from 6% in children with newly diagnosed leukemia to as high as 50% in children with stage 1V neuroblastoma.[4]

It is believed that certain types of treatments by themselves promote PEM, e.g. major surgeries, irradiation of the head, neck, esophagus, abdomen or pelvic surgeries, or an intense course of chemotherapy. Besides this, intake is decreased due to complications like pain, fever and frequent recurrent infections.

That nutritional status has a prognostic effect upon outcome of children with cancer, is well established. Patients with solid tumors and lymphomas who are malnourished at diagnosis have a poor survival when compared to their nourished counterparts.[5] PEM in a cancer patient may also be associated with lethargy, irritability and lack of interest in playing. It is therefore crucial to take measures to prevent this PEM to improve outcomes and minimize the function of various organ systems affected like the hemopoietic, gastrointestinal and immunological.

Nutritional Assessment

The first step to determine the extent of malnutrition in a child with cancer is nutritional assessment on which is based successful management. There are different criteria described for assessing PEM in children, but the one generally accepted and used at diagnosis involves weight for age and weight for height. (Table 40.1). In growing children these criteria are conservative estimates of true depletion (especially in those with large abdominal masses), since the tumor itself may weigh as much as 3% of the child's weight.[6]

Serum albumin concentrations of 3.2 g/dl or less are considered as an indicator of PEM. Weights,

TABLE 40.1: Criteria for nutritional staging of children at the diagnosis of neoplastic disease

Stage	Criteria
Nourished	<5% weight loss
	>5th percentile weight for height
	>3.2 g/dl albumin
Malnourished*	≥5% weight loss
	<5th percentile weight for height
	Height is <5th percentile for age†
	≤3.2 g/dl albumin

Refer. Rickard KA, Grosfed JR, Coates TD, et al. The value of nutritional support in children with cancer. Cancer 1986;58:1904-10.

*A child meeting any one of these criteria is staged as malnourished.

†Patient considered chronically malnourished when both weight for age and height for age are <5th percentile

heights and weight for height measurements plotted sequentially on growth charts[7] are well accepted tools for assessing the growth of a child. For ongoing nutritional assessment albumin is a useful indicator of protein malnutrition in some patients.[8] Table 40.2 illustrates indices used for nutritional assessment of children.[6]

Cachexia in Cancer

In cancer cachexia indicates a state of tissue wasting, weakness, anemia, hypoalbuminemia, hypoglycemia, impaired liver function, glucose intolerance, accelerated gluconeogenesis, skeletal muscle dystrophy, visceral organ atrophy and anergy.[9] In contrast to uncomplicated steatorrhea, cachexia in patients with cancer is an advanced state of wasting marked by excess depletion of skeletal muscle mass and adipose tissue relative to total body weight.[10] There are various contributing factors to cachexia in children with cancer like disturbances in metabolism of macronutrients, increased requirements, inadequate intake or chemotherapy as shown in Table 40.3.[11]

The consequences of malnutrition on the child has adverse effects on the child with cancer, some of them being short-term or long-term as illustrated in Table 40.4.[12]

TABLE 40.2: Ongoing nutritional assessment measures which identify real or impending nutritional depletion in children with cancer

Measurements	Risk criteria & implications
Nutrient intakes Energy, kcals/kg (% of healthy children)	80% of median intake Low intake
Anthropometry Height Height for age	<5th percentile. Growth stunting (may be due to chronic PEM)
Weight %change	>5% loss. Acute PEM (with adequate hydration state
Weight for age	<5th percentile. Acute or chronic PEM
Weight for height*	<5th percentile. Acute PEM when height forage is >10th percentile.
Skinfold thickness measurements*†	<10th percentile. Depleted body stores
Triceps Subscapular absolute change	>0.3 mm decrease : sub clinical PEM
Biochemical Albumin‡ (%change)	<3.2 g/dl#. Acute/chronic PEM >10% decrease
Transferrin‡ (% change)	>200 mg/dl:subclinical PEM >20% decrease: subclinical PEM

Refer. Rickard KA, Coates TD, Grosfed JR, et al. The value of nutrition support in children with cancer. Cancer 1986;58:1904-10.

*Inaccurate when child had has edema, pleural effusion or excess fluids for chemotherapy administration.

†Steroid therapy may increase fat deposition.

‡May be decreased in presence of severe liver dysfunction.

#May be increased in presence of infection or iron deficiency.

TABLE 40.3: Contributory factors to cacexia in cancer

Abnormal host metabolism of macronutrients
Tumor consumption of nutrients for tumor growth
Host requirements of adequate nutrients for normal growth
Anticancer therapy
Inadequate intake of nutrients to meet expenditures

Refer. Kern KA, Norton JA. Cancer cachexia. J Pareneter Enter Nutr 1988;12:286-98.

TABLE 40.4: Short and long-term consequences of malnutrition on the cancer survivor

Short-term consequences	Long-term consequence
Wasting of muscle and fat mass	Growth impairment, reduced height
Decreased tolerance of chemotherapy	Decreased long-term survival in several types
Unfavorable response to chemotherapy	Impact on motor, cognitive nad neurodevelopmental impairment
Treatment delays	Risk for metabolic syndrome
Fatigue	Risk for secondary causes
Bio-chemical disturbance (anemia, hypoalbuminemia)	Risk foraging
Delayed recovery of normal marrow function	Increased mortality rate
Changes in body composition	Retardation of skeletal muscle
Drug dose alteration	Abnormal bone mineral density
Decreased quality and productivity of life	Decreased quality of life
Greater levels of psychological distress	
Higher susceptibility to infections	

Refe. Bauer J. Jurgens H and Frukwald MC. Important Aspects of Nutrition in Children with cancer. Advances in Nutrition 2011 (July).

Adverse Effects of Cancer Therapy on Nutritional Status in Children

Since children with cancer are administered multimodal therapy comprising chemotherapy, radiotherapy or surgery, there is an additional risk of adverse effects on their nutritional status as shown in Table 40.5.[7]

Chemotherapy

Most chemotherapeutic agents have adverse effects on the nutritional status due to various side effects caused by different agents since they not only act on the tumor cells, but also affect the normal cells, especially the gastrointestinal (GI) system. The duration of the drug administered, dosage and rate of metabolism may affect the degree of the GI functioning. A list of chemotherapeutic drugs used for treatment of various neoplasms and their adverse effects are highlighted in Table 40.6.[13]

TABLE 40.5: Types of neoplastic diseases of childhood associated with high and low nutritional risk

High nutritional risk	Low nutritional risk
Advanced diseases during initial intense treatment Stages III and IV Wilm's tumor and unfavorable histology Wilm's tumor stages III and IV neuroblastoma Pelvic Rhabdomyosarcoma Some non Hodgkins's lymphoma* Ewings sarcoma Acute nonlymphocytic leukemia Some poor prognosis lymphocytic leukemia Multiple relapse leukemia Medulloblastoma	Good prognosis acute lymphocytic leukemia (ALL). Non metastatic solid tumors. Advanced diseases in remission during maintenance treatment.

*Tumor which significantly impairs gastrointestinal function. Refer.[6]

Surgery

Some children with cancer might require surgical intervention for removal of tumor, or a radical surgery for head and neck or a massive intestinal resection for head. In such circumstances there is a decrease in intake for a prolonged period which may affect the nutritional status. Surgeries of the head and neck can cause chewing or swallowing problems, while intestinal resection may lead to malabsorption of vitamin B_{12} or bile acids, thus adversely affecting their nutritional status.

Radiation

Along with the two modalities of chemotherapy and surgery for treating cancer in children, some of them may require radiation too, which again is not without its own complications.[14] These could vary depending upon:

- The region of the body irradiated.
- Dose, fractionation, length of time and field size of radiation administered.

TABLE 40.6: Chemotherapeutic agents and toxicity affecting nutritional status

Drug	Antitumor spectrum	Toxicities
Mechlorethamine	Hodgkins brain tumors	N&V, muositis, NT (HD)
Procarbazine	-do-	N&V, NT, rash, mucositis
Lomustine	Brain tumors, lymphomas	N&V, renal & pulmonary toxicity
Antimetabolites		
Methotrexate	Leukemia, lymphoma, osteosarcoma	Mucositis, rash, hepatic, renal (HD), NT
6-Mercaptoprine	Leukemias (ALL, CML)	Hepatic, mucositis
6-Thioguanine	Leukemia (ANL)	N&V, mucositis, hepatic
Cytarabine	Leukemia, lymphoma	N&V, mucositis, ocular, skin (HD)
Antibiotics	Leukemia (ALL, ANL), lymphoma, most soild tumors	N&V, mucositis, cardiac, pulmonary, skin
Plant alkaloids		
Vincristine	Leukemia (ALL), lymphomas, most solid tumors	NT, constipation, hypotension
Vinblastine	Histocytosis, Hodgkins, testicular	Mucositis, mild NT
Etoposide	Leukemia (ALL, ANL), lymphomas, neuroblastoma, sarcomas, brain tumors	N&V, mucositis, mild NT, hypotension, allergic
Miscellaneous		
Prednisolone (orally) Prednisolone (IV) Dexamethasone L-Asparaginase	Leukemias, lymphoma Leukemia, lymphomas Leukemias, lymphomas, brain tumors ALL, lymphomas ALL, lymphomas	↑appetite, centripetal obesity, myopathy, osteoporosis, pancreatitis hyperactivity, hypertension, diabetes, growth failure, impaired wound healing, atrophy of sub cutaneous tissue N&V, acute pancreatitis, ↓serum albumin, insulin and lipoproteins
Alkylating agents		
Cyclophosphamide	Lymphomas, leukemias, sarcomas, neuroblastomas	N&V, cystitis, water retention, cardiac (HD)
Ifosamide	Sarcomas	N&V, cystitis, NT, renal
Cisplatin	Testicular and other germ cell osteosarcoma, brain tumors, neuroblastoma	N&V, mucositis
Busulfan	Leukemia, used inc oditioning regimen in marrow transplant	Avoid eating 1 hour prior and after taking drug
Decarbazine	Neuroblastoma, sarcomas	N&V, flulike syndrome, hepatic
Melphalan	Rhabdomyosarcoma, sarcomas, neuroblastomas, leukemia	N&V, mucositis, diarrhea (HD)

Refer. Balis FH, Holenberg JS, Poplack DG. General principles of chemotherapy. In: Principles and Practice of Pediatric Oncology. Pizzo DH and Poplack DG. Eds 1984, Lippincott Williams and Willams

***Note*:** ALL(acute lympholymphatic leukemia), ANL (acute non lymphocytic leukemia), CML (chronic myelogonous leukemia), AML (acute myeloid lymphoma), N&V (nausea and vomiting), NT (neuro toxicity), HD (high dose)

TABLE 40.7: Radiation effects in pediatric patients

Head and Neck • Nausea, anorexia • Mucositis, esophagitis • Decreased taste and smell • Damage to developing teeth • Decreased salivation→thick viscous mucus • Decreased motility
Thoracic • Pharyngeal and esophageal inflammation and cell damage • Sore throat, dysphagia • Abdominal or pelvic • Nausea vomiting, diarrhea • Ulceration • Colitis • Malabsorption • Fluid electrolyte imbalance
Total Body • Nausea, vomiting, diarrhea • Mucositis, esophagitis • Decreased taste and salivation • Anorexia • Delayed growth and development

Refer. 1, 14, 15

- Concurrent use of other antitumor therapy, e.g. surgery or chemotherapy.
- Child's pre-existing nutritional status.

The impact of radiation on various organ systems and how they affect the nutritional intake are summed up in Table 40.7.[1,14,15] As can be appreciated from the table, due to various side effects of radiation on different organs, like nausea, mucositis, vomiting, diarrhea, colitis, esophagitis, etc. the intake can be drastically compromised leading to severe malnutrition and delayed growth and development.

Nutritional Support for Children with Cancer

The goal for any nutritional support to be implemented for a child with cancer is:

- To enable tolerance to chemotherapy or radiation and minimize side effects
- To facilitate growth and healing
- To maximize quality of life
- To gain, maintain or lose only a minimal amount of weight.

Feeding a child with cancer can be quite a challenging task, keeping in view the complications associated with the treatment as mentioned earlier. Anorexia, nausea, mucositis and gastrointestinal disturbance can deter the child to consume optimally. During phases of chemotherapy, the child is able to eat very minimally due to complete aversion to eating. But this phase is mostly a transient one lasting till such time chemotherapy is continued. Subsequently, the appetite improves and it is during this period that maximal effort should be made to make the child eat optimally. Nutrient dense foods may be encouraged which can be given in smaller portions. Energy requirements can be based on the age and weight of the child and suitable increments can be planned to meet the increased needs. The requirements of these children are almost 20% higher than the normal dietary allowances. Protein needs are equally important for these children to maintain positive N balance and serum albumin levels at or above 3.2 g/dl, besides that required for optimal growth and development.

The energy density of foods may be enhanced by the use of fats like butter or cream on various preparations (Table 40.8). Due to the presence of anorexia, it is recommended that they have small feeds in greater frequency, rather than having fewer large sized portions of foods. Proteins can be enhanced by use of skimmed milk powder (36% protein) which is also calorie dense (360 kcals/100 g). Most important is to introduce maximum variety since mostly children liking a particular food on one day may refuse the same on another occasion.

The sense of taste and smell are greatly altered due to the side effects of chemotherapy or radiotherapy. These changes can affect the appetite and consequently optimum intake. Parents and care givers are advised to follow certain guidelines by which the child can be helped and encouraged to accept maximally as outlined in Table 40.9.[16]

Route of Feeding

Oral Feeding

As far as possible, it is recommended to encourage oral feeding. Due to the side effects of drugs, problems of nausea, vomiting or altered taste and smell as mentioned earlier may pose limitations in adequate nutrition being provided. This may be

TABLE 40.8: Tips to enhance energy density of diets

- Add finely cut cottage cheese to soups, vegetables or rice
- Add skimmed milk powder to chapatti, rice, milk, curd or any other milk based preparation. Use full cream milk
- If desired, hardboiled egg may be added to the vegetables or rice preparation
- Butter, cream or ghee may be added to the preparations to enhance flavor and energy
- Add raisins, dates, almonds or walnuts (chopped finely), into the preparations like milk, porridge or rice
- Beverages like sweetened drinks and fruit juice should be encouraged
- Small amounts of meals should be served rather than large meals per day
- Milk can be served with added cream
- Calorie dense sweets (from khoya) can be used to make puddings, desert, etc.
- Milk shakes with different flavors can help build up energy density
- Cooked peas, beans tofu may be used in preparations like rice, upma, etc.
- A protein based snack can be offered at bed time

TABLE 40.9: Guidelines for managing common nutritional problems of pediatric oncology patients

Problems	Ways to tackle
Tooth decay	If weight loss not a problem, limit sugars in the diet. Avoid sticky foods like candy, caramels, etc. Avoid bottle feeding to prevent baby bottle syndrome
Dysphagia (Taste alterations)	Flavor foods like milk, yoghurt, beverages Use herbs, spices to enhance taste Use highly aromatic foods Maintain good oral hygiene. Use mouth wash Blend fresh fruits into shakes, smoothies, ice cream, etc. Avoid too hot foods/beverages
Xerostomia (oral dryness)	Moisten foods. Use more of semi liquid foods Sucking of lemon/flavored sugarless candy can be helpful Encourage liquids with meals Add vinegar/pickles/chutneys to foods Extra sauces, gravies, butter and broth may be used Use commercial saliva substitutes Maintain good oral hygiene
Mucositis (oral/esophageal inflammation of mucosa)	Soft pureed texture or blenderised liquid diets Smooth blended moist foods (custard, soups) Use straw to drink beverages and liquids Frequent mouth washing to be done
Xerostomia (oral dryness)	Moisten foods, and use of liquids with meals to be encouraged Add vinegar/pickles/chutneys to foods Extra sauces, gravies, butter and broth may be used Use commercial saliva substitutes Maintain good oral hygiene
Thick viscous saliva	Adequate fluid intake to be ensured
Nausea and vomiting	High carbohydrate foods and fluids (crackers, toast, gelatin) Small frequent feedings Cold, clear liquids and solids Avoid very sweet of high fat foods Encourage sipping liquids through a straw Encourage rest periods after meals Avoid caffeine Ensure adequate fluids to maintain hydration

Condt...

Condt...

Problems	Ways to tackle
Diarrhea	Low fat, low fiber foods advised Low lactose foods recommended Avoid caffeine Adequate fluids to prevent dehydration
Constipation	Encourage adequate fluids Encourage high soluble fiber based foods Regular exercise if tolerated Avoid apple juice Avoid fizz drinks and chewing gum
Anorexia	Encourage small frequent meals of foods high in calories and proteins Use carbohydrate supplements and protein powders Avoid strong odors Avoid forced feeding Relaxation techniques and light exercise before meals can help
Heartburn (Reflux)	Limit high fat rich foods Avoid highly seasoned foods Avoid caffeine, chocolates and peppermint
Early Satiety	Encourage smaller frequent foods Limit high fat foods Avoid liquids at meal time Encourage regular exercises if tolerated

Refer. 16

especially so during the period of chemotherapy. In such conditions the care givers can be a little relaxed and feed whatever the child accepts for the duration of the chemotherapy period. But subsequently it is generally observed that the child is able to accept and tolerate orally. During the chemotherapy period effort should be made to maximize the density of the food or dishes the child is particularly fond of (Table 40.8), so that the lean period is compensated. For some children lactose load may cause gastrointestinal (GI) intolerance. In such cases, milk free based soya foods like tofu and soya flour or milk can be made use of to provide adequate proteins in the diet. There are certain lactose free supplements available commercially which can be incorporated in their feeds or other preparations to further enhance the nutrient density of the foods.

Enteral Feeding

In children where oral acceptance is minimal for a prolonged period of time, enteral route is the next option to be considered. These may be given through nasogastric route which is the most common technique of feeding in children with cancer. The benefit of such feeding is that one can ensure the desired amount to be fed as per the nutrient requirements in a given volume which can be evenly distributed over the whole day and night. This also eases the stress on the part of the care givers to ensure adequate feeding, especially when the child is very irritable or refusing to eat at all. However, older children initially might resent this mode of feeding because of psychological trauma associated with the insertion and maintenance of tubes, but over a period of time they do get accustomed to it and get fairly comfortable with it.

An alternative to nasogastric feeding is gastrostomy feeding which is known to provide more effective nutritional support as compared to other modes and is also found to be a safe and cost effective method of reversing malnutrition in very malnourished children.[17] This mode of feeding is particularly effective where nasogastric feeding may be difficult or unsuitable in conditions of nausea and vomiting or delayed gastric emptying.[18]

In children who are unable to tolerate enteral nutrition in the form of nasogastric feeding, gastric or jejunal tube feeding is also another alternative, which can bypass the nasopharynx route. Percutanous endoscopic gastrostomies (PEG) have been used successfully in patients with cancer, which can increase the intake and also reduce stress of feeding on family members.

Parenteral Nutrition

Parenteral route of feeding is usually used as the last resort, when the patient cannot ingest, digest or absorb food via the GI route.[9] The decision to use PN depends on factors like the existing nutritional status, expected duration of therapy, availability of peripheral veins and most important the cost involved.

Partial PN may be resorted to till such time the child is able to tolerate oral or enteral feeding. Complete PN should be reserved for shorter periods in children with failure of enteral absorption and no response to dietary supplements. However, the potential complications of PN do exist which include risks of infection, metabolic disorders, hepatotoxicity and reduction of oral intake.

It has been shown that there is a positive role of glutamine supplementation by reducing the detrimental effects of anti cancer drugs on the gastrointestinal mucosa.[19] In addition carnitine supplementation too has been shown to improve the 'cancer fatigue syndrome' by influencing nutritional and immunological parameters.[20] A summary of various feeding strategies used for feeding children with cancer are presented in Table 40.10.[12]

TABLE 40.10: Feeding strategies In children with cancer

Nutritional strategy	Indications
Enteral Route	In all patients with functional GI meeting >95–100% of estimated energy needs.
Tube Feeding (Nasogastric)	Inability to ingest full energy needs (>90%) through oral diet for 3–5 days.
PEG Jejunostomy	Inability to meet full energy needs through tube diet for 3–5 days Weight loss despite tube feeding
Parenteral Nutrition	Altered GI absorption for 3–5 days Severe vomiting and diarrhea Severe pancreatitis Intestinal manifestations of graft vs host disease Paralytic ileus

Refer. 12

MARROW TRANSPLANT

Marrow transplant (MT) is becoming a practice in an increasing number of children with hematology and oncological problems. Children with various conditions like those of hematologic malignancies which include acute lymphoblastic leukemia (ALL), acute myelogenous leukemia (AML), recurrent lymphomas are all suitable candidates for MT. Other conditions include those of solid tumors, neoplastic disorders of the bone marrow, like severe a plastic anemia, genetic storage disorders like niemann pick disease, infantile osteoporosis and certain immunologic disorders, which merit considering MT.

Before the process of MT, there is a period of conditioning regimen which is initiated preceding any multimodal chemotherapy or high dose radiotherapy over a period of 4–10 days. This is done to remove any active and residual malignant cells and also improve immunosuppression of the patient for favorable response of marrow graft.[21]

Post-Transplant Course

Patients after the transplant period are highly susceptible to bacterial and fungal infections till the period the marrow is completely engrafted. This may take almost 2–6 weeks and this is why in most dedicated centers, patients are placed in isolated areas with all precautions of barrier nursing. Complications interfering with nutrient intake may be mucositis, esophagitis, altered taste, nausea and vomiting. Diarrhea and steatorrhea may also add to the complications.

It may be necessary to use EN or PN in the earlier 5–6 days, if oral intake is compromised due to the above mentioned factors. As soon as oral intake is established and the child is able to consume adequately, high calorie and high protein based diet can be initiated. Since these children are at risk of infections and may be immunocompromised, care should be taken to advise neutropenic precautions (Table 40.11), which involve a slightly modified

TABLE 40.11: Foods to be restricted on a neutropenic diet

- Raw and undercooked vegetables, salads, fruits
- Raw and undercooked meats, eggs, fish
- Unpasteurised milk and milk products like curd, paneer
- Tofu, sausages, cold or smoked fish
- Ripened cheese or cheese based salad dressings
- Any stale, moldy vegetables or fruits
- Untoasted bread/buns/pastries/cakes
- Herbal food supplements
- Honey if not processed and sealed. Mushrooms
- Untreated water from any source

Refer. 22

diet than normal home based one.[22] The child after discharge needs to be followed up regularly for continues counseling and reinforcement to avoid a state of malnutrition. Table 40.11 lists the foods to be restricted on a neutropenic diet.

Complications of Marrow Transplant

Graft vs Host Disease

Patients who have undergone a marrow transplant, usually are at risk of developing GVHD, which is an immunologic reaction leading to multi-organ damage. In this condition there is an immunologic response by the newly engrafted marrow to the host cells which it does not recognize.[23]

The GVHD may manifest through different organ systems like the gastrointestinal, skin or liver, which may result in symptoms like diarrhea with bleed, anorexia, dyspepsia and cramps in the abdomen. In such conditions, the patient is given bowel rest initially and later gradually progressed to a normal diet, taking care to begin with one food at a time. This transition is also termed as 'refeeding',[24] which implies slow and gradual progression from a liquid to solid foods in small frequent amounts. The diet should be energy dense and high in proteins, but low in fiber. Some high energy and protein foods which can be incorporated are:

- Full cream milk and milk products
- Butter, oil, ghee
- Soups with creamy base
- Boiled eggs
- Dips , made with cream cheese
- Protein based supplements may be used
- Low fiber foods like melons or peeled fruits
- Use of refined cereals/pulses, white bread, rice, etc.
- Low lactose products like yoghurt may be used if milk intolerance is indicated.
- Small frequent feedings, are advised, every 2–3 hourly (liquid to semi solid feeds initially), followed by more solid foods in greater amounts as tolerated.

REFERENCES

1. Rickard KA, Grosfeld JL, Coates TD, Weetman R, Baehner RL. Advances in nutrition care of children with neoplastic disease: a review of treatment, research and application. J Am Diet Assoc. 1986;86:1666-76.
2. Meadows AT, Friedman DL, Neglia JP, Mertens AC, et al. Second neoplasms in survivors of cancer: findings from the childhood cancer survivors study Cohort. J Clin Oncol. 2009;27:2356-62.
3. Ham Markey T. Nutritional considerations in pediatric oncology. Semin Oncol Nurs. 2000;16:146-51.
4. Coates TD, Rickard KA, Grosfeld JL, et al. Nutritinal support in children with neoplastic diseases. Surg Clin North Am. 1986;66:1197-12.
5. Donaldson SS, Wesley MN, De Wys WD, Suskind RM, et al. A study of nutritional status of pediatric cancer patients. Am J Dis Child. 1981;135:1107-12.
6. Rickard KA, Grosfed JR, Coates TD, et al. The value of nutritional support in children with cancer. Cancer. 1986;58:1904-10.
7. Hamill PV, Drizd TA, Johnson CL. NCHS Growth Curves for children birth to 18 years, US Vital and Health Statistics Series 2. National Center for Health Statistics. 1977.
8. Stead RH, Brock JF. Experimental protein and calorie malnutrition: Rapid induction of protein depletion signs in early weaned rats. J Nutr. 1972;102:1357-66.
9. Alexandar HR, Rickard KA, Godshall B. Nutritional supportive care. In, Pizzo PA, Poplack DG, Eds. Principles and Practice of Pediatric Oncology. Philadelphia: JB Lippincott Co. 1997:1167-82.
10. Elia M. Hunger disease. Clin Nutr. 2000;19:379-86.

11. Kern KA, Norton JA. Cancer cachexia. J Pareneter Enter Nutr. 1988;12:286-98.
12. Bauer J. Jurgens H and Frukwald MC. Important aspects of Nutrtion in children with cancer. Advances in Nutr. July 2011.
13. Balis FH, Holenberg JS, Poplack DG. General principles of chemotherapy. In: Principles and Practice of Pediatric Oncology. Pizzo DH and Poplack DG. Eds. Lippincott Williams and Willams. 1984.
14. Donaldson SS, Lexon RA. Alterations of nutritional status. Impact of chemotherapy and radiotherapy. Cancer. 1979;43:2036-52.
15. Coates TD, Rickard KA, Grosfeld JL, et al. Nutritional support of children with neoplastic diseases. Surg Clin North Am. 1986;66:1197-1212.
16. Charuhas PM. Introduction to marrow transplant, Oncology Nutrition, Dietetic Practice Group Newsletter, vol 2, No. 3, pp.2-9.
17. Aquino VM, Smyrl CB, Hagg R, et al. Enteral nutritional support by gastrostomy tube in children with cancer. J Pediatrics. 1995;127:58-62.
18. Holden D, Sexton E, Paul L. Enteral nutrition. Pediatr Nurs. 1996;8:28-33.
19. Kuhn KS, Muscaritoli M, Wischmerger P, Stehle P. Glutamine as indispensable nutrient in oncology: experimental and clinical evidence. Eur J Nutr. 2010;49:197-210.
20. Hockenberry MJ, Hooke MC, Greguirch M, Nc Carth K. Carnitine plasma levels and fatigue in children/ adolescents receiving cisplastin, ifosfamide or doxorubicin. J Pediatr Hematol Oncol. 2009;31:664-9.
21. Peterson FB, Bearman SL. Preparative regimens and their toxicity. In: Forman SJ, Blue KG, Thomas ED eds. Bone Marrow Transplantation. Boston. Blackwell Scientific Publications. 1994.
22. Moe GL. The low microbial diets for patients with granulocytopenia. In: Bloch A ed. Nutritional management of the cancer patient. Gaithersburg. MD Aspen Publisher. 1990:125-34.
23. Pichel D. Bone marrow transplant in children. J Pediatr. 1993;122:331-41.
24. Lenssen P. Bone marrow and stem cell transplantation. In: Matarese LE, Gottschlich MM, eds. Contemporary Nutrition Support Practice: A Clinical Guideline. Philadelphia. WB Saunders Co. 1998;561-81.

41 The Ketogenic Diet in Management of Epilepsy

The treatment of epilepsy has been described since the era of Hippocrates in 400 BC,[1] when it was considered as a prophetic curse. He refuted this belief and advocated 'purging and fasting' as a cure for the disease. Detoxification method was also used by earlier workers in 1911 by Guelpa and Marie[2] by reducing vegan diet and fasting and purging.

HISTORY OF KETOGENIC DIET

In 1920, Russel Wilder at Mayo Clinic proposed that the benefits of fasting would be obtained by producing high levels of ketones in the body (ketonemia) through excess of fat and lack of carbohydrates. This led to the coining of the new term 'ketogenic diet'. In 1921, Geylin first reported about fasting as an alternative treatment to anti-epileptic drugs (AED) for controlling intractable seizures. In the 26 patients who were fasted for 15–25 days, 18 of his patients showed marked improvement. This was attributed to a neutralization of the deleterious effects of toxins from the Peyer's patches in the intestines.[2]

Wilder's colleague pediatrician Myne Peterman later formulated the 'classic diet' with a ratio of 1 g of protein per Kg body weight and 10–15 g carbohydrates (CHO)/day and the balance calories to be obtained from fat. This diet was seemingly supposed to mimic the metabolic effects of fasting. This was akin to the 4:1 ratio keto diet used today.

In 1938, Dr Merritt and Petrmann discovered dilantin and subsequently in 1939 phenytoin became the drug of choice in the management of epilepsy. Susequently there was an advent of a series of AEDs like carbamazepine in 1950s, clonazepam in 1974, sodium valporate in 1978 and clobazam in 1979. As a result fewer children were placed on KD, leading to a steady decline in the use of KD. In 1971, Dr Huttenlocher introduced the MCT diet in an attempt to retain the beneficial effect which was less restrictive and easier to administer. This diet was found to be too rigid, too unpalatable and difficult to prepare and maintain.[3]

The Story of Charlie

Charlie was a young boy of 2 years and half, who first developed seizures on March 11, 1993, which could not be controlled and by 1994, he had as many as 100 seizures a day. None of the drugs worked for him and it was then that his father Jim Abraham, a TV producer heard of John Hopkins Hospital and the KD. Charlie was put on KD and within a few days he stopped having seizures. He continued on this diet for 2 years, remaining totally seizure free and then stopped. Within a few days seizures again recurred and he was back on KD. Subsequently, he became seizure free and went off the diet and medication for many years. It was then that Jim started the 'Charlie Foundation. He produced a video about Charlie's story and sent it to every pediatric neurologist in the US in 1955, Charlie Foundation started the first multicentric study on KD.[4] In 1997, he produced a movie 'First do no harm', starring Meryl Steep and Millicent Kelly, a dietician at John Hopkins Hospital.

Mechanism of Action of KD

The KD is a diet with high fat content, which causes conversion of fats to ketones, which are further utilized for energy instead of glucose. This diet allows incomplete oxidation of fatty acids by the liver resulting in the accumulation of ketone bodies in urine and blood. The body uses these ketones instead of glucose as a source of energy. When carbohydrates are deprived to the body by prolonged fasting, the body begins to utilize fats and proteins for fuel. As fats are oxidized for energy, they are not oxidized completely thereby resulting in a buildup of residues or waste products of acetone and ketone bodies. These ketone bodies build up in the blood and spill over into the urine, resulting in a state of ketosis. This has an anticonvulsant effect, thereby inhibiting seizures.[4] Others put forth the theory that certain changes occur at the neurotransmitter level which improves cerebral energy.[5]

While on a ketogenic diet, the body does not solely rely on stored fat and ketones as the primary fuel source. It will also rely on dietary fats. This is the major difference between starvation and ketogenesis. This is also why one cannot consume unlimited calories on a ketogenic diet and expect to lose weight. The body will use dietary fats as a primary fuel source along with the subsequent ketone bodies from oxidation of dietary fats and then will use adipose, only if the calories are maintained at a level below that required to maintain body weight. If calories are maintained at suboptimal level on KD, the body is forced to begin lipolysis. This becomes the primary energy source with other physiological mechanisms stepping up to allow normal and efficient functioning while on KD.[6]

Selection of Patients for Ketogenic Diet

Type of Epilepsy

The response to KD is largely based on the type of seizure of childhood, like myoclonic, where good response has been reported.[7] Those with tonic clonic (grand mal) epilepsy may be helped, but in other types of seizures this diet may not be effective. Children with refractory epilepsy were found to benefit more with the diet as compared to any alternative anticonvulsant drug.[7]

For patients who benefit, half will achieve a seizure reduction within 5 days. If the diet starts with an initial fast of 1–2 days, three fourths achieve a seizure reduction within a fortnight and 90% achieve reduction within 23 days. If the diet does not begin with a fast, the time achieved for about 50% of the children could be longer, but the long-term seizure rates are unaffected. Since fasting increases the risk of acidosis and hypoglycemia, it is recommended only in some medical emergency. A carbohydrate wash out regimen is a better alternative before initiating KD. If no improvement is seen within 2 months, it indicates failure of the diet.[8]

Age of the Patient

Ketogenic diet has been found to be most effective in children between ages 2–5 years old. These children become ketotic soon and maintain adequate levels of ketosis with the diet. The diet seems to get less effective with each progressive year and by adolescence, is rarely found to be successful.[9] On the other hand very young children rarely produce ketosis and hence not indicated.[10] Infants are at greatest risk from nutritional deficiencies of the dietary regimen and therefore should be avoided in this age group.

Motivation/Compliance

The KD can be successful and adhered to only if there is a complete rapport between the parents and the patients and the dietetic and metabolic team. If the diet is not complied with rigidly, the ketotic effect disappears thus nullifying the benefit effect of going through the whole exercise. Accidental lapse or pilfering of carbohydrates based diet if taken at any point even in minute amounts can negate the ketosis, thereby bringing back the seizures which may falsely implicate failure of the diet.

Failure of AEDs

The KD is initiated only after at least 2–3 medicines have failed, as it is not very easy to administer and maintain on this diet. Moreover the diet is comparatively rigid and demands lifestyle changes.

Literacy and Socioeconomic Factor

Following a KD involves some expenditure in terms of dietary products to be procured, which need to be labeled for all the nutritive values. This therapy involves measuring urine ketones daily to ensure adequate ketosis and this requires use of keto diastix to measure ketosis. These diastix are not very cheap and regular use entails recurrent expenditure. It may not be financially possible for families with limited resources. Literacy level of parents/care givers too is crucial since the diet maintenance requires careful weighing of all ingredients and reading all food labels before preparing the diet.

Other factors

Patients with infantile spasms who respond poorly to medication should also be considered for KD. According to Dr Nathan, since there is 90% improvement in children with infantile spasm on KD, it is recommended to initiate this diet as first line of treatment.[11] Children who are retarded, or are fed by gastrostomy tube or on Ryle's tube, may also be suitable candidates for KD, as it is easier to use and be more effective than trying medications.

Initiating Ketogenic Diet

Initiating ketogenic diet involves 4 phases as follows:[11]

Phase 1

Prediet counseling: Before a patient is put on KD, it is very important that the parents be counseled regarding all the details of the therapy and need to be explained the rationale behind this mode of therapy in a scientific way:

- It has to be impressed upon them that they should not expect miracles from the therapy. However, they can be reassured regarding the goal of this type of management, even though results may be appreciated not before 4–6 weeks of initializing the diet.
- The importance of actually weighing the food ingredients and use of only instructed food items in prescribed portions should be explained and impressed upon them for the therapy to be successful. If possible, a list of recipes and their demonstration of preparing them will create a greater impact.
- Demonstration of urine testing for ketones needs to be done and a ketone chart should be maintained. This helps both parents and the dietician and the keto team to obtain a fair feed back of the efficacy of the diet.
- Parents need to understand that the yardstick of success of the diet is gauged by reduction/control of seizures.
- Reduction of AEDs comes secondary and may be found in about 30%, another 30% may be totally free of seizures while the rest 40% may not show any reduction.
- Most children may show generalized mental alertness and increase in intelligence.
- Care givers/parents need to be explained regarding the history of dietary management, which can help them adhere and comply strictly to the diet.
- All medications have to be sugar free, even to the extent of the tooth paste used, which can contain some sugar.
- Sugar free toothpastes like Vicco or Meswak should be used only.
- While using IV fluids, only saline should be used instead of dextrose based.
- Keto diets may be with held for sometime during periods of acute illness or infections.

Initiating of the KD

Managing a child with KD requires the following steps:

1. ***Personal history:*** This includes details relating to the patients contacts, family physician, family members at home, grandparents and other members in a joint family who also need to be counseled regarding the significance of the KD, meticulous planning and execution of the diet.
2. ***Anthropometry:*** Recording of the weight and height of the patient is the primary step before planning a KD, since the calories fixed are based upon the ideal body weight (IBW) and involves a formula using both parameters. However, height recording may be problem in children with presence of spaticity and contactures.
3. ***Medical history:*** History regarding any pre-existing problems of allergies has to be considered,

other chronic ailments like asthma, diabetes mellitus, tuberous sclerosis should be also accounted for while planning the diet. Other AEDs prescribed need to be recorded.

4. ***Diet History:*** While planning a diet for the child, it is worthwhile to extract certain details of the eating patterns likes/dislikes, the number of meals taken over the day, preferences, and religious issues, e. g. vegetarian or nonvegetarian and any other relevant ethnic background information.
5. ***Investigations:*** Some common investigations required are serum proteins, CBC, Lipid profile, serum electrolytes, serum calcium, uric acid, serum creatinine, blood sugars, and liver enzymes along with blood for gas values. EEG and psychometric examinations need to be done at the beginning and once annually thereafter.

Phase 2

Carbohydrate wash out or pre keto diet: In the earlier days before initializing the KD, the patient was made to fast for 1–2 days to enable to produce ketosis easily. But gradually the practice of fasting was rarely followed and instead a carbohydrate wash out is administered to achieve a ketosis of 4+ within 3–4 days. The advantage of this diet is that it does not require any exact weighing of food or fixing timings of meals. The major constituents of this diet are fats and proteins and negligible carbohydrates. A list of foods that can be given during the carbohydrate wash out phase are listed in Table 41.1.

Certain points need to be borne in mind while following a CHO wash out diet like:

- Offer small frequent feeds
- Check urine ketones
- Free foods to be given in between like sugar free jelly, sugar free sherbet
- Offer water unrestricted
- No calculations or weighing of foods needed
- Follow a diet for a minimum of 2–3 days to achieve 4+ ketones
- No hospitalization required.

Prerequisite of a ketogenic diet: Before the actual KD is initiated, during the CHO wash out phase, parents are advised to procure the following items to actually prepare and monitor the diet:

TABLE 41.1: Foods allowed and restricted in CHO wash out phase

Not allowed	Allowed moderately	Allowed liberally
All cereals/pulses: Chapati, rice, suji, dals Gram flour, corn flour	Tomato, cucumber-5g	All non vegetable foods: Chicken, fish, eggs, homemade mayonnaise
Sugar and sweets: All sweets, honey, jaggery, all bakery products	Amul/Britannia cheese/paneer - 1 cube	All soya products: Soya flour, soya dal, soya rawa, soya granules, soya milk (Godrej-Sofit/Natural Staeta)
All processed foods, aspartame, sugar free tabs	Amul cream - 50g	Beverages-water, plain soda (color, essence, sugar free natura tab)
Vegetables-all root vegetables Fruits-Banana, mangoes, chikkoo	Almonds, walnuts, groundnuts – 5-	Fats and oils-butter, ghee
Medicines-syrups or any sugar coated pills, toothpaste, IV dextrose		Sugar free toothpaste- Vicco/ Meswak, IV Saline

- Digital weighing scale with ± 1 g accuracy
- Other kitchen items like measuring cups, glass, spoons, airtight containers, non-stick pan, fiber spatula rubber and wooden spatula
- Urine keto diastics for measuring ketones.

Phase 3

Once the ketone levels of 4+ are achieved on a CHO wash out diet, or even if not, and on the diet for at least 3–4 days, the ketogenic diet is calculated and planned by the dietician. The ratio of the keto diet has to be fixed, i.e. 2:1 or 3:1 or 4:1 depending upon the age, severity of seizures, etc. and then the ideal body weight (IBW) for the child is derived from his height and weight.

Diet Calculations

The steps involved in the calculations are as follows:

a. To begin with the IBW is derived for the given child which works out to be- 50th centile of IBW÷50th centile of height × actual height.
b. The calories required are then derived which should be 75% of the RDA for the given child as per his age (Table 41.2).
c. Next the keto ratio has to be decided, which is the ratio of grams of fat to the sum of grams of carbohydrate and proteins, e.g. 2:1, 3:1 or 4:1. In a ratio of 2:1, it implies that 2g of fat to 1 g of protein and carbohydrates combined. For instance 2 × 9 (cals per g from fat) = 18 and 1 × 4 (cals per g from carbohydrate and protein), i.e. 18 + 2 = 22. So, the Dietary Unit Composition (DUC) = 22.
c. Next Dietary Unit Quotient (DUQ) is calculated as Calories ÷ DUC
d. Fat Allowance = DUQ × 2 (keto ratio)
e. CHO + Protein allowance (C + P) = DUQ × 1(C + P ratio)
f. Protein Allowance: This is calculated for a given age group based on the RDA (Table 17.3) which may range from 1 – 1.5 g/kg/d.
g. CHO allowance = C + P – P
h. Meal Order: This is the number of meals the child would consume per day, e.g. 4, 5 or 6. meals/d. This number divided by the total fats, carbohydrates and protein allowance is the per meal distribution for fats, carbohydrates and proteins.

Planning of Recipes

It is important that each recipe is calculated based on the derived fat, carbohydrate and protein for that specific patient. For this, the dietician needs to be aware of and have a list of all commercial food products available locally, so as to be able to calculate the exact values. A table of nutritive values of different foods per 100 grams should be at hand for ready reference.[12] Knowledge of all the locally available commercial foods is essential, which can be used in various recipes and parents need to be encouraged to use those products only for preparing the KD. Vegetables and fruits are divided into A and B groups depending upon their carbohydrate content as given in Tables 41.2 A and 41.2B.[12] There are some free foods which can be given to the child in unrestricted amount and any time of the day. These are:

- Sugar free, flavored sherbet, juices (sugar free) should be sucrolose based only, e.g. naturla gold
- Sugar free jelly, ice candy
- Gelatin, jelly
- Plain soda

The food groups that can be given in a ketogenic diet are as listed in Table 41.3

TABLE 41.2A: Food exchange list for vegetables*

Vegetable A group (4% CHO)-20g	Vegetable B group (8% CHO)-10g
Amaranth (Chaulai), Bitter gourd, bottle gourd, brinjal, capsicum, cucumber, green papaya, tomato, parwal, French beans, ridge gourd, snake gourd, spinach, tinda, white radis	Onions, broad beans, cauliflower, cluster beans, cabbage, carrots, fenugreek

*Veg. Group B =1/2 of Vegetable Group A
Refer.[12] ICMR values

TABLE 41.2B: Food exchange list for fruits*

Fruit A (10% CHO) -15g	Fruit B (15% CHO) -10 g
Figs, guava, sweet lime (mausambi), muskmelon, watermelon, orange ripe, pears, papaya, plums, raspberry, strawberry, rose apple (jambool)	Amla, apple, ramphal, cashew fruit, red cherries, grapes (blue and green), lichi, mango ripe, pomegranate (anar), prunes

*Fruit B = 2/3rd of Fruit A
Refer.[12] ICMR values

TABLE 41.3: List of foods to be given in a ketogenic diet

	Foods restricted	Foods unrestricted
Carbohydrate Source	Given in less amounts (CHO foods)	Vegetables, fruits, cereals, pulses, milk, some spices
Fats	Given in liberal amounts (fats and protein foods)	Fats, oils, cheese, paneer, cream, chicken, fish, egg, soya products
GO	Free foods	Sugar free, jelly, zero calorie drinks, zero tab salt

Considerations or Special Categories of Patients

a. ***Overweight children:*** In case of overweight children, it is recommended to reduce and achieve desirable weight, which can be done by reducing 100 calories from the calculated 75% of the RDA for the given age group. It is essential that the child burns the excess body weight. A brief diet history can give an idea of the pre diet intake. The activity level of the child also will determine the required calories.

b. ***Underweight children*:** In case of underweight children, if calories are inadequate, there is risk of the proteins being utilized for energy, therefore it is recommended to add 100 calories to the derived 75% of the RDA for the given child.

c. ***Fluid allowance*:** The fluid allowance for a child on KD is generally 1 ml/cal.

Fine Tuning of Ketogenic Diet

Once the KD is planned, there may be many questions the parents /caregivers might come across in the days to day routine. Therefore it should be kept in mind that just planning a diet does not end the task of the dietician's task. A lot of fine tuning may be required on individual basis and from time to time. Following are the general principles to be followed:

- Make only one change at a given time—either calories (usually 100/d) or ratio (usually 0.2–0.5).
- It might take 15–30 days to assess the effect.
- Urine testing should be done regularly (3–4/d) and around the same time.
- Ensuring charting to be done immediately.
- The warning signs of excess ketosis should be explained to the parents.

Some of the problems which may arise at initiation of KD would revolve around the following factors which need re adjustment:

- Calorie intake
- Keto ratio
- CHO ratio
- Use/misuse of free foods
- Recipe preparation
- Recipe presentation
- Fastidious eaters
- Fluid intake
- Processed food content
- Proper calculation of recipe
- Proper food values
- Intercurrent illness.

Tube Feeding of KD

In children where tube feeding is required the following points need to be considered:

- Plan the feed based on the IBW and calories required. The recipes however would be different.
- Same precautions of weighing ingredients are required as for other KD.
- Oil/butter/ghee should not be pre-mixed in the recipe but done so just before feeding.
- The mixture should be brought to room temperature or made slightly warm before feeding.
- After feeding the tube should be flushed with 10–15 ml of sterile water.
- The vitamin supplements if required should be added to the feeds.
- Rest of the precautions required for any tube feeds, apply to feeding KD too.

Phase 4

After the child is initiated on the KD, it is essential to follow them up at regular intervals. The follow-up involves:

- Anthropometry: Weight and height at every visit.
- Check ketone charts which are to be maintained by patients.
- Recheck of ketone testing should be done at every visit.
- Weighing scales to be evaluated for accuracy.
- A variety of recipes to be planned and given to patients.
- Problems of constipation/diarrhea or urine frequency to be addressed at every follow-up.

Side Effects on KD

As this diet is not as per the typical normal diet, certain side effects may occur in some patients, but all of them can be handled 3 with the required adjustments. Side effects may be short-term or long-term as shown in Table 41.4.

Hypoglycemia: Generally seen in children who begin with fasting, especially in small babies. But currently fasting the child is not practiced. To manage the effect of hypoglycemia, blood sugars should be checked

TABLE 41.4 Side effects of ketogenic diet

Short-term early side effects	Long-term side effects
Hypoglycemia	Growth retardation
Drowsiness	Anemia
Dehydration	Hypomagnesemia
Nausea, vomiting	Zinc deficiency
Constipation	Osteopenia
Hyperuricemia	Hypercarotenemia

every 4 hours. In case the child is very sleepy, 30 ml of sugar free orange juice may be given. A carbohydrate wash out diet should be initiated rather than fasting before a KD.

Drowsiness: This can happen due to possible change in binding of certain anticonvulsants allowing higher concentration of these into the brain, causing lethargy or drowsiness in some children.

Dehydration: Fluid intake may be suboptimal, as in patients on KD, thirst is decreased and the child becomes more sedated. Therefore one should look for signs of dehydration. To manage this problem, plain water or soda with sugar free tablet with flavors like orange or sweet lime may be offered. Normal saline can also be given.

Nausea/Vomiting: When patients are fasted before starting on KD, followed by a high fat diet with ratio of 4:1, there may be excess of ketosis and acidosis which can cause vomiting. In some children long-term used of foods like eggs, soya and excess of oil/ghee in the diet could cause vomiting. To manage the problem, fasting should be avoided and a lower keto ratio of fats to carbohydrates and proteins may be planned. Sucking of ice cubes before and after meals can reduce this problem. Plain soda with flavors (sugar free) before and after can help reduce the effect of vomiting. High ketosis causing vomiting may be managed by offering some orange juice (sugar free) before meals.

Constipation: *This may occur due to a small volume of food which is very low in carbohydrates. A very low fiber and restricted fluids intake can also contribute to the problem. To manage this problem, fiber content may be increased by adding vegetables from Group A (Table 37.2 a) in the diet. Laxatives which are sugar free can help alleviate the problem.*

Crystalluria: A high protein intake and restricted fluid intake can lead to formation of crystals in the urine. This can be corrected by increasing water or fluid intake and also reducing intake of purine rich foods like meats, pulses, beans, etc.

Long-Term Side Effects

Growth retardation: Most children do lag behind the normal growth velocity due to restricted calories and proteins but once they are off the diet, they do catch up with expected growth pattern.

Nutritional deficiency: Since the diet is not a normal diet, it tends to lack in some essential micronutrients, resulting in deficiency of some essential micro nutrients, resulting in anemia, hypomagnesemia, selenium deficiency, zinc deficiency and osteopenia. It is therefore important to supplement these vitamins and minerals in their feeds.

Hyperlipidemia: The ketogenic diet being very high in fats, risk of hyperlipidemia cannot be ruled out. However, the adverse effects can be minimized by a judicious use of various fats and oils. The combination of fats is vital and also the ratio of various fats, rather than any one single fat, like groundnut oil and sunflower oil and ghee in the ratio of 2:1 in a 4 meal day (monounsaturated, polyunsaturated and saturated). Use of soybean oil is advocated due to its hypocholesterolemic effect. Good amount of fiber through fruits and vegetables can also help.

In general all complications of the KD are transient and can be managed easily with various conservative treatments. However, life threatening complications need to be monitored closely during follow-up.[13]

Important Factors to be Considered on KD

- Offer small/frequent meals (2–3 hourly).
- Use liberal fats /oils.
- Use a combination of groundnut oil and sunflower oil in alternative recipes.
- Use sugar free medications/tooth paste.
- Supplement vitamins and minerals as required.
- Soya pack once opened should be consumed within 24 hours.
- In case of vomiting/decreased appetite, seek medical aid.

The MCT Keto Diet

This type of diet uses medium chain triglycerides (MCT) based fat in combination with the KD. The advantage of this is that the energy distribution is done as 30% from MCT, 30% from fat and 40% energy from combined natural foods which will provide proteins, carbohydrates and additional dietary fats. It could be 19% carbohydrates and 10% proteins and 11% other fats. Sources of MCT used are butter, ghee, mayonnaise olive oil, margarine, coconut oil and commercially available formulations (Simyl MCT). Success rate with use of MCT oil along with classified KD in some percentage to help achieve ketosis and also to increase the bulk of the diet. The advantage of MCT is that it allows more protein intake, includes more micronutrients and has fewer incidence of kidney stones or constipation. But there are certain disadvantages too of this diet as it was found to be very unpalatable thereby having lower compliance. Problems of abdominal cramps, severe diarrhea or nausea and vomiting may occur on this diet. Moreover it is more costly than the other diets.

Therefore it is recommended that MCT based KD be used in patients who:

- Are not on valporate or epival anticonvulsant as it may interfere with these drugs.
- Are not on gastric tube feeds.
- Have no problem of aspiration or diarrhea.
- Are picky eaters.
- Have large appetites.
- Are older than 1 year especially adolescents.

Lastly MCT diet can be used in any ratio, based on individual tolerance and the need to improve seizure control.

Discontinuation of Diet

The diet may be weaned off or discontinued after 2–3 years on the diet, or after 6 months of seizure free period. This should be done gradually over a period of 2–3 months by lowering the keto ratio, till urinary ketosis is nil. Thereafter a free diet without any calorie restriction is allowed. But the rate of recurrence of seizures is expected in about 20% of the cases, over varying periods averaging 2 years. At certain centers this diet can be carried out for as long as possible or till the child is able to accept and tolerate it well. The policy may vary from one center to the other.

Modified Atkins Diet

If the classical KD or the MCT based diets are too difficult to follow or too restrictive, the modified Atkins diet is an easier alternative to help control seizures. Although mAD was basically introduced for inducing weight loss, it has found a reasonable acceptability as an alternative to the classic KD. In this type of diet a consistent level of ketosis may not be achieved, but in older children, who may not comply with restrictions of a classical KD, mAD may be a more tolerable option.[14] It is typically a high fat, low carbohydrate diet, the advantages of which are:

- No fasting/hospitalization is required
- No calculations/weighing is required
- No limit to the amount and timings of eating.
- Wider variety
- Does not require constant supervision of a doctor/ dietician.

Table 41.5 highlights the major differences between the original and modified Atkins diet.

The list of foods allowed in mAD is as given in Table 41.6. There are certain points to be instructed to the care givers while preparing the mAD like:

TABLE 41.5: Modified Atkins diet versus Classic ketogenic diet

Modified Atkins diet	Classic ketogenic diet
High fat foods strongly encouraged	High fat foods are allowed
Amount of carbohydrates: 0–2 years—5 g 2–12 years—10 g >12 years—15 g	Carbohydrates 20 g/d for just 2 weeks
Weight loss not the goal Eat ad lib	Weight loss is the main goal

TABLE 41.6: Foods allowed in modified Atkins diet

Carbohydrates	Given in prescribed amounts	Vegetable/ fruits, milk/milk products, nuts
Fats/Proteins	Zero carb foods given freely (fats and protein foods)	Fats, oils, chicken, fish, eggs, soya products, homemade mayonnaise
Go (Ad lib)	Zero calorie foods/free foods	Sugar free jelly, zero calorie drinks, zero tab salt

- Chop vegetables in small pieces and deep fry chicken, eggs, fish, mutton, etc.
- Make cubes/toffees of butter. Freeze it and then grate or top it on recipes or use as garnishing.
- Use ad lib oil/ghee for recipe preparations.

The amount of carbohydrates permitted varies on the age of the child:

2–12 year olds—allowed any 4 items/d, each containing 2.5 g CHO from the listed foods rich in CHO (vegetables, fruits, milk/milk products, nuts)

>12 year olds—allowed any 3 items/d each containing 5 g CHO.

The CHO exchange list to be used in mAD is as shown in Table 41.7.[11]

The Low Glycemic Index Treatment

In the LGIT diet, stable blood glucose levels are attempted to be achieved, using a restricted diet. This is based on the hypothesis that blood glucose may be involved in achieving ketosis. This allows for greater freedom to use carbohydrates up to 40–60 g/d, which is more than in either the classic or the modified Atkins diet. The only restriction is the limit the carbohydrates of low glycemic index foods, i.e. up to 50 or less. Quite a few centers offer both the types of regimen—mAD and LGIT despite their limited trials, they have shown to be more accepted by adolescents.[15]

Table 41.7: Carbohydrate exchange list in mAD

Fruits	For children 2-12 years (any 4/d)	For adolescents and adults >12 years (any 3/d)
Fruit A (Apples, papaya, pear)	1 cup	2 cups
Fruit A (Orange, sweet lime)	3 pcs	6 pcs
Fruit A (Pomegranate)	3/4th cup	1.5 cups
Fruit A (Grapes)	6 pcs	12 pcs
Milk (Milk Products) Soya Milk (Natural Staeta)	2.5 cups	5 cups
Cow's Milk/Buffalo Milk	1 cup	2 cups
Paneer/Cheese	1–5 cubes	3 cubes
Cream	1 cup	2 cups
Nuts Almonds/Ground nuts	20 pcs	40 pcs
Walnuts	1 cup	2 cups
Coconut	1.5 tbsp	3 tbsp

Source: J. Nathan[11]

REFERENCES

1. Ries LAGSM, Gurney JG, Tamira T, et al. Cancer incidence and survival among children and adolescents. United States SEER Program 1976-95. National Cancer Institute, SEER Program NIH Pub Bethesda, MD. 1999. pp.17-34.
2. Jensen C. New study suggests link between maternal diet and childhood leukemia risk. Science Daily. Aug 24, 2004.
3. Marilyn l Kwan, Gladys Block, Steve Selvin, Stacy Month and Patricia A Buffer. Food consumption by children and the risk of childhood acute leukemia. Am J Epidemiology. Vol 160, No. 11. pp.1098-1107.
4. www.cureepilepsy.org/psas/charlies_story.asp
5. John WL. Puntis. Nutritional challenges in special conditions and diseases, Hemato Oncology In: Pediatric Nutrition in Practice, Ed. Koletzko B. Karger. 2008. pp.244-47.
6. Oeffinger KC, Mertens AC, Sklar CA, et al. Obesity in adult survivors of childhood acute lympoblastic leukemia: A report from The Childhood Cancer Survivor Study. J Clin Oncol. 2003;21:1359-65.
7. Bower BD, Schwartz RH, Eaton J and Aynsley Green A. The use of ketogenic diet in the treatment of epilepsy. In: Topics in Perinatal Medicine (ed) Wharton BO. 1982.pp.136-40.
8. Kossoff EH, Lau LC, Blackford R, Morrison PF, et al. When do seizures usually improve with ketogenic diet? Elipelsia. Feb 2008;49(20):329-33.
9. Wheless JW. History and origin of ketogenic diet. In; Stafstorm CE. Rho LM editors, Epiepsy and the ketogenic diet. Totowa: Humana Press. 2004.
10. Livingston S. Dietary treatment of epilepsy. In: Comprehensive management of epilepsy in infancy; Childhood and Adoescence. Springfield, Illinois: Charles C Thomas. 1972.pp.378-405.

11. J Nathan. Epilepsy and Keto Research Trust, Mumbai.
12. Gopalan C, Rama Sastri BV, Balasubramanian SC. Nutritive Value of Indian Foods. National Institute of Nutrition, ICMR, Hyderabad. 2008.
13. Zhou W, Mukherjee P, Kiebish MA, et al. The calorie restricted ketogenic diet, an alternative therapy for malignant brain cancer. Nutrition and Metabolism (London). 2007;4:5.
14. Kang HC, Lee HS, You SJ, Kangder C, Ko TS, Kim HD. Use of a modified Atkins diet in intractable epilepsy. Epilepsia. Jan 2007;48(1):182-6.
15. Kossoff EH, Zupec-Kania BA, Amark PE, et al. Optimal clinical management of children receiving the ketogenic diet. Recommendations of the International Ketogenic Diet Study group. Epilepsia. Sep 23. 2008.

Index

Page numbers followed by *f* refer to figure and *t* tefer to table